SUBSTANCE ABUSE ASSESSMENT, INTERVENTIONS AND TREATMENT

BATTLING THE OPIOID EPIDEMIC

SUBSTANCE ABUSE ASSESSMENT, INTERVENTIONS AND TREATMENT

Additional books and e-books in this series can be found on Nova's website under the Series tab.

SUBSTANCE ABUSE ASSESSMENT, INTERVENTIONS AND TREATMENT

BATTLING THE OPIOID EPIDEMIC

VINCENT HARDY

EDITOR

snova
New York

Library of Congress Cataloging-in-Publication Data

ISBN: 978-1-53615-548-8

Published by Nova Science Publishers, Inc. † New York

CONTENTS

PREFACE

America is in the middle of an epidemic it has never seen before. The opioid crisis knows no bounds. It is affecting individuals and families in every congressional district. Its consequences, ranging from personal health to the economy, are devastating. The opioid epidemic represents the convergence of the abuses of opioids, heroin, and synthetic drugs like fentanyl.

Chapter 1 is a hearing before the committee on the Judiciary of the House of Representatives on challenges and solutions in the opioid abuse crisis.

Chapter 2 reports on the Subcommittee on Oversight and Investigations' hearing on the DEA's role in combating the opioid epidemic.

Drug cartels operate out of countries in the western hemisphere, and they do so by using sophisticated distribution systems that move narcotics into and across the United States. Heroin supplied by these cartels has created a public health epidemic and fueled drug violence across the United States as reported in Chapter 3.

Chapter 4 provides an overview of heroin trafficking into and within the United States. It includes a discussion of links between the trafficking of heroin and the illicit movement of related substances such as controlled prescription opioids and synthetic substances like fentanyl. The chapter also outlines existing U.S. efforts to counter heroin trafficking and possible congressional considerations going forward.

Chapter 5 evaluates the extent to which DOD has strategy and implementing guidance for the National Guard counterdrug program, and assesses DOD's processes to approve states' counterdrug plans and distribute funding to the program, among other things.

In: Battling the Opioid Epidemic
Editor: Vincent Hardy

ISBN: 978-1-53615-548-8

Chapter 1

CHALLENGES AND SOLUTIONS IN THE OPIOID CRISIS*

The Committee on the Judiciary

Tuesday, May 8, 2018
House of Representatives
Committee on the Judiciary
Washington, DC.

The committee met, pursuant to call, at 10:00 a.m., in Room 2141, Rayburn House Office Building, Hon. Bob Goodlatte [chairman of the committee] presiding.

Present: Representatives Goodlatte, Sensenbrenner, Smith, Chabot, King, Gohmert, Marino, Collins, DeSantis, Buck, Ratcliffe, Gaetz, Johnson of Louisiana, Biggs, Handel, Rothfus, Nadler, Lofgren, Jackson Lee, Cohen, Johnson of Georgia, Deutch, Bass, Richmond, Cicilline, Swalwell, Lieu, Raskin, Jayapal, and Demings.

Staff Present: Shelley Husband, Staff Director; Branden Ritchie, Deputy Staff Director; Zach Somers, Parliamentarian and General Counsel; Anthony Angeli, Counsel, Subcommittee on Crime, Terrorism, Homeland Security, and Investigations; Joe Graupensperger, Minority Chief Counsel on Subcommittee on Crime; Monalisa Dugue, Minority Deputy Chief Counsel, Subcommittee on Crime, Terrorism, Homeland Security, and Investigations; David Greengrass, Minority Senior Counsel; and Veronica Eligan, Minority Professional Staff Member.

Chairman GOODLATTE. Good morning. The Judiciary Committee will come to order, and, without objection, the chair is authorized to declare recesses of the committee

* This is an edited, reformatted and augmented version of Hearing before the Committee on the Judiciary, House of Representatives, One Hundred Fifteenth Congress, Second Session, dated May 8, 2018.

at any time. We welcome everyone to this morning's hearing on challenges and solutions in the opioid abuse crisis. I will begin by recognizing myself for an opening statement.

America is in the middle of an epidemic it has never seen before. The opioid crisis knows no bounds. It is affecting individuals and families in every congressional district. Its consequences, ranging from personal health to the economy, are devastating. The opioid epidemic represents the convergence of the abuses of opioids, heroin, and synthetic drugs like fentanyl. Individuals suffering from addiction often switch between using opioids and heroin, based on a variety of factors including cost and purity.

Drug traffickers are further exploiting personal misery by adding deadly fentanyl analogues to the heroin and the illicit opioid supplies to increase their profits. Sadly, unwary and unsuspecting users are suffering deadly results. More frequently, pure fentanyl analogues in the illicit drug supply are resulting in overdose deaths and injuries to first responders. Since these analogues can be deadly in quantities as little as two milligrams, police and other first responders can unknowingly inhale airborne fentanyl or have it come in contact with their skin, causing them to overdose and suffer other severe reactions.

Tragically, more than 64,000 Americans died from drug overdoses in 2016. The sharpest increase occurred among deaths related to synthetic opioids, with over 20,000 overdose deaths. Not only has the total number of opioid pain relievers prescribed in the United States skyrocketed in the past 25 years, but recently studies have shown that over half of chronic prescription drug abusers receive the pills from friends or family. In 2018, more than 2 million Americans will suffer from addiction to prescription or illicit opioids.

Over the past 2 years, the House Judiciary Committee and Congress have passed several bills to address the opioid crisis. These bills include the Comprehensive Addiction and Recovery Act, or CARA, enacted in July of 2016, and the Stop Importation and Trafficking of Synthetic Analogues Act, or SITSA, approved by the House Judiciary Committee in July of 2017. While much work has been done, we must redouble our efforts to turn the tide in this crisis.

We know now more than ever that a crisis like this requires dynamic and outside-of-the-box solutions. Today's hearing will examine what is working and what needs to be looked at again in the opioid crisis. We will learn about best practices in international and domestic enforcement, and promising solutions in treatment and prevention. We will also hear about the devastation ravaged by this epidemic from a firsthand perspective.

I want to thank all of our witnesses for appearing today and I look forward to hearing their responses to our questions. And it is now my pleasure to recognize the ranking member of the Judiciary Committee, the gentleman from New York, Mr. Nadler, for his opening statement.

Mr. NADLER. Thank you, Mr. Chairman. I welcome today's hearing as an opportunity to explore ways in which we can best address the crisis of opioid abuse in our country. I believe it is critical that we do so in order to identify what works and what does not work, so that we do not repeat mistakes we have made in the past.

In the United States, drug overdoses are the leading cause of accidental death. With opioids being involved in nearly two-thirds of overdose deaths. Overall, the number of drug overdose deaths has nearly quadrupled over the past 20 years. Although effective for the treatment of pain, prescription opioids are highly addictive, and nearly half of all U.S. opioid overdose deaths involve a prescription opioid. Deaths related to heroin have similarly increased, as individuals often transition from more expensive prescription opioids to cheaper heroin.

As this crisis has intensified, Congress has contemplated various responses, and, in some instances, adopted legislation. In 2016, 2 years ago, we enacted the Comprehensive Addiction and Recovery Act, a law that included a wide array of provisions advanced by many of our committees. The provisions in the jurisdiction of this committee included a number of worthy initiatives, such as programs to expand treatment as an alternative to incarceration. It is impossible not to see the contrasts without Congress' response to the opioid crisis in comparison to their responses to some other drugs, particularly crack cocaine.

While I agree that we should develop and implement the comprehensive strategy with respect to opioids, with the emphasis being on preventing and treating abuse, we did not take this approach with crack cocaine. There, focusing our response on the enactment of lengthy, mandatory minimum sentences, and treating the use of crack as a law enforcement issue.

That approach was wrong and continues to be wrong, disparately impacting African-American communities while fueling mass incarceration. We must not make that same mistake with any of the drugs classified as opioids, and we must reverse and rectify the mistakes we have made in other drugs such as crack, through an increased emphasis on prevention and treatment and by changing our counterproductive and unjust sentencing laws.

Certain opioids, such as heroin and fentanyl, are already subject to mandatory minimum penalties, and these penalties have not prevented the current crisis, and increasing them would also not be effective. We also do not need more "get tough" rhetoric from President Trump or Attorney General Sessions about imposing the death penalty for drug crimes, and we should not be telling prosecutors to ratchet up criminal charges and penalties for drug offenders. None of that solves the problem. Instead of doubling down on failed policies that do nothing more than proliferate misery, we need real leadership, involving a commitment to increase resources for alternatives that we know are actually effective.

There are a number of proven alternatives that are being implemented in the States, and we must commit to supporting them. For instance, law enforcement assisted diversion programs, known as LEAD, allow law enforcement to divert appropriate arrestees from criminal court, instead providing treatment and other services that address addiction and reduce recidivism.

Developed and initially implemented in Seattle, the LEAD approach is now being used with success in other areas. We should support efforts such as LEAD, as well as other approaches at the local level, including medication-assisted treatment, supervised injection facilities, expanding the availability of overdose reversal drugs, and better education of doctors and the public about the proper prescription and use of opioids as pain medication.

We will not be able to arrest and incarcerate our way out of a drug abuse problem that has many causes. Instead, we must support the development and implementation of a variety of solutions. I hope this will be the path of the committee as we consider our contribution to addressing this crisis. I yield back the balance of my time.

Chairman GOODLATTE. Thank you, Mr. Nadler. Without objection, all other opening statements will be made a part of the record.

We welcome our distinguished witness on our first panel. And, Mr. Patterson, if you would please rise, I will begin by swearing you in.

Do you swear that the testimony that you are about to give shall be the truth, the whole truth, and nothing but the truth, so help you God? Thank you very much. Let the record show the witness answered in the affirmative.

Mr. Rob Patterson is the acting administrator of the U.S. Drug Enforcement Administration. He is the principal advisor to the Attorney General on international drug control policy and related operations in the United States.

Mr. Patterson, welcome. Your entire statement will be entered into the record in its entirety, and we ask that you summarize your testimony in 5 minutes. There is a timing light on the table that will indicate when 4 of those 5 minutes have gone, and then, when it turns to red, your 5 minutes are up. We thank you for indulging us, and Mr. Patterson, you may begin. Thank you.

STATEMENT OF ROBERT PATTERSON, ACTING ADMINISTRATOR, DRUG ENFORCEMENT ADMINISTRATION

Mr. PATTERSON. Thank you, sir. Chairman Goodlatte, Ranking Member Nadler, and distinguished members of this committee: thank you for holding this hearing on the opioid crisis. Our Nation has been devastated by opioid abuse, an epidemic fueled in part, and for a significant period of time, by a change in prescribing practices. This has helped create a generation of opioid abusers presently estimated at more than 3 million Americans.

Effectively combating this crisis requires addressing it from multiple angles: enforcement, education, and treatment. DEA's enforcement strategy utilizes a full spectrum of criminal, civil, and administrative tools to attack the trafficking of illicit and the diversion of licit supply.

We know that most new heroin users continue to begin their cycle of addiction with prescription pills, so we are constantly evaluating ways to ensure that our more than 1.7 million registrants comply with the law. Leveraging traditional enforcement methods with diversion authorities, DEA has established 77 tactical diversion squads and two mobile teams solely dedicated to investigating and dismantling criminal diversion schemes. In curbing diversion, we continue to integrate and strengthen our intelligence and enforcement efforts.

For example, in January, we analyzed DEA data alongside HHS and some State PMP data to identify prescribers and pharmacies whose activities warranted investigation. This analysis identified more than 400 leads, which were then provided to our 22 field divisions.

The resulting surge led to 188 active investigations, 28 arrests, 283 administrative actions, and removing the ability of 147 registrants to handle controlled substances. The complex nature of the epidemic requires data sharing and deconfliction, and fully committed to doing this better across the board.

Over the last 6 months, DEA has developed information sharing agreements with our State counterparts to share ARCOS data. Likewise, we need all States to find paths forward to share their PMP data, a vital piece of this puzzle.

Through a number of efforts we will discuss today, combined with an increased public awareness of the opioid epidemic, DEA has seen a corresponding decrease in prescriptions for opioids. While this is a very positive step, we still face many challenges. As an example of these ongoing efforts, we continue to review proposed changes to our quota program with a goal of utilizing multiple data sets thoughtfully to assess production needs while avoiding shortages for patients.

We are, however, seeing a dramatic and disturbing shift from licit opioids to the illicit market. Criminal organizations have filled this void by producing and distributing cheap powder heroin, often mixed with illicit fentanyl and related substances, and then selling it in powdered form or pressed into counterfeit pills resembling licit pharmaceuticals.

The changing chemical composition of synthetics makes it difficult to intercept these deadly substances before they hit our streets, and prosecutions are hindered by labor-intensive court proceedings. For example, to meet standards set forth in the Federal Analogue Act, prosecutors must prove in each case a substance substantially similar in chemical structure and pharmacological effect to a schedule I or schedule II substance.

DEA has moved aggressively to place temporary schedule I controls on new and emerging synthetic drugs, including 17 fentanyl analogues. Unfortunately, the temporary emergency scheduling process of a substance is reactive, requiring us to first observe the deadly consequences of synthetic drug abuse before initiating control.

In February, DEA proactively placed temporary emergency controls on the entire class of fentanyl-related substances, in the attempt to help curb fentanyl-related overdose deaths. This is an aggressive step to combat an unprecedented threat.

The logistics of how this poison reaches the U.S. is yet another challenge. Movement of fentanyl varies from the direct mailing of small amounts to cartels moving bulk quantities through their already-established transportation networks.

Complicating the issue, especially on the direct mailing, is technology that allows sellers and purchasers to conduct seemingly endless and relatively anonymous transactions on the web. However, with agencies working together, FBI, U.S. Postal, HSI, CBP, and others, and our critical international partners, no issue is insurmountable. The seizure of the dark web marketplace AlphaBay and subsequent darknet cases are prime examples demonstrating that no criminal network is untouchable.

While DEA's top priority is enforcement, there is also a natural fit for us in education. We have partnered with leaders in prevention and education to provide direct outreach to young people and parents on the dangers of prescription and illicit drugs. Simultaneously, DEA has worked to improve communication and cooperation with the registrant community, offering year-round free training to doctors, pharmacists, distributors, importers, and manufacturers. Ultimately, to fundamentally change this epidemic, we must decrease demand for these substances, working collaboratively on all fronts.

I am extremely appreciative of your commitment and support to tackling this epidemic. DEA has reviewed more than 60 pieces of pending legislation and appreciates the opportunity to provide technical assistance wherever appropriate. Thank you for the invitation to be here before you, and I look forward to your questions.

Chairman GOODLATTE. Thank you, Mr. Patterson. We will now proceed under the 5-minute rule with questions, and I will begin by recognizing myself.

Mr. Patterson, I have been watching with interest the investigation currently ongoing at the Energy and Commerce Committee about the distribution of opioids to West Virginia. As you may know, my district is just across the border, and I have no doubt that some of the opioids from pill mills in West Virginia have ended up on my side of the border. Earlier this year, you testified about some of the DEA's historical failures to identify and stop these pill mills. What did the DEA learn from these failures, and what are you doing differently today as a result?

Mr. PATTERSON. Sir, I appreciate that question, mainly because, as we talk about the period of 2006 through 2010, which is where a lot of those events really started and blossomed in West Virginia, we and others did not do a great job with the data that we had. Part of that was how we got the data, and part of that was our responses to certain things that we saw, right. There was not a real-time look on these things. The compliance with the industry was also problematic.

I think the huge difference that we see now is that we understand more than ever, especially working with the States, how to use the various data sets that we have. And as I just explained, you know, the HHS data that we are able to obtain—DEA's ARCOS data, the State PMP programs, where they are participating with us—all essentially allow us to see the outliers. The key piece to us doing enforcement actions and trying to hold distributors and others accountable really comes from us being able to find where those pills ultimately end up on the streets. The key to that is that PMP data set, and when we move back from that.

So, we have got a ton of lessons learned. I know both you and Mr. Nadler started this way, and I think we are all growing and expanding from what works as opposed to what has not worked in the past, and important lessons learned.

Chairman GOODLATTE. Thank you. In a recent press release, the Department of Justice highlighted the DEA's continued efforts to reduce drug quota, the ability of approved manufacturers to make certain quantities of controlled substances, including powerful ones like opioids.

Could you please explain the proposed rule, and how this will help with preventing diversion? And, also, give us some assurance that when drugs that are used as means of getting people off of, other drugs like methadone and so on, to make sure that supply is still available to those who are prescribing it for people who are trying to overcome their addiction.

Mr. PATTERSON. No, I understand. And thanks, again, for that question, sir. So, quota is a delicate balance. The reality is that DEA, for a long time, essentially bumped quota up to ensure that there would be full access for manufacturers to produce X amount of product.

In hindsight, looking back on how we dealt with quota, the more you allow manufacturers to produce, it is a business. They have more incentive to sell additional, which then drives more usage. So, what we have done over the last handful of years is to try and pull slack space out of that, for lack of a better word.

And now, the proposals that we put forward and that we are making are out there, and we just got comments back on, to take a look at other factors as we develop quota. And this is more on the prescribing side, as to the medical-assisted treatment side, but it has to deal with us taking in additional data sets, how we look at that, understanding the diversion in what we see.

And, quite frankly, I give credit to a lot of the States who have enacted legislation, and prescribers that have changed their methodology of a 5-day or a 7-day supply up front, which, all is pulling down how much pharmaceutical needs to be made. DEA has to be aggressive with essentially making sure that number is where it needs to be, with a heavy emphasis, though, on making sure that patients that need access to medicine have that access.

Chairman GOODLATTE. In your written testimony, you state that DEA is witnessing the transition from controlled prescription drugs to heroin and fentanyl and related synthetic analogues. What efforts is the DEA making to address this fundamental shift?

Mr. PATTERSON. So, I think, look, this trend has changed over the last couple of years, and we are trying to be much more aggressive on where our problem set really is. Fentanyl accounted for approximately a third of our overdose deaths, so the transition has really happened. As we see again, the licit market, or the pharmaceutical market, continues to come down. It creates a natural void where these criminal organizations will fill that void with their product for people that are truly addicted. And that is the struggle that we have.

Fentanyl, like I said, comes, essentially, to the United States in two forms: one is through smaller, much higher-percentage purity packages coming out of China, and then what we see coming across our southern border with the traditional organizations that have shipped heroin and methamphetamine and other drugs into this country for years, much lower concentration, although the volume is much higher. These are struggles that we are dealing with. The good piece of this is that all of your law enforcement agencies in this country are centering their efforts on the illicit market as we see this continuing to be the problem set moving forward.

Chairman GOODLATTE. Thank you. The chair recognizes Mr. Nadler for 5 minutes.

Mr. NADLER. Thank you. Mr. Patterson, in February of this year, the Department of Justice announced it would emergency schedule all illicit fentanyl. In its public announcement, the Department of Justice noted that this emergency scheduling action would mean that, "Federal agents and prosecutors can take swift and necessary action."

The Department of Justice has highlighted difficulty with prosecuting individuals for offenses under existing analogue control laws involving a suspected analogue of a controlled substance. Has this emergency scheduling action by the department facilitated the prosecution of individuals with suspected analogues of a controlled substance?

Mr. PATTERSON. Specific to fentanyl, sir? Specific to fentanyl, yes. So, the key for this, and I think this is where the struggle sits, is this is an aggressive use of scheduling on the fentanyl class.

And, again, when we talk about the balancing, HHS and others, you know, and their desire to do research and find actual medicines out of these medicines, when before we took the scheduling action, we went in and sought to see if anybody was looking at any of these classes of fentanyl that already existed.

Remember, this scheduled fentanyl that had not even come onto the market yet, as well. But, to look to see if anybody was trying to do research, and that answer was no, to the best of their ability to do that search. In addition, since we scheduled it in February, I am unaware and I have not been told by anybody about the efforts to do research in that class.

Mr. NADLER. Sorry, so, you are saying you are unaware?

Mr. PATTERSON. Unaware, sir.

Mr. NADLER. Of research?

Mr. PATTERSON. Of anybody asking to do research on the existing class of fentanyl that we see. The key to this really comes down to, sir, is the ability to charge criminal organizations that are importing the fentanyl as a substance. Using the Analogue Act, it is difficult, right? It is a time-consuming process for prosecutors and the reality is that this was the only way we could try and balance that out. And, again, balance being the key word here.

Mr. NADLER. Okay. Now, do you think that drug manufacturers should have more of a role in ensuring compliance with the Controlled Substance Act?

Mr. PATTERSON. Should drug manufacturers?

Mr. NADLER. Yes.

Mr. PATTERSON. Have more control.

Mr. NADLER. Have more of a role in ensuring compliance.

Mr. PATTERSON. Absolutely. I mean, one of the frustrations, I think, with the manufacturing population, so manufacturing and distributing somewhat lumped together, they are aware of the problems. They have been aware of the problems.

Frankly, we have done a lot of civil fines, but when you look at major businesses, civil fines seem to have little impact. And I think that is part of the frustration. In cases where we have not seen this behavior yet fixed, and we are talking about behavior that we have seen for the last decade, I think we have to hold them more accountable.

And that is why DEA, I think, is also taking a posture of, "Make sure that they are best informed." We have to work with them, which sometimes feels a little bit contradictory to do, as you are also investigating them. But we have to work to make sure that they understand their role in this place.

Mr. NADLER. And what is the total budget for the DEA for the current fiscal year?

Mr. PATTERSON. 2018 was just under $2.2 billion.

Mr. NADLER. Just under 2.2?

Mr. PATTERSON. Yes, sir.

Mr. NADLER. And how much Federal money is allocated for drug treatment this year?

Mr. PATTERSON. I actually do not know, ultimately. I know that at one point, though, there were conversations. I do not know what is allocated, sir. I know there were conversations about, I believe, $6 billion.

Mr. NADLER. All right, six. Okay. Now, in the past, you have stated that prescription monitoring programs, which involve State- to-State data sharing and mandatory prescriber registration, are important to helping create a clear image of where opioids are being distributed to the population. Can you discuss further the benefits of States participating in PMPs?

Mr. PATTERSON. So, I think that vast majority of States, and as we have gone and talked to people, I think doctors feel the same way, want to be able to do right in this space and be able to see what their patients are doing and what pharmacists are doing and prescribing, or what is going out. I should say, ultimately, to the user population, right, or the patients, in this case.

I think the key to it is where States either do not have the ability to connect with each other, or the systems actually are not being used, is highly problematic. So, you know, as I talked about in the opening, ARCOS is a critical first step for us to be able to take a look at where pills are going in, and we should take a look at that to understand where they are going into pharmacies. The key piece, frankly, is where you are seeing that diversion happening from the pharmacy area and from doctors, in some cases, out into the general public.

Mr. NADLER. Okay. I have one more quick question, thank you. Since 2011, the number of immediate suspension orders, which allow the DEA to free suspicious shipments of controlled substances when there is an imminent danger to public health or safety has significantly declined. Can you explain why this has happened in the midst of the opioid epidemic?

Mr. PATTERSON. Yes, sir. I would be happy to do so. So, there is two factors on this, and as I have gone around and spoken to a number of the members, one is that tool is an aggressive use of the tool against distributors. It is not a tool that was generally used against distributors. The case of using that only had happened a handful of times in the previous number of years prior to 2011, 2012.

The other piece of it is when the bill did change, the Ensuring Patient Access bill changed, it raised that standard to where the conduct would have to be much more egregious for us to be able to prove at the distributor level.

I understand, in talking to a number of folks, you know, again, through the various members, that there was confusion in the industry. And I think the importance here is to strike a healthy balance of making sure the industry understands exactly where the rule is in giving us a tool back that we can then use to essentially work forward.

Mr. NADLER. Thank you.

Chairman GOODLATTE. The chair recognizes the gentleman from Wisconsin, Mr. Sensenbrenner, for 5 minutes.

Mr. SENSENBRENNER. Thank you, Mr. Chairman. We have heard an awful lot about fentanyl analogues in the two previous series of questions. I have a bill in to schedule fentanyl analogues. Does the DEA support this legislation?

Mr. PATTERSON. So, let me do it this way to keep myself out of trouble, which is: we have emergency scheduled the entire class of fentanyl analogues, and we need a legislative fix to keep this and have this remaining in schedule I.

Mr. SENSENBRENNER. How long does the emergency schedule last?

Mr. PATTERSON. So, it started in February. It will go for 2 years, and we can extend that for 1 year.

Mr. SENSENBRENNER. So, at the end of 3 years from February— which puts us at February 2021—you cannot do anymore without legislation?

Mr. PATTERSON. That is correct, and we will be back to the same problem of having to do one at a time and go through a decision.

Mr. SENSENBRENNER. Is it hard for a prosecutor to obtain a conviction based on an emergency schedule, rather than having this schedule done by legislation?

Mr. PATTERSON. I think it poses risks, as we get closer and closer to that 2021 date with how prosecutors would charge their cases. Because, in theory, they would have to charge both under the Analogue Act, as well as using fentanyl as a schedule I, because the balance would then come in to: if they charge a case and it has not gone to trial, my understanding is that, come February of 2021, that fentanyl drops off or we have not yet been able to do our emergency scheduling, it would be unscheduled. So, the answer is yes, it does pose challenges.

Mr. SENSENBRENNER. All right. I hope we can get this bill passed this year, because I think there is an urgency, rather than having to start over after the election of the next Congress. And I yield back the balance of my time.

Mr. PATTERSON. And if I could just add one other thing, sir. We look forward to providing any technical assistance on that, because it does require a legislative fix.

Mr. SENSENBRENNER. Thank you.

Mr. PATTERSON. Thank you.

Chairman GOODLATTE. The chair recognizes the gentlewoman from California, Ms. Lofgren, for 5 minutes.

Ms. LOFGREN. Thank you, Mr. Chairman. I was very interested in your testimony starting on page two. And I think trying to understand what is going on here in our communities is important to coming up with the proper solution.

You say that in 2016, almost 3.4 million Americans aged 12 or older reported misusing prescription pain relievers in the last month. And that prescription misuse is more common than use of any category of illicit drug, absent marijuana, which has now been legalized in half the States for one purpose or another. And that 75 percent reported non-medical use of prescription opioids before initiating heroin use.

Now, you go on to say that the reasons an individual may shift from one opioid to another will vary, but it is less expensive than the prescriptions. So, I am getting a picture, not just from you but from other witnesses at other hearings, that most people do not just start using heroin. For one reason or another, often times they are prescribed or over-prescribed for some remedy an opioid, and they get hooked. And then they go on to use and overuse, and then when they cannot get the opioids, to go to the illegal provisions. Is that your understanding? Or, if I am wrong, correct me.

Mr. PATTERSON. No, I think that is a completely accurate understanding. And if I could add, you know, it always feels odd, but for me to be efficient in our law enforcement efforts, we have to understand the back-end problem of this, which is treatment, and what these people, or addicts, go through.

Ms. LOFGREN. Oh, absolutely.

Mr. PATTERSON. Frankly, when we go out and speak with them and understand their problems, I hear the same story over and over again, which is at some point, this opioid high that you get from it, and sometimes it is very quickly, becomes an issue of not being sick. And that is what then drives the switch from licit opioids, which they, you know, run into a problem of not being able to afford, and then, into the world of heroin.

In 2011, 4 out of 5 people started, prior to heroin, by misusing opioids. That number dropped down, I think, in 2016, to 3 out of 5, but that is still a stunning number, that 60 percent of your people started with a licit pill.

Ms. LOFGREN. Well, you know, if that is the case, it seems to me one of the most effective things we could do would be to focus on why people are using so much prescriptions. I mean, if you compare the use. You know, I am not one who says the cancer victim, you know, should die in agony. You know, that is not really what we are talking about.

But we had a witness in an immigration subcommittee hearing a few months ago who said that some of these companies were providing so much opioids, it would be enough for, you know, 10 pills for every adult in the town that was sent to the pharmacy. Obviously, someone must know that that is not a proper use.

And so, the question is, "What are we doing about that?" We have got companies that should know—they must know—that what they are developing is fueling this opioid crisis, and they are doing it anyhow, to make money. What is our strategy on that?

Mr. PATTERSON. So, again, I think this gets back to the education of Americans. The companies are not going to change their behavior.

Ms. LOFGREN. Well, let me interrupt if I may, because I believe in the education of Americans. I think people, you know, who break a leg, can say, "I do not want 50 opioid pills, you know, I want two." You know, but that does not get to the root of the problem, which is you have got people profiting, companies—real companies, not drug dealers—incorporated companies profiting out of starting this addiction. What is our strategy to go after that?

Mr. PATTERSON. So, the strategy, again, is to work with industry, and try and make them understand their role, whether they change their practice or not. But I will give you another fact that you can add to that toolbox of the argument of overprescribing. So, DEA has done these take back events for the last, you know, number of years. In total, it has been just about 10 million pounds we have taken back. So, in April, we took back——

Ms. LOFGREN. If I may interrupt? I do not mean to be rude, but we only have 5 minutes, and I have got 10 seconds left. I will just say that I am for educating people, I am for buybacks, but to allow certain companies to profiteer by addicting wide swaths of the country, and our action is, "We are going to work with them," I think that is insufficient. That is lame.

And I do not blame you; you are administering the law, but we need a very different strategy than we appear to have now. And I know my time is up, Mr. Chairman, so I yield back, and I thank you, Mr. Patterson, for being here.

Mr. PATTERSON. Could I just finish one thing real quick, sir? Chairman GOODLATTE. Yes.

Mr. PATTERSON. So, I agree with you, ma'am. It has to start there. My point on bringing back the take back: every 6 months, we take in about 1 million pounds of pharmaceutical drugs. That is a conversation that has to be had. If we are returning that every 6 months, what are we doing wrong?

Ms. LOFGREN. Thank you, sir.

Chairman GOODLATTE. The chair recognizes the gentleman from Pennsylvania, Mr. Marino, for 5 minutes.

Mr. MARINO. Administrator, I have never worked with a finer agency than the DEA, and I see the positive move under your leadership.

In October 2017, the Washington Post and 60 Minutes put out a joint report on the Ensuring Patient Access and Effective Drug Enforcement Act, a bill which I was the House sponsor, because I heard from seniors and pharmacists in my district that they were not able to get prescriptions, especially for terminally ill patients.

This report was filled with falsehoods that completely misrepresented the law and its effects. After my legislation passed the House by unanimous vote, the Senate introduced their version of the bill, where my language of "foreseeable risk" was changed to "substantial likelihood," which is a much higher burden for the DEA to satisfy.

But this was language the DEA had asked for, and in Senate Judiciary hearing last year, when asked about the language, Ms. Demetra Ashley stated that the DEA supported the legislation and the version that passed. The bill then passed the Senate by unanimous consent, passed the House, again, by unanimous consent, was signed into law by President Obama at the recommendation of DOJ and DEA.

The DEA has now testified twice that the bill has in no way stopped the DEA from doing its job. In October 25, 2017 energy and commerce hearing, Mr. Neil Doherty, the deputy assistant administrator of the Office of Diversion Control testified, in court, it did not stop the DEA from doing its job in the diversion space.

In December 12, 2017 Senate Judiciary hearing, Ms. Demetra Ashley, the acting assistant administrator in the Office of Diversion Control stated that, "I agree wholeheartedly that it did not stop us from doing our job." She later stated, "Has it impacted our ability to issue ISOs? No, sir, it has not."

Since 2012, the DEA did not issue an Immediate Suspension Order, or ISO, against a drug distributor until 4 days ago, using the new "substantial likelihood" standard. Ensuring Patient Access and Effective Drug Treatment Act was signed into law in 2016. So, for 4 years, the DEA did not issue an ISO under the prior standard. Taking all this into account, it would appear that the DEA shifted to using other tools to go after the opioid epidemic, rather than using ISOs against manufacturers, that the law did not hamper or stop the DEA from doing their job in any way, and that, very recently, the DEA used ISOs against a manufacturer, effectively showing that this language does not stop you from using an ISO.

The DEA now says they want to change the law and would like to see the "substantial likelihood" that the Senate passed, at the request of the White House, language to "probable cause." My language that was in the original bill and passed in the House was "foreseeable," which is a lower standard than either "probably cause," and much lower than "substantial likelihood."

I understand that the DEA is still advocating for probable cause, but I would be willing to consider a lower standard that would give DEA an even more flexible use of what you are currently asking for.

As I mentioned, my original language that passed the House was "foreseeable risk," which is the lower standard. During the Senate Judiciary Committee hearing, Senator Blumenthal asked, "But you had to show some likelihood before?" and this was Ms. Ashley, the assistant administrator.

Her response was, "We were aiming to prevent diversion because it is foreseeable. If drugs are diverting, they get to someone who should not have them. It is foreseeable that there will be harm." From reading that, it certainly seems that the DEA was also using a foreseeable standard before, in regards to the ISOs. That is the standard that was in my legislation.

I want to explain something here as far as "foreseeable." The courts have ruled an act must be sufficiently likely before it may be foreseeable, in the legal sense. That does not mean simply imaginable or conceivable. Now, I am going to switch to probable cause.

What the Supreme Court says were, "the facts and circumstances within the officers' knowledge, and of which they have reasonable trustworthy information, are sufficient in themselves to warrant a belief by a man reasonably cautioned that a crime is being committed." That definitely is a higher standard. Would you agree with me, sir, that "foreseeable" is a lower risk than "substantial," "probable" cause, and that is the lowest hurdle that you would have to get over?

Mr. PATTERSON. So, "foreseeable" is certainly lower than "probable" cause, and as I have discussed with you and others, I appreciate the ability to get that level as low as possible. The reason why we have picked "probable cause" is it is a well-defined, essentially, standard for our agency. As we looked as all of these issues, we found that we could meet probable cause every time. So, I appreciate your effort to go to "foreseeable." At the same time, I think that using "probable cause" strikes a balance between the industry and understanding where that is.

Mr. MARINO. And I will support that, if that is what the agency wants. With that, I have run out of time. Mr. Chairman, could I enter some things into the record?

Chairman GOODLATTE. What do you have?

Mr. MARINO. I ask unanimous consent, I would like to place in the record the transcript from the House Energy and Commerce hearing on Wednesday, October 25, 2017, as well as the transcript from the Senate Judiciary Committee hearing on December 12, 2017 and December 17, 2017, a 60-minute transcript of David Schiller, a former DEA supervisor who said, "With the opioid epidemic getting worse year by year, special agent Schiller and his team wanted to send a message to the pharmaceutical industry. They wanted to fine the company a billion dollars to revoke registration distribution."

On to say that he was asked, "Did the DEA attorney actually tell you that they were not going to pursue that case because they had lawyers who went to Harvard and Yale?" Schiller said, "they told me those exact words because the case would take too much time and too much effort, by the way, and what if we lost," and this was a statement that came from the DEA and the Department of Justice back in 2014.

Chairman GOODLATTE. Without objection, they will be made a part of the record.

The chair recognizes the gentleman from Tennessee, Mr. Cohen, for 5 minutes.

Mr. COHEN. Thank you, sir. Mr. PATTERSON, first, welcome. The DEA has always been a position, I think, of great importance, and it is important that the DEA administrator stay current with what the people have shown, by their actions and their statements, what they believe is the right priorities for DEA.

And it has been pretty clear, as Ms. Lofgren mentioned, that 29 or 30 jurisdictions, in some way or another, have legalized marijuana for one purpose or another. And yet, because of the inaction of the DEA, marijuana is still a schedule I drug, along with heroin and ecstasy and acid. Do you believe that marijuana should be classified as the same as LSD, ecstasy, and heroin?

Mr. PATTERSON. So, the reason why it remains in schedule I is because of the science.

Mr. COHEN. The science?

Mr. PATTERSON. The science. So, FDA does its eight-factor analysis, DEA does its review, and therefore, it remains in schedule I.

Mr. COHEN. Before we talk about the science, and I am happy to hear that you believe in science, that is refreshing. What do you think? Do you think marijuana should be schedule I? Based on your knowledge of the harm that marijuana causes, as distinguished from the harm that heroin causes the public and society?

Mr. PATTERSON. So, I am going to give you my honest opinion. And this actually does not shape how we do enforcement at DEA, because our priorities are the biggest priorities that we face, which is the opioid issue, methamphetamine, cocaine is now on the resurgence.

So, marijuana, obviously, is lower on the scale of what we do. And where we look to deal with that is in States where we see the importation of crime into those States from other States that are growing to distribute it back out, or exportation from those States, groups that are violent, other actions that are going on. So, that is where DEA prioritizes.

I fear—and I am just giving you my honest opinion—that we are going down a bad path with marijuana. And I will tell you the reason why I say that. This is not from, necessarily, the law enforcement person, because if I give you the law enforcement version, it is discounted as law enforcement. All of the driving conversations of this generally go around revenue. And that is unfortunate to me.

And I think 10 years ago we would sit here, and we could have this debate as to what is better, what is worse, you know? Is heroin worse than marijuana? And I am not going to debate that because I think, to me, they are two completely different things. Right?

I think the concern we see is we now have a body of evidence in States that have run what I call "the social experiment" for 10 years. Right? So, Colorado is a great one. And if we have an honest conversation about what we are starting to see in Colorado, my fear is that in 10 years, and I will not be sitting here, but you will all have someone here from DEA or some other agency saying, "Why was no one saying something?" I see that path coming.

And frankly, if you look back 20 years ago on the pharmaceutical world, people were screaming into the wind. It was a small percentage of people really concerned about what they were seeing. You have extremely high THC and, putting all the other things aside, right, property values in Colorado, or the fact that revenue is not essentially making up for what the costs are, issues with children, all these other things.

If you take that all and just put it aside, and simply ask the question to the adults in this country, which is, "At what point did we determine that revenue was more important than our kids?"

Mr. COHEN. Mr. Patterson, I appreciate your statements, and I can see where you have a different perspective than some previous DEA administrators, at least your honesty. Because I think the last one under Obama, I think, thought like you did but did not talk like you did.

I think most adults do not see it as dollars and cents. Most adults see it as a freedom issue and taking somebody's liberty from them for smoking marijuana.

And the fact that three and a half times more African-Americans than Caucasians are arrested and lose their liberty, and possibly their hope in the future, for educational Pell Grants or education scholarships or public housing if they need it, is taken away from them because of smoking a plant that is legal and that does not cause people to die. I look at it, most adults look at it as a freedom issue and, as you put it as beneath three other drugs, I think. And I am sure you put meth above it, as well.

Mr. PATTERSON. Probably farther down than that.

Mr. COHEN. Yeah. And I mean, meth kills people. Crack can kill people. You get addicted. Opioids, you get addicted, and heroin, you die, kill people. Marijuana is not the same thing. So, there is a limited amount of resources the DEA has, police officers have, judicial law enforcement, everybody, and there is an opportunity cost. And when you spend time dealing with marijuana, all you are doing is taking time away from drugs that kill people and cause crimes.

Mr. SENSENBRENNER [presiding]. The gentleman's time has expired.

Mr. COHEN. So, I thank you for your honesty and appreciate the time, and you can answer some more, if you would like.

Mr. PATTERSON. If I could just add one comment on the end. So, DEA does not expend its resources on users of marijuana. And quite frankly, I am not sure what State is. So, I think that you see, even States where it remains illegal, I do not see a huge enforcement presence. That is a good conversation to have, but I hear this statistic all the time, that there is mass incarceration of users, not just of marijuana but of drugs in general, and I do not see it. So, it would be a conversation I would like to have further, to be honest with you.

Mr. COHEN. Thank you, sir.

Mr. SENSENBRENNER. The chair recognizes the gentleman from Florida, Mr. DeSantis.

Mr. DESANTIS. Thank you, Mr. Chairman. Good morning, Mr. Patterson. So, if you look at the opioid crisis, what is the driving force right now? Because I know that, you know, there is a history of the prescription medications and the addictive qualities of that. But I look at what is happening with the fentanyl and some of this stuff pouring into the country. This stuff is poison. It is very lethal. And it seems to me, prescriptions are down for some of the pain killers, and I know they are all important. But is it more being driven right now on the prescription side, or on the street drug side?

Mr. PATTERSON. No, I think, and we had started off by having that conversation, we have crossed the paths, of where the licit, or the prescription side, is now the leading problem. Fentanyl and heroin and other adulterants out there are our problem. And frankly, what drives this now is an abuser population of 3-plus million people that we have to work with, and that then comes hand in hand with treatment and other issues that we have to deal with there. But, as we have seen with every other illicit drug, there are cartels and groups that are willing to fill this space to meet that need.

And you know, we are here on an opioids conversation. We have a massive methamphetamine problem in this country, too, that most of your States are struggling with, that does not get a lot of conversation. But we have a drug abuse problem in this country, and it occupies the illicit space, and these organizations will continue.

Mr. DESANTIS. And that is being driven by organizations that are bringing it across the southern border, primarily?

Mr. PATTERSON. Certainly. Southern border and off into the areas of China and India.

Mr. DESANTIS. That is an interesting thing, because we did a bill, President signed it a couple months ago, to try to let the Post Office intercept some of this stuff that gets mailed in. If they try to mail it Federal Express, FedEx will stop it, but the Post Office just kind of comes in.

So, have you seen any change of the Post Office's ability to interdict some of the stuff that is being shipped from China in the last, you know, month or two, since this bill has been in effect?

Mr. PATTERSON. So, I do not know if it is specific to the bill, because I am not familiar with that bill, sir, but the U.S. Postal Service has done an amazing amount of work with trying to get additional data to help them. We are trying to fuse that as a law enforcement body with all the data that we have.

So, in other words, where we see issues and problem spots coming up, so that they can be more nimble. But the reality is that you have a volume problem, when we talk about the logistics of packages coming in. So, that is not a southern border problem. The southern border problem is the roots that we have always dealt with, the Mexican cartels. Really, when you get into U.S. Postal's lane, that has to do more with the packages that are coming out of China and other places around the world, and that is a pure volume problem.

So, we have to be smarter, as an overall group, as to how we target and use those resources the best way. I do not know if we will ever get to a point where we will be able to scan through every piece of mail. And remember, you know, ounces, right? Not even ounces, right? You know, grams of fentanyl produce thousands of dosage units. And if you can think about that, that means that I am just putting, you know, a couple of grams, or a sugar pack, in an envelope, and asking U.S. Postal to find that as it comes in. It is highly problematic.

Mr. DESANTIS. Now, what is the typical profile? And I know these things vary. But, so, someone overdoses on fentanyl. Is this somebody who was starting to do prescription drugs and then ended up going to street drugs? Did they start with marijuana and then go? I mean, I am sure it varies, but just give me a sense of how it gets to the point where we have users of a very highly lethal, highly addictive product.

Mr. PATTERSON. Right. So, I think when you look at the overdose population, and there are probably better people than myself to speak to this. The unfortunate thing is it can be one of a host of things, right? So, you have your heroin user where it is adulterated with fentanyl. We are seeing it now in cocaine, as well. In fact, there was just a recent article that came out on all these cocaine users, that the ones that survived had no idea that there was fentanyl in the cocaine. That is also a disturbing trend we see. But you also have the people that go out and believe they are buying a licit pill, right, that is nothing more than binder and fentanyl. And I think this is the problem.

And as you listen to the stories, I stopped using the number of overdose deaths a long time ago. Because, to me, the individual stories are what is critical here. And they all have the same kind of feeling, right? "I did not understand that it was happening in my family," "did not understand the addiction of my loved one," but it happens in so many various ways, and that is part of the challenge that we have here.

Mr. DESANTIS. What can States do to help what the DEA is doing?

Mr. PATTERSON. So, look, again, the continued number to drive down is that population that is using or abusing opioids. And that still comes on the prescription side. So, I see States being very aggressive in that space.

I am happy that groups like ADA, the American Dental Association, has come out and talked about prescribing rates. We have to fix that problem. And although it is a good trend down, we cannot let that continue any other way than down. And we see a handful of States where it is either flat or still continuing to go up. That is where we are putting our efforts in on the prescription side.

On the illicit side, it is going to be essentially, again, an educational problem mixed with law enforcement.

Mr. DESANTIS. Thank you. My time is up.

Mr. SENSENBRENNER. The gentleman's time has expired. The gentlewoman from Texas, Ms. Jackson Lee.

Ms. JACKSON LEE. Mr. Patterson, welcome. Thank you and your men and women for the work that you do. In particular, let me acknowledge the team you have in Houston, Texas, and the "bring your drugs in" or "bring your drugs back" day that you had all over the country, I believe, just a week or so ago, if I am clear on the one that we had here in Houston, or forthcoming. So, thank you for that kind of work.

Let me just remind you of the ways of different drugs from the crack cocaine, heroin, of course, fentanyl is something that this committee has addressed, and it is a sensitive issue when you begin to think of mandatory minimums and the impact. You all are the enforcers, but you know what happened with mandatory minimums. Sick people went to jail, if you will, or people that were using small amounts, and we do not know if it benefitted or not.

So, let me just ask you this question: with respect to people being incarcerated who are addicted or users and they were caught up, probably may have had a mandatory minimum, do you think it is on the recidivism side of it, because you see those individuals back in your cycle, that there should be a major component of drug treatment in the incarceration mode, in the prison system? That that should be an aspect for those individuals, as relates to recidivism?

Mr. PATTERSON. So, thank you for that question, and I go back to what I just said a few minutes ago. So, I think DEA predominately sees—and I should not even say predominately, I mean, we deal with the distribution end of this. I think a State and local approach is a very different feel, right? They are dealing with people that are generally impacted. And I am not saying that people that we want to arrest in the distribution stream also do not have substance abuse problems.

I think there is a host of programs out there where States are trying. I am probably not the right guy to speak to that. I think that I am certainly a person, though, that believes that people that are impacted by drug abuse need help.

And, you know, there are times and I have had conversations with, you know, first responders, EMS, State and local police, local prosecutors, in which, frankly, the arrest is saving certain peoples' lives. Right? Because it puts them down a path of treatment. But you have to want to be treated, as well. I think this is one of the delicate balances and I do not feel comfortable speaking for the States as they look at that, because we do not necessarily deal in that space, if that makes sense to you.

Ms. JACKSON LEE. No, it does make sense. We do have that problem in the Federal system, though. There are people in the system that are addicted. But I appreciate the thoughtful response.

Let me ask you, as relates to distributors: do you think there are adequate consequences? Or, well, let me just say this: under the Controlled Substances Act, the applicable regulations require the distributors to report orders of an unusual size, orders deviating substantially from a normal pattern, and orders of unusual frequency, to the DEA. Is that correct? Are they supposed to do that?

Mr. PATTERSON. That is correct. Suspicious activity reports.

Ms. JACKSON LEE. Thank you, and I like it in that context: suspicious activity. Do you think there are adequate consequences for distributors that fail to report orders of unusual size, orders that deviate from the norm, redundancy, and orders of unusual frequency?

Mr. PATTERSON. So, I do not believe that is happening as much as it should be in the distribution world. We are trying to make efforts at DEA to get additional information out there to help in this.

Ms. JACKSON LEE. But do you think there are consequences for those entities that are engaged who fail to report unusual size, and sales that deviate from the norm, and orders that are unusual frequency? Are the consequences strong enough?

Mr. PATTERSON. The consequences have traditionally been fines, civil fines. And you recognize that there are certain companies out there, certainly when you look at the bigger manufacturers, those fines have, unfortunately, become the price of doing business. There has to be more accountability in that space, but DEA also needs to do a better job in terms of how we look at those and hold people to that level of accountability.

Ms. JACKSON LEE. Let me ask you this final question: in the landscape of drug containment, or responding to the vast drug world, where are we in 2018? Staffing, with DEA, and as well, success.

Mr. PATTERSON. So, staffing is a challenge, has always been a challenge for us. The good news is that we have a healthy influx of State and local partners that come on to our task forces. We just announced recently that we got funding, and I appreciate the funding that we did get, to bring on an additional 400 State and local task force officers. That is our true quick force multiplier, is we try and ramp up. But staffing, I think, will always be a problem.

Mr. SENSENBRENNER. The gentlewoman's time has expired.

Ms. JACKSON LEE. Thank you very much. Thank you for your service.

Mr. SENSENBRENNER. The gentleman from Texas, Mr. Gohmert.

Mr. GOHMERT. Thank you, Mr. Chair, and we appreciate your being here, Mr. Patterson. It has been several years ago, but Steve Chabot and I had journeyed down to Colombia and met with DEA officials there and went out into the jungles, basically, and looked at all the efforts we had at trying to help Colombia combat cocaine. And it was a huge problem at that time, and the FARCs were pretty much running things when we were there. But it made a great deal of impact and seemed to dramatically cut the amount of coca that is raised and cocaine that is sent up.

We were told that two-thirds of the cocaine came up by fast boats on the Caribbean side, Gulf of Mexico side, and about a third went up to California. And then, they put in in Mexico—and I asked why they did not just go ahead to the beach in Texas or California, and our eight DEA agents said it was because they are business people, and the odds of getting it across the Mexico-U.S. border were so much better than if they landed even on an abandoned beach.

Back then, we did not have drones that could be used, and my understanding, and I want to know if it is correct, is that we have dramatically impacted the amount of cocaine coming up from Colombia, is that correct?

Mr. PATTERSON. I think, for a period of time. I think with the peace process with the FARC—and this is a relatively long answer and I think you may have more that you want to talk about—I mean, I would be happy to come and sit down with you. There is a real issue with the production of cocaine in Colombia, yet again, that I think we have to wrestle with. We have had these conversations with the government of Colombia and our counterparts in the law enforcement world. There are a lot of challenges in this space, in what they were dealing with, with the FARC, but it is problematic, in terms of production, again.

Mr. GOHMERT. Is it still true that most of what they send north to United States goes across the water, puts into Mexico, and comes across our Mexico-U.S. border?

Mr. PATTERSON. Yeah. Central America into Mexico, Mexico up, or directly into Mexico. Correct.

Mr. GOHMERT. Yeah. Do they skip most of the Central American countries and just come in at Mexico?

Mr. PATTERSON. I think it depends on the organization, sir. So, I mean, regardless, it is coming across our southern border.

Mr. GOHMERT. Okay. Now, I know there has been great issue raised in recent years about the disparity in Federal penalties for possession for crack cocaine as opposed to powdered cocaine. And Dan Lungren that was here had pointed out that in the 1980s, most of the Republicans were following the lead of the Congressional Black Caucus members who were saying, like Charlie Ran-gel, that this crack cocaine is a scourge on the African-American community.

And if you are not willing to really come down with powerful punishments even more so for crack than for powder, then, you know, you are discriminating against the black community. And for that reason, people like Dan said, "We voted for it because that is what they said was best for the black community." Obviously, since then, we have found there really should not be a disparity.

And I realize I have just got 1 minute, so let me just go directly to this question: we now have drones. How much help do you think you could use from drones? Have you made a specific request for a fleet of drones to help patrol both our Mexico-U.S. border and the Gulf of Mexico and Pacific?

Mr. PATTERSON. So, sir, we have not specifically.

Mr. GOHMERT. Do you not think they would help?

Mr. PATTERSON. I know that we work well with, obviously, CBP. So, I view it more as we would pass actionable intelligence to CBP to work on that particular issue on the border.

Mr. GOHMERT. You would not want a fleet of drones for DEA's own use?

Mr. PATTERSON. That is a good question. I think, in terms of border security, we are going to leave that to CBP and others to work on that.

Mr. GOHMERT. Well, I understand, but you have got the Gulf of Mexico and you have got California.

Mr. PATTERSON. Right. It is something I would certainly think about and come back to you.

Mr. GOHMERT. We would encourage that. Thank you. I yield back.

Mr. SENSENBRENNER. The gentleman from Georgia, Mr. Johnson.

Mr. JOHNSON of Georgia. Thank you, Mr. Chairman. Sir, of the 64,000 drug overdose deaths in 2016, you are familiar with that figure, right? 64,000. What percentage of the 64,000 were for nonprescription opioids; in other words, heroin and fentanyl?

Mr. PATTERSON. So, fentanyl alone makes up for about 20,000, so roughly a third. And where heroin and fentanyl came, combined, I do not recall. Overall, "opioids" was 44,000 of that 64,000.

Mr. JOHNSON of Georgia. And, of the 64,000, how many deaths came as a result of overdosing on marijuana?

Mr. PATTERSON. I do not recall even seeing that on the chart.

Mr. JOHNSON of Georgia. So, in other words, you do not have any information that there is any death that marijuana is responsible for, within that 64,000?

Mr. PATTERSON. I am aware of a few deaths from marijuana.

Mr. JOHNSON of Georgia. You are aware of a few deaths from overdosing on marijuana?

Mr. PATTERSON. I do not recall if it was overdosing, but deaths attributed to the use of marijuana.

Mr. JOHNSON of Georgia. Deaths attributed, okay. What do you mean by that?

Mr. PATTERSON. I do not recall whether it had been adulterated with something else. I would be happy to go back and look.

Mr. JOHNSON of Georgia. I would love for you to do that.

Mr. PATTERSON. I understand the issue here, which is, one is not comparable to the other, I think is what you are asking me.

Mr. JOHNSON of Georgia. How many drug arrests throughout the country in 2016 for all illegal substances, drugs?

Mr. PATTERSON. I do not know.

Mr. JOHNSON of Georgia. According to a Washington Post article, which I just had here, which is dated September 26 of 2017 by Christopher Ingraham, he notes that more people were arrested last year over pot than for murder, rape, aggravated assault, and robbery combined. About 800,000 arrests for pot in 2016.

Now, you stated, in response to Mr. Cohen's question, you pretty much intimated that marijuana arrests were not that profound, not too many. But 800,000 is quite a big number, is it not?

Mr. PATTERSON. Again, I am referencing what I see in the space we work at.

Mr. JOHNSON of Georgia. And that is just for marijuana.

Mr. PATTERSON. Right. But again, the task forces that we participate with, DEA as a whole, these are certainly not our numbers and what we see.

Mr. JOHNSON of Georgia. Yeah. The ACLU did a study which determined that African-Americans are 3.73 times more likely than whites to be arrested for marijuana. Do you agree or disagree with that number?

Mr. PATTERSON. I have no reason to dispute the number.

Mr. JOHNSON of Georgia. Do you believe that marijuana being listed under schedule I has anything to do with Federal, State, local law enforcement policy, with respect to those 800,000 arrests?

Mr. PATTERSON. Well, again, I would go back on the Federal policy. I just do not see those arrests happening in the Federal space, and I would not be the person to address State and local arrests.

Mr. JOHNSON of Georgia. Okay. I am going to yield the balance of my time to Mr. Cohen.

Mr. COHEN. Thank you, Mr. Johnson, I appreciate that. Mr. Patterson, you said the science had to be looked at, and it does, but I think the science has got to be faulty. The basis to list a drug in the schedule is likelihood of propensity to making someone addicted. Marijuana does not cause addiction, does not cause addiction.

And the second thing is uses that can be seen in medicine, for health, and there are lots of people, veterans in particular, who say that the pain relief that marijuana gives them is so much better than opioids, and it keeps them off opioids, that it also helps people with their appetites, et cetera, et cetera. So, the science is wrong, and I hope you could try to see a new scientific study that reflects the science that is real and that reflects today's values.

And as far as you said of Colorado, do you think marijuana is worse than alcohol for Colorado, as far as traffic deaths, domestic violence, assaults, murders?

Mr. SENSENBRENNER. The gentleman's time has expired.

Mr. COHEN. Can he respond?

Mr. SENSENBRENNER. The gentleman's time has expired.

Mr. COHEN. But the answer has not expired.

Mr. SENSENBRENNER. The gentleman's time has expired. Welcome to Rome. We will now hear from the gentleman from Colorado, Mr. Buck.

Mr. BUCK. Thank you, Mr. Chairman. If the witness would like to answer the last question, please feel free to do so.

Mr. PATTERSON. So, sir, to wrap up on your question, I do not like getting into the comparison of one being better than the other. I think we have a substance abuse problem in this country and to add to that is problematic.

Mr. BUCK. Good morning. First of all, thank you very much for meeting with me a few months ago. I am concerned about sanctuary city policies and their effect on the opioid crisis. When I was at the U.S. Attorney's Office in Denver, Denver was a hub city for heroin and cocaine and other serious drugs that were imported into the country, and from Denver, drugs were transported all the way to the Canadian line and Nebraska, Kansas, Utah. And I contacted some friends in law enforcement just recently, within the last couple of months, and they tell me that Denver is still a hub city for heroin in particular. Heroin is not grown in this country, am I correct?

Mr. PATTERSON. That is correct.

Mr. BUCK. And is it your opinion that Denver is still a hub city for the distribution of dangerous drugs like heroin?

Mr. PATTERSON. Yes, sir.

Mr. BUCK. And the importation of those drugs like heroin comes from other countries and then goes into Denver. And how does that transportation happen?

Mr. PATTERSON. You are talking about the routes that go into Denver? Predominately, I would say through vehicles, right? Trucks or smaller passenger vehicles.

Mr. BUCK. Okay. So, it typically comes across the southern border?

Mr. PATTERSON. Yes, sir.

Mr. BUCK. It may come in by sea, but typically comes across the southern border, and is transported by human beings in vehicles to a place like Denver.

Mr. PATTERSON. Right. When you are talking about the traditional cartels, that is correct.

Mr. BUCK. And typically, those individuals that are transporting the heroin are illegal immigrants. They are illegally in this country. Is that fair to say?

Mr. PATTERSON. I think that is a fair statement.

Mr. BUCK. Okay. So, a city like Denver, that gives sanctuary to illegal immigrants that are involved in the drug trade, is in fact aiding and abetting—or, I will let you use your words, but my words, "aiding and abetting"—the opioid epidemic that we have in the Rocky Mountain region.

Mr. PATTERSON. I think that where this really becomes problematic is the ability for State and locals to impact and work those types of cases. Obviously, on the Federal level we still can, but it impacts our partners in that fight. And as I just talked about before, the State and local population and how we worked those cases is a critical piece.

Mr. BUCK. You were former law enforcement, before you got a cushy desk job, as I might put it. You actually worked the streets. And you knew, and I am hearing this from narcotics officers with the Denver Police Department, and I say "cushy" with tongue in cheek, please.

Mr. PATTERSON. It does not feel that way most days.

Mr. BUCK. Especially now, I would guess. But they tell me that in a typical drug transaction, you have one person that accepts the money from the buyer. You have another person who delivers the drugs to the buyer. And you have one or two lookouts who are making sure that if they see anything suspicious with the police, they can signal the other two people.

So, in a drug transaction like that, with four individuals, you have two individuals that you can arrest and prosecute for the crime of distributing a dangerous drug. You have two other people that are very difficult to prosecute unless they actually get involved in the hand to hand in one way or another.

And so, typically, what would happen in that drug transaction is ICE would be called in, and the two individuals that were lookouts could be deported if they were in this country illegally, but maybe not prosecuted. And I will give you the remainder of my time here, but in that situation, is it important in the fight against the opioid crisis?

Is it important in the fight against heroin distribution for State and local officials to be able to work with the Federal Government to disrupt drug organizations, so that we are safer in our communities and we stop hub cities from spreading this poison throughout the region?

Mr. PATTERSON. Absolutely. It is not really a long answer, right? Our ability to work with those partners and the intelligence and evidence that they gather at the State and local level, is critical to how we do our job.

Mr. BUCK. And I guess my point is that it is not always prosecutable cases that disrupt organizations, right?

Mr. SENSENBRENNER. The gentleman's time has expired. The gentleman from Louisiana, Mr. Richmond.

Mr. RICHMOND. Thank you, Mr. Chairman, and thank you, Mr. Patterson for being here. I asked you a series of questions and you have been very kind today in answering, either in your professional opinion or your life experiences being a law enforcement officer. And I would like to just keep doing that, but just let us know when you are answering as DEA administrator and, too, from just your life experiences. But let me give you some stats first and ask if you have any reason to disagree.

At the height of the crack cocaine epidemic, you had maybe 2,500 deaths associated with crack cocaine, only in terms of the health aspect of it, not with the crime associated with it. Would you have any reason to disagree with that?

Mr. PATTERSON. No, I believe that is consistent with what I have read in the past.

Mr. RICHMOND. And I think what we heard today, overdose numbers are somewhere around 64,000 in the U.S.

Mr. PATTERSON. For all drugs, correct.

Mr. RICHMOND. Correct. And fentanyl and other opioids, I think, is somewhere around 20,000?

Mr. PATTERSON. Opioids, in total, is 44,000.

Mr. RICHMOND. And the other research shows that about 80 percent of the opioid deaths are white, 10 percent black, 8 percent Hispanic. Any reason to dispute that?

Mr. PATTERSON. Honestly, sir, I do not know the breakdown of what that is. I know it goes across all spectrum of people.

Mr. RICHMOND. And do you think that our addiction substance abuse treatment infrastructure in this country is adequate?

Mr. PATTERSON. No.

Mr. RICHMOND. Do you think that if we, in 1980, when we first had a drug epidemic, if we would have answered that with the substance abuse treatment model that we are trying to do now, that we would be ahead of the curve in terms of creating that substance abuse infrastructure, so that today we would not find ourselves in such an inadequate manner to treat the substance abuse we have in this country?

Mr. PATTERSON. So, I am going to give you my personal opinion here, which is, the infrastructure is important. I think, in dealing with the opioid issue, you have a much different issue than cocaine or crack cocaine, sir.

Mr. RICHMOND. Well, if you can briefly tell me the difference, I would love to hear it.

Mr. PATTERSON. So, the opioid path to recovery, in talking to treatment folks, is amazingly hard, and a long-standing problem that they are going to have to deal with for years to come. I think there is a more treatable solution when you talk about cocaine.

Mr. RICHMOND. Which actually stuns me because, if you are telling me it is a lot easier—well, you did not say a lot, but you said it was easy—to break the cocaine addiction, or at least treat the cocaine addiction. Then it would just make sense to me, instead of the path we took, which was mass incarceration, mandatory minimums, to take a health approach, which is what we are doing now in terms of the public health crisis, and treat the addiction as well as fight the violence and the distribution.

But we did not treat the addiction. And I just believe that, had we treated the addiction in the 1980s, we would actually have some addiction treatment infrastructure in this country that would help us become the framework for how we save all of these lives that we are losing today. Am I wrong for drawing that conclusion?

Mr. PATTERSON. I would not say you are wrong. I think, look, there is obviously an evolving process of all best practices as we move forward. And I think, look, hindsight is always, you know, a good thing to go back on. I do not dwell, necessarily, in the past, but we learn lessons every day. So, to your point, you know, look, if things had been different in the '80s, would they be different in 2018? It is very conceivable that the answer is yes.

Mr. RICHMOND. And I do not want to dwell on the past, but I think that we have to learn from the mistakes in the past, and part of our mistakes in the past, some of those people are still incarcerated today. And every dollar we spend on incarceration actually makes every neighborhood, every mother, every father, every grandmother less safe, because it is money that could go to something that would actually prevent a crime.

For example, we do not call opioid-addicted children "crack babies." I mean, there is just a difference, and I will just close with this. I have 10 seconds left. But with the crack epidemic, when we found a grandson in public housing with cocaine, law enforcement pushed to evict the mother, we passed Federal law to do that.

Mr. SENSENBRENNER. The gentleman's time has expired.

Mr. RICHMOND. Are we doing that with opioids?

Mr. SENSENBRENNER. The gentlewoman from Georgia, Mrs. Handel.

Mrs. HANDEL. Thank you, Mr. Chairman, and thank you, Mr. Patterson, for being here. This has been very, very helpful. I wanted to touch on neonatal abstinence syndrome. As you can imagine, with the opioid crisis, we are seeing an increase in babies born with addiction. Yet, DEA does have a policy where it is maintenance only for an addicted mother, versus being able to move that mother off so that the baby is not born with that syndrome.

There has been some compelling research out of the Medical College of Georgia, Augusta University, looking at being able to do programs to move that mother off of addiction. That has significantly reduced the neonatal abstinence syndrome. Is that policy something that DEA is looking at to, perhaps based on some additional research, you might adjust?

Mr. PATTERSON. I would be happy to go back and go through the details with you on the policy and any implications it has. I mean, my exposure to this has been primarily in people I talk to in treatment more than anything else, in terms of the issues related to pregnancy and addiction, and the concerns, quite frankly, of bringing addicted people off during their pregnancy.

Mrs. HANDEL. Could I follow up with your office and share this new research with you? Maybe I could work with someone.

Mr. PATTERSON. Absolutely. I would be happy to read it, because, like I said, me being better educated helps us make better decisions in this space.

Mrs. HANDEL. Great. Wonderful. I wanted to also follow up; my colleague, Representative DeSantis was talking a little bit about fentanyl coming in from China. And I know that last month, the Justice Department arrested 55 indictments in international opioid and fentanyl trafficking rings. Can you just give us a sense of what degree of a dent, small, medium, large, that is even making? And just really the bigger picture about China and the influx of fentanyl.

Mr. PATTERSON. So, I think the critical thing to understand here is that our efforts with DEA and our other law enforcement counterparts in the United States, working with especially the Ministry of Public Security in China, kind of the DEA of China—we are learning more and more not only about the fentanyl itself but the precursors that are then going down into the South and Central America for not just this but methamphetamine and other drugs.

So, there is a good and healthy relationship in terms of how we are trying to work together, recognizing the challenges. The DEA is putting additional people in China, in Guangzhou and looking at some other places to try and leverage better where we can share information back and forth.

I think the key to this is, you know, we have a demand problem that is always going to continue to pull drugs, and so, as we work better with China, we are going to have to then deal with India or other places. So, you know, as you squeeze one part of the balloon it goes someplace else. Demand is a critical piece of this.

I would love to tell you that law enforcement, you know, this could sit at the feet of us, and we could get this fixed, but that is why I always go back to it is got to be a three-piece approach to this.

Mrs. HANDEL. And one last question. If right now, today, you could have two pieces of legislation, additional authority resources, two things that you could say to us in this room that if you had this today or tomorrow it would help you in your effort, what would that be?

Mr. PATTERSON. SITSA is one. The second is, as I stated off by starting with this, we have to deal with this fentanyl issue, so, whatever piece of legislation ultimately we come up with, we have to permanently schedule that in Class I.

Mrs. HANDEL. Great. Thank you very much. Mr. Chairman, I yield back.

Mr. PATTERSON. Thank you.

Mr. SENSENBRENNER. The gentlewoman's time has expired. The gentleman from California, Mr. Swalwell.

Mr. SWALWELL. Thank you, Chairman. Mr. Patterson, first, thank you and your agents for the work that they do in our communities, putting their lives in harm's way every day. It does mean a lot to me and my constituents. You have a presence in our district, and you have worked very closely with our local law enforcement, and I do appreciate that.

There are a number of different, I think, tracks to take to address opioids in America and what we can do to reduce addiction. And I also want to associate myself with Mr. Richmond and a lot of his concerns about just some of the issues and lessons that we should learn from the past. But I want to focus on teenagers.

I have met with families in my district who have lost a teenager, a high schooler, to opioid addiction, and, you know, for many of them, as you described earlier, they describe the same symptoms; they describe the same pattern of behavior. And then, oftentimes it is too late, and the loss, you know, is quite overwhelming to go back and fully understand what they could have done differently.

But what can we do differently with high schools, with the physicians and dentists to these young men and women? I fear that, you know, there is an over-prescription, particularly with young people who do not necessarily appreciate the effects, and then they are down a rabbit hole that they can never get out of. So, if you could first just talk about what we could do with the teenage population as far as awareness, you know, whether it is in the schools, local communities, or the physician community.

Mr. PATTERSON. I will say, I appreciate that. And so, DEA has a program called Operation Prevention which is in the schools, it was done in public-private partnership with Discovery Channel. The key to this, and I think to your point, is we have to start with education and not at high school. It has got to be before high school. I think we all recognize that kids that are now 10 or 11 are probably where we were maybe when we were in our early 20's.

I mean, they are bombarded with technology, they understand things in a much different way, and they have grown up much quicker than we did. So, the key is to get to that age. And I hate to do this, but I am going to do it to you, and this is what concerns me about marijuana. Right? Because those same stories I hear all the time, I generally hear marijuana introduced.

And again, I am not going to compare what is better, what is worse. I am not going to say it is a gateway; I am not—the problem is that these things all seem to dovetail together, and my concern is—and again, I will take my DEA hat off for a second—as a person in the United States, what message do we send as we try and navigate this space in terms of that? And I think that is problematic. So, the education of our youth is important.

Where it really seems to hurt, and more than anything else, is we have these pharmaceuticals that all sit in our house. And I recognize I am going to run you out of time here, and you probably have other things. But we have to get those out, because, like I said, every one of these stories generally sounds the same, and they all hurt. For me, they personally hurt, because it is something that has happened yet again that we feel like we talk about all the time, and for some reason it does not get heard.

Mr. SWALWELL. And Mr. Administrator, can I just ask—when I say teenagers I also include 19-year-old, and the issue I have seen there—even into the early 20's—is that many parents—you know, they still consider the 19-year-old or the 20-year-old, you know, their son or daughter, and they lose their rights, you know, to make healthcare decisions for them, obviously, at 18. And so many parents have told me, "There has to be a way that I can fight for my kid, even though they are 19, 20 years old. I see that they are incapable of, you know, making healthy choices for themselves."

And I understand, like, you know, it is the law, for very good reasons, that you are an adult at 18. But is there—do you have any ideas on what we can do if a parent sees a 19-year-old struggling with addiction, and they are now incapable of, you know, being a part of healthcare decisions or, you know, getting them, you know, the treatment that they need? I do not know if you have encountered this at all.

Mr. PATTERSON. I mean, look, we have, I think, an enormous problem in that college range. It is the big experimentation. Your parents are not over your shoulder every day; you are now amongst your peers. We see this especially in the issue with pharmaceutical pills. And there have been some very public stories about people buying what they believe is a Xanax or something else, and it is not.

So, this space is important and critical. And again, this gets back to an ongoing dialogue, and we in this country tend to like to put a blame on someone and fix it that way, by them being the problem. We all have to admit that this is a nationwide problem, and we have to stop looking at it: "It is this person, or it is that person, or it is this group." And maybe this is now the time.

Mr. SENSENBRENNER. The gentleman's time has expired. The gentleman from Pennsylvania, Mr. Rothfus.

Mr. ROTHFUS. Thank you, Mr. Chairman. It is good to see you, Mr. Patterson. The last time we spoke, you and your colleagues were hosting me for a briefing at DEA. I appreciate your participation here today and trust my colleagues are giving your testimony the way the weighty consideration that I think it deserves.

There are some scary portions of your testimony regarding fentanyl and other similar synthetic drugs. You also mentioned increased trend of fentanyl being mixed with heroin and traffickers now making counterfeit pills that appear like other pharmaceuticals, primarily CPDs, but actually contain fentanyl and other synthetics. What can Congress do to stop pill presses from coming into Mexico and the U.S. to illicitly produce such counterfeit pills?

Mr. PATTERSON. So, sir, we had put out a regulation some time ago, I guess probably about 9 or 10 months ago now, on pill presses that I think we are still trying to evaluate how helpful this is in trying to get people to acknowledge pill presses coming into the United States. I think there is space here, that the question is: how much are we able to impact through legislation these folks that are importing them?

I think that the production of counterfeit pills is a problem that we are going to struggle with for some time, and pill presses certainly are part of that equation. So, legislation that would be proposed and that we can offer technical assistance on I think would be great.

Mr. ROTHFUS. So, you think there might be some room for some additional legislation to address this issue?

Mr. PATTERSON. I do, sir.

Mr. ROTHFUS. Well, we look forward to following up with you on that. Are we seeing a corresponding trend of increased overdoses from counterfeit pills with fentanyl?

Mr. PATTERSON. That is correct.

Mr. ROTHFUS. As far as, you know, looking where this is heading, do you see this getting significantly worse with these counterfeit pills?

Mr. PATTERSON. So, again, as the licit market; as we tighten that and make it harder and harder for licit pills to be there, I think that it naturally pushes and makes the potential for counterfeit pills to become much more of a problem for us.

Mr. ROTHFUS. Given the demand that is out there for fentanyl— and actually, I hear from back home where people look for tar- fentanyl—given how cheap these are to transport and produce, do you see criminal organizations switching from heroin to these substances?

Mr. PATTERSON. I do. The profit margins make them appealing to organizations that are willing to participate in selling.

Mr. ROTHFUS. You referenced Mexico-based transnational criminal organizations in your testimony like Sinaloa and how they are extremely violent, sophisticated, and with large networks. I am also very concerned about the growing interconnectedness of these TCOs globally and potential overlaps with terrorist organizations. Is the administration giving DEA and other agencies the resources and support you need to confront this interconnectedness?

Mr. PATTERSON. I think it is incumbent upon all the agencies that work under this administration to ensure that they are sharing information. We have good centers to do that that are already established, but I think, to your point, the world has gotten very small for these organizations, and the interconnectedness is there. That also gives us opportunity, though, as well.

Mr. ROTHFUS. Now, you know, when I started looking at this a number of years ago I was surprised to learn that the heroin that we are seeing, that it predominately is coming from Mexico; almost all of it. Is that still the case?

Mr. PATTERSON. It is. More than 90 percent of our seizures come from heroin produced in Mexico.

Mr. ROTHFUS. Well, internationally, in the world, 90 percent of the heroin is coming from Afghanistan. It is coming from Afghanistan, across the world, not just the United States, but worldwide.

Mr. PATTERSON. Certainly we do not see the presence in the United States, but they do produce a good portion of the rest of the world's heroin.

Mr. ROTHFUS. Does the supply coming out of Afghanistan impact the price in United States?

Mr. PATTERSON. Probably not.

Mr. ROTHFUS. We do have resources in Afghanistan, DEA resources, yes?

Mr. PATTERSON. We do.

Mr. ROTHFUS. Not nearly what we used to have, correct?

Mr. PATTERSON. No, sir.

Mr. ROTHFUS. Are there sufficient resources, in your opinion? Because I understand last fall we started targeting sites for manufacturer in Afghanistan—our forces did.

Mr. PATTERSON. Right. So, again working with the assets that we have and the resources we have, the best we can do is put intelligence out to that region for them to take action. I think part of the problem is other agencies, and the military has pulled out. It became much harder. You reference it; we are down obviously substantially in our people there. It is much harder for us to work in countries——

Mr. ROTHFUS. Well, given that, you know, most of the heroin in our country is coming from Mexico, do you think other countries that have heroin problems originating in Afghanistan are stepping up enough? Could they be doing more—other countries—with respect to interdiction efforts in Afghanistan?

Mr. PATTERSON. You are talking about internal, in their own country?

Mr. ROTHFUS. Well, also internationally, deploying resources to Afghanistan.

Mr. PATTERSON. No, I do not think that most countries are putting the resources they need to when they are production countries. Mr. ROTHFUS. I yield back.

Mr. SENSENBRENNER. The gentleman from California, Mr. Lieu.

Mr. LIEU. Thank you, Mr. Chair. Thank you, Mr. Patterson, for being here. Thank you for your public service. You have an important job, and this is an important topic. I apologize, I was not here earlier as I at another hearing, so if I ask questions you have answered before, it is because I have not heard them.

When I was in California State Senate before Congress I worked on the opioid issue, and I helped put in the prescription drug monitoring program that California has, and you have put in your written statement that you view that as important for States to have these. I have a question. What happens if someone is in Nevada and gets a prescription, then crosses into California? Do those two databases talk to each other? How does it work when people cross State lines?

Mr. PATTERSON. I do not know specifically the State-to-State connections. That is probably the most critical piece of any PMP, that States, especially where they have borders, are able to see each other's. Because that is what we see all the time in the licit diversion of pharmaceuticals: People crossing State boundaries to essentially go pick that up. I was just out in California and speaking to our office out there; that is one of the better PMP programs that is out there.

Mr. LIEU. Is there any movement towards a national database that would prevent that, or is that too complicated to do?

Mr. PATTERSON. It should not be too complicated, and it is absolutely necessary.

Mr. LIEU. Would that require legislation, or could the DEA start doing that? What would be needed if we wanted to -

Mr. PATTERSON. Look, it could come in a couple of different forms. One, obviously—probably the easiest—would be legislation.

We have tried to push the States to have more interconnectivity. I think there are a number of people that have already put this forward, and again, we would be happy to provide assistance in what we see on that. I think the key is we hear this all the time from pharmacies and doctors as well, is that inability to see these patterns impacts them being able to make good decisions. So, where States fall short on this; this is the place that for me is highly problematic.

Mr. LIEU. Thank you. I also work on the issue of people able to buy opioids on Craigslist and other internet websites. Has that increased, decreased, or remained the same the last few years?

Mr. PATTERSON. I think, unfortunately, it is probably increased. I think you still see it across the spectrum of the internet. We are looking at, obviously, the darknet and Clearnet as to these locations, in essence for information that we can then use to target some of these folks. It would be nice if we could work better with the industry in having all of these sites pulled down. They recognize the challenges with that, but I think from a governmental standpoint, from a law enforcement standpoint, I think at some point we have to start dealing with known crimes that are occurring over the internet.

Mr. LIEU. If you have any ideas, let this committee and let us know regarding the internet trafficking. It is a hard issue. At the time, I was working on it, Purdue Pharma said they made oxycontin a different form that made it hard to use it legally. Did that work?

Mr. PATTERSON. I believe people figured out how to abuse that as well.

Mr. LIEU. Okay, so that did not really work.

Mr. PATTERSON. People with problems find ways to abuse drugs when they need to abuse drugs.

Mr. LIEU. In your written testimony you stated that there was a 70 percent increase in emergency visits related to opioids in the Midwest. You had some other regions; it was 20 percent in the Southwest. Why was there such a large spike in the Midwest?

Mr. PATTERSON. I think there are a couple things that factor into why we see spikes, and I do not necessarily know if it has changed it. Now, obviously, with emergency room visits we have seen a shift. We look at States that traditionally have not had this problem. I look at New Mexico, Utah, some of some of those States that have all of sudden had kind of a pick-up in this area, and it is incumbent upon us to be able to react and pay attention to that. That is why we are, unfortunately, tracking overdoses, overdose deaths, so that we can position ourselves to help those communities as it goes.

As we look at the Northeast and see some promise there, we have to be nimble enough to move our resources around to where we are seeing problems. But I think you see pockets showing up all over, and I know, certainly in terms of overdose deaths, sometimes those spikes end up being additional work that is being done in the ME or the coroner offices.

Mr. LIEU. Thank you. It also seems part of problem are patients who get prescriptions for doctors who treat pain, and then they get addicted to opioids. Do you know if doctors are being trained to recognize this more broadly, or is there continuing medical education or medical schools are onto this? Are they trying to train their doctors in a different way than, let's say, 10 years ago?

Mr. PATTERSON. I hope. I mean, look, we strongly support CME, or continuing medical education, in this space. I think that is a critical piece of what we see. DEA does outreach on a voluntary issue with the doctors, and I think the other thing that we are doing is trying to communicate much better with the 1.7 million registrants through the ability that we have to send them notifications and things; again, all voluntary. But I go back to the fact that I look at the vast majority of doctors: 99.99 percent are all trying to do right by their patients. So, I think the key is to, again, keep working on it educational process.

Mr. SENSENBRENNER. The gentleman's time has expired. The gentleman from Arizona, Mr. Biggs.

Mr. BIGGS. Thank you, Mr. Chairman, and thank you, Mr. Patterson, for being here today. It has been a very informative hearing. If I understand right, the vast majority of fentanyl and its derivatives are coming from China through Mexico across the southern border. Is that a fair takeaway?

Mr. PATTERSON. There are two different trends. So, you have bulk, you know, the larger quantities coming across the southern border. I think you have much more smaller packages coming directly in through China into the United States.

Mr. BIGGS. And I think in the second panel there will be a lady testifying of a young man who received it directly from China. But in this instance, I was curious about the role of Phoenix and the Tucson corridor for both transfers across the border. Can you elaborate on that a little bit, and also the efforts to interdict?

Mr. PATTERSON. All of those points of entry into our country have been blitzed with not just opioids but methamphetamine and other drugs coming across the southern border. Our border offices—so, you know, Texas, certainly Phoenix, or Phoenix division, San Diego, and El Paso, where these places are—it is the bulk of our work trying to deal with the mass quantities coming across the border, and that is where those folks primarily focus their efforts.

Mr. BIGGS. You talked about China, and then, as you squeeze the balloon, you are seeing that there is a potential moving to India, trying to fill a void if you are able to suppress China. And in your written testimony you elaborated quite a bit about China, and you talked about DEA liaison in in China. Can you tell me, what does that liaison do exactly, and how is that helping to slow the flow?

Mr. PATTERSON. So, our personnel that sit in China currently— the key is that intelligence sharing back and forth and an ongoing dialogue of things that they can do to help us in our process, and, frankly, training each other. So, we have had a number of them come over to understand from a chemistry side how to look at things that we are seeing. And a lot of this goes back to them trying to schedule the various analogues over in China, because we do see that when they do scheduling actions it has an impact in that country, which ultimately impacts us and what we are seeing here.

Mr. BIGGS. I am glad you said that, because that was my next question. Have the joint efforts produced some kind of positive reduction?

Mr. PATTERSON. They have, but again, these are chemists, and they will constantly change structures to avoid that. Part of the reason for us scheduling fentanyl as a class the way we did was to try and persuade China to do that in kind, to do the similar type of thing, and we are continuing to work through that effort. And they have done a number of fentanyl analogues and precursor chemicals, which is critically important.

Mr. BIGGS. Okay, so, if they open up the schedule or regulation of the schedule to a broader segment of fentanyl and its analogues, that is one way. But are they doing anything else to physically interdict shipments to the U.S., either through, like you are talking about, both the small transfers—direct mail, if I can put it that way—and bulk?

Mr. PATTERSON. Yeah, there have been seizures made over in China, and I think the key for us is being able to share data back and forth in a productive way of understanding the targets where those folks are shipping to the United States, and there has been a good pass of information back and forth in that realm.

Mr. BIGGS. Okay. You mentioned in your written testimony that in 2015 there was enhanced collaboration, and I am wondering what the next steps are with China. And what do you see the next steps working with China would be?

Mr. PATTERSON. I think the key for us is to get more resources there. We have a limited staff in China. Like I said before, you know, we are going to put additional personnel in Guangzhou, which is a big shipment point out of China, to try and really deal with these issues. But there is a willingness, certainly, at the agency level to participate and work fully in doing that.

One of the other huge pieces that we are trying to do is the precursors that are leaving China, going down into Central America, into Mexico, because that is a huge piece of not just the opioid side or what potentially could be an opioid problem, but the methamphetamine piece that we are dealing with in this country.

Mr. BIGGS. So, if we are successful in the Chinese interdiction, or at least to slow that down, and you anticipate maybe someplace like India or someplace else. What are the anticipated efforts that that are going to be necessary in those future countries?

Mr. PATTERSON. It will be taking that playbook that we learn from in China on how to work, essentially, the chemicals, which are the critical piece of this, and into India and other regions.

Mr. SENSENBRENNER. The gentleman's time has expired. The gentleman from Maryland, Mr. Raskin.

Mr. RASKIN. Thank you, Mr. Chair. Mr. Patterson, thank you for your service and your testimony today. Sixty-four thousand overdose deaths in 2016, which is more than the number of Americans who died in the entire Vietnam War; two-thirds of those 64,000 deaths opioid-related. Are we winning the war on opioid abuse? Are we losing it? Is it a stalemate? What is the report to the American people today?

Mr. PATTERSON. I think the issue that we have is, one, it is not a win. So, I mean, again, the number is problematic for me. I think what we see is that we are going to have to deal, you know, whether it is for the year or for in the next couple years, with a population that has been abusing opioids and what that will mean for us as a Nation.

Mr. RASKIN. And, you know, in your effort you reported a huge number of Take Back drugs that DEA receives. What percentage of the Take Back drugs are opioids?

Mr. PATTERSON. So, we do not break those out, sir. I will tell you that I think, you know, most of us in our homes have had those bottles of opioids sitting around, so there is a percentage of it. You know, you could even put it at a small percentage and realize that we have a problem with overprescribing in this country in terms of the volume that we prescribe.

Mr. RASKIN. Okay. I found one academic article online just as you were speaking, because it sounded promising, that there were tons of Take Back drugs, but this one article says that only 0.3 percent of Take Back drugs are opioids, and most of them are aspirin or Flintstone vitamins. Is that right?

Mr. PATTERSON. I would find that statistic to probably not be accurate, sir.

Mr. RASKIN. What would you estimate it as?

Mr. PATTERSON. I do not know.

Mr. RASKIN. They are saying it is less than 1 percent.

Mr. PATTERSON. Even if you put it at 2 or 3 percent, it is still a pretty dramatic number of opioids. And we do not go through that and count up which it would be; our quest is to get the volume of prescription drugs out of the homes. And I do not know if we have any analysis, but if I find out that we do I will get back to you.

Mr. RASKIN. Please. I would be very curious to know. So, I was interested in your colloquy with my colleagues Johnson and Cohen about science, and I was glad to hear you testify in favor of science. Do you favor a rigorous and comprehensive scientific study about the addictiveness, the lethality, and the negative and positive health effects of marijuana?

Mr. PATTERSON. So, I think we have been pretty vocal about our belief in the research towards the medicine that could come from marijuana. I think our application process that we put in August of 2016 showed that we were trying to help the industry in terms of understanding where that research may go with giving additional growers.

Mr. RASKIN. So, you would favor a comprehensive scientific health study on the effects of marijuana?

Mr. PATTERSON. Absolutely.

Mr. RASKIN. Okay. Let me ask you. We are in such a terrible situation with the opioid crisis as well as with drug abuse generally, as you are saying. Tell me how America's experience with liquor prohibition informs your analysis of the most effective strategies we can be using in order to address this public health crisis.

Mr. PATTERSON. I am not your person to talk about liquor analysis, so I cannot help you on that topic, sir, in terms of how that correlates with, I think, the drug issue in the United States.

Mr. RASKIN. Okay. I ask this question not rhetorically but seriously: do you favor, speaking either as the head of the DEA or personally, the 21st Amendment and the repeal of prohibition of alcohol? Obviously, there remain tens of thousands of people who die every year from alcohol abuse, both in terms of health effects but also because of drunk driving on the highways. Do you have a position on that?

Mr. PATTERSON. To repeal it?

Mr. RASKIN. Well, the 21st Amendment repealed prohibition, the Eighteenth Amendment. Do you support the 21st Amendment, or do you think we made the wrong decision then? Would it have been better to continue with prohibition of alcohol?

Mr. PATTERSON. I think this goes back to it is a personal use decision to be made. So, I mean, I would not sit here and tell you that I think that was a bad decision. I do think that all these factors, like I said, we all have to be the adults in the room.

Mr. RASKIN. And I appreciate your answer very much, because I certainly tell my kids that I think using alcohol is a bad decision. We have a relative who was killed by a drunk driver; I feel very seriously about it. On the other hand, I think that our experiment with prohibition failed because there was a public demand for it for the reason you say, that people like to experiment with their consciousness in different ways. Do you think that, after decades of criminalizing marijuana, that experiment in prohibition has proven to be a failure, and it is time to call it off?

Mr. PATTERSON. So, I will give you my personal opinion on this, which is I think over the last decade my opinion has changed on this. Ten years ago, I may have told you yes, and I think now, more than ever before, as I see what fuels some of our addiction problems in this country, starting with marijuana, I have gotten a much more stronger opinion as to that. I believe that we are now in a dangerous environment in terms of what we are doing with legalization.

Mr. ROTHFUS [presiding]. The time of the gentleman has expired. The chair recognizes the gentleman from Louisiana, Mr. Johnson, for 5 minutes.

Mr. JOHNSON of Louisiana. Thank you, Mr. Chairman. Mr. Patterson, thanks for being here. As you know, an ISO was issued on Friday afternoon against a large distributor in my district, accompanied by a DEA press release. And I just have two kind of categories of questions related to that, one with regard to the patients that are affected by this ultimately, and second, with regard to process.

Regarding the patients, by Monday I had already received multiple constituent inquiries about all this, including a local hospital who said that this was creating a serious situation for them and an affidavit from the Louisiana Independent Pharmacy Association expressing the immeasurable impact this decision is going to have on the many hospitals and pharmacies and patients throughout my State, and really the Nation, because this distributor serves many States around the country. Mr. Chairman I would like to ask unanimous consent to enter into the record a copy of this affidavit.

Mr. ROTHFUS. Without objection.

Mr. JOHNSON of Louisiana. Thank you. The affidavit is from the CEO and president of Louisiana Independent Pharmacy Association, and he says in a three-page affidavit—the most important language, I think, is at the end. He says, "This suspension has already caused a disruption in the supply chain for our members"—all the independent pharmacies—"and is currently impacting the delivery of care to the patients those members serve.

Affiant believes that continued suspension will worsen the problem, causing patients served by independent pharmacies to have their care delayed and perhaps be denied. The most significant impact is to the patients who are unable to find the pharmacy healthcare and necessary prescription drugs in their community and to find the continuity of care to help maintain and improve their health and health outcomes."

The question is: when an immediate suspension order is issued, is there any consideration at all given to the patients that rely on these lifesaving drugs that are effectively left without access to critical medication overnight?

Mr. PATTERSON. There absolutely is.

Mr. JOHNSON of Louisiana. I mean, what did you do in this situation, by way of example?

Mr. PATTERSON. So, again, as we spoke about earlier, the issue for us here is we have not heard from these same hospitals that have now provided—and I have not seen that affidavit—an affidavit, obviously for the temporary restraining order that is going to be filed today, and there is a process by which the company down there can go and go about that. We have not heard the same concerns, as——

Mr. JOHNSON of Louisiana. Let me stop you, because I am short on time. Let's just apply common sense here. Let me assume, for the record, that you have not heard since this happened Friday afternoon, and we are here on Tuesday morning; you have not had time to hear from a lot of these folks. Would you take my word for it that many are affected? And if you do not take my word for it, use common sense.

This distributor, for example, supplies hundreds of hospitals in Louisiana and the surrounding region, hundreds of Louisiana pharmacies totaling hundreds of millions of doses per year. So, is it safe to say that that puts patients affected, I mean, at least in the numbers of tens of thousands, if not hundreds of thousands of patients, in some immediate jeopardy? Some of those are lifesaving medications, are they not?

Mr. PATTERSON. I understand that, and simply what I will counter with you is that the hospitals or pharmacies that we have talked to have secondary supplies, as most generally do.

Mr. JOHNSON of Louisiana. How many have you spoken to on this case?

Mr. PATTERSON. I do not know. I think less than 10 have reached out to us. So, every one of those people that have the ability to distribute narcotics or distribute schedule I or schedule II, in this case, have backup sources, and those that do not have already reached out to DEA to seek remedy.

Mr. JOHNSON of Louisiana. Well, this affidavit from the Louisiana Independent Pharmacy Association, they have at least 85 pharmacies, about 82 million prescriptions filled each year, and they are directly affected. So, you might want to consider that. I am concerned about going forward in other cases, before you issue an ISO, which I understand is a rare occasion, there ought to be some regard paid to all these patients.

I have a lot of constituents who are literally some on their death bed today; I am not using hyperbole. They cannot get their necessary medications because the DEA decided to do this. I am concerned about the process. And let me ask you, in a case like this, would the DEA consider, as they have in the past, this example? This company, for example. Will they have an opportunity to offer a remedial plan rather than just instantly removing access to millions of doses a year for all these patients? Are they going to have a chance to correct?

Mr. PATTERSON. There is. There is a process in which they will have the chance to correct. But I go back to the fact of if you have a company that shows woeful neglect and continued bad behavior, we have to hold these folks accountable.

Mr. JOHNSON of Louisiana. Well, it is not for you and I to litigate the specific facts of this case.

Mr. PATTERSON. I agree.

Mr. JOHNSON of Louisiana. That is for the court. But is it a normal process, a normal procedure, for the DEA to allow an alleged offender to present a remedial action plan?

Mr. PATTERSON. The corrective action plan is part of the process. Mr. JOHNSON of Louisiana. And would they be afforded that in this case?

Mr. PATTERSON. Yes.

Mr. JOHNSON of Louisiana. I am almost out of time. One more question about process: if it comes to light that the DEA acted prematurely or that evidence did not support the claims in this case, for example, are there processes in place to offer restitution? So, for example, if a company goes out of business because of this delay, what remedy do they have against the Federal Government? I am out of time, but you can answer.

Mr. ROTHFUS. The gentleman's time has expired. The chair recognizes the gentlewoman from California, Ms. Bass, for 5 minutes.

Ms. BASS. Thank you. I actually want to follow some of the questioning of my colleague here. And I know, you know—excuse me— we are back and forth; we all have hearings the same time, and some of these questions you might have been asked before.

But I really wanted to talk about the drug manufacturers, even before they get to the point of distributing it. You know, this problem has not existed forever. I mean, it has been many years since I worked in the medical field, but when I was working in the medical field we did not have this problem.

And so, before the drugs are even distributed to individual pharmacies, what relationship do you have with the manufacturers to begin with? Because one has to question why they are manufacturing millions and millions of opioids when they were not needed before? So, how do you work at the point of manufacturing with the manufacturer?

Mr. PATTERSON. I think this is really where the rubber meets the road on this issue. We can fight this downstream, right, with doctors and pharmacies and diversion of pharmaceuticals, but you have to elevate this conversation back to the prescribing practices the United States.

Ms. BASS. Well, the prescribing practices, absolutely. I agree with you. But I am talking about even before the prescribing practices.

I mean, the companies that make these drugs: does the DEA put pressure on them for producing and manufacturing the volume that they do?

Mr. PATTERSON. So, under the quota process we do, but what I was going to finish up on that last sentence is the prescribing practices cannot be driven by industry. They need to be driven by the medical community, and I think that is where the disconnect is there.

So, DEA has done more and more education with distributors, and even in the manufacturing space, to explain the problem, but where this has to change is in the prescribing practices, because there are corporations that are making pills. As long as that continues to get put out in the same manner, we have a problem.

Ms. BASS. But you do know the relationship, right? So, you know that the distributors go to doctors' offices and promote the prescribing practices? I mean, when I listen to my colleague there talk about the tens of thousands of people that need opioids in his district, I really have to raise the question: do they really?

Mr. PATTERSON. You are asking the wrong guy that question, because I will give you the law enforcement answer, which is no. I mean, it does not need to be. And there are some good studies out there to show that opioids—the VA just did one where opioids had the same impact that Tylenol did when you do blind studies. So, I mean, there is science out there, again, to go back to that word.

Look, we have to change our culture, and that is why I said this is not a one-size-fits-all answer to anything. We have to change a culture in this country. But it goes across all of us. Right? So, whether it is legislation capabilities to fix this problem; whether it is, you know, the pharmaceutical industry ultimately recognizing the harm that is being done; whether it is law enforcement and their efforts; I mean, we all have to work collectively together on this problem.

Ms. BASS. Yeah, I agree with you, but at some place we have to figure out how to hold the companies responsible, because they push the medication on the doctors. They hand out free supplies; they put on lunches and dinners. I mean, I worked in many medical offices before, and I also have a hard time understanding.

And I hear about—I do not know that this exists in Los Angeles, but I do think it exists in a number of your districts—where you have these "pharmacies," and people will get off the freeway offramp and go pick up huge volumes of opioids that there is no way in the world you can say that that has a medical use, and that is allowed. And I do not understand that. I do not understand how those type of pharmacies can even exist.

Mr. PATTERSON. No, and that is where law enforcement does have to step in. So, once you have moved from the manufacturing into the distributor and then the pharmacies and the doctors and that relationship there, we have to do a much better job. And I know you had not been here earlier, but where we interact with States and then using HHS data and others to find these in a real, efficient, and timely manner to stop that harm, because that is ultimately where those pharmaceuticals get introduced to the general public.

Ms. BASS. Right, but they would not have those if the manufacturers were not producing it at such a volume. Thank you.

Mr. PATTERSON. Thank you.

Ms. BASS. I yield back.

Mr. ROTHFUS. The gentlewoman yields back. The chair recognizes the gentleman from Iowa, Mr. King, for 5 minutes.

Mr. KING. Thank you, Mr. Chairman. First, Mr. Patterson, I want to thank you for your direct testimony, and my sense of your testimony here today is you came here to help inform this Congress of the job we all have ahead of us. Sometimes we get evasive witnesses, and you are not one. So, thank you. Maybe I would start with this. Do we have a decent idea on how many drug misusers we have in America?

Mr. PATTERSON. Overall, or for in the opioid space?

Mr. KING. Overall.

Mr. PATTERSON. Overall, it is obviously in the millions, probably, you know, 10 or so million, 11 million.

Mr. KING. Okay. And I am looking at a number around 11.5 million, so that is in the zone. And I am not going to ask you to answer the components of this now, but is it something you could put together for us to build us a pie chart that would tell us the overall population of drug misusers, and then break it down by the different types of drugs so we could get a better handle on the scope of this drug abuse problem we have in America?

Mr. PATTERSON. I would be happy to do that, sir.

Mr. KING. Good. I appreciate that, and I will be looking forward to seeing that. Do we know what the street value is of the illegal drugs consumed in America? The illegals?

Mr. PATTERSON. Yeah. Across, again, the platform of all narcotics, yes, we do.

Mr. KING. What is that number? The street value?

Mr. PATTERSON. The street value?

Mr. KING. Yes.

Mr. PATTERSON. Maybe I am misunderstanding your question. I thought you meant like what someone would pay for a dose of a certain thing. You are talking about the total off——

Mr. KING. No, I am interested in how many dollars out of our U.S. GDP are spent on illegal drugs? What does it do to our economy?

Mr. PATTERSON. It is a massive drain on our economy.

Mr. KING. Do you have to guess at that, though? I mean, I saw a number reported by Fox about 4 years ago of $40 billion; I saw a number reported, $60 billion. We have got $60 billion or more that are transferred south of the border for some reason. Some of that is laundered money. So, do you think that number is up from those estimates I am seeing?

Mr. PATTERSON. I do, but part of the issue here is whenever you see these numbers it depends on what is being factored into it. Right? A lot of them do loss of wages; loss of productivity; cost to, you know, Medicare, Medicaid, and prescription; all these other things. So, I would be more than happy to come back and give you some real numbers as to what we see.

Mr. KING. I would very much like that, and we can flesh that question out in a little more detail, perhaps, off the panel. Let's see. What percentage of the illegal drugs consumed in America come from or through Mexico?

Mr. PATTERSON. I would suggest that, for the bulk number, probably of the vast majority.

Mr. KING. If I remember a previous discussion with DEA some years ago, their estimate was between 80 and 90 percent. That would be in the zone that you understand today?

Mr. PATTERSON. I think that is certainly a fair estimate.

Mr. KING. Okay. And then, what percentage of the illegal drug distribution chains include at least one link that is an illegal alien? Mr. PATTERSON. One link that is an illegal alien?

Mr. KING. Yes.

Mr. PATTERSON. I would assume almost all of them.

Mr. KING. That has been consistent with the responses I have gotten with others as well. And so, then, do we have any data? I know some of these estimates you mention address the American productivity, so we can flesh that question out a little bit more, too. I want to get a better scope on what it does to our economy; what it does to our families; the impact on our children. I do not see very good estimates of that that are quantified, and that might fall in the line of sound science.

But you made a statement here that—first, I want to put another thing into your ear. If I do the math on this, 11.5 million drug misusers in America; 64,000 of them died in the year 2017. So, if I just divide the 64,000 into 11.5 million, I come up with a number one out of 180 drug—I call them drug abusers—die to overdose in any given year. If they are going to use drugs for 10 years, they have got a 1-in-18 chance rather than a one-in-180 chance. In 20 years, it is one in nine. That is the scope of the devastation that we are seeing in our society.

But you made a very important point here, and I think it is the most important one of the whole panel, and it says, "We have to change the culture in this country." That really does, I think, ring the bell as close to the center of the truth that we are dealing with here, as complex as it is. And so, I want to pose an approach to this, and then it is this: if society were determined to solve this problem, I believe we would do this.

First, we would test in the workplace, then we would test in education, and we would test certainly in government as well, and then we would test in welfare. And if we did that, theoretically, we would dramatically reduce the drug abuse in each of those arenas. Those left would be the dealers and stealers, and they would be the ones that law enforcement would contend with, and we should be able to handle that if that is the only ones left out of the universe.

And so, I pose that, but the big question still is, how do we get the culture change to accept such a change? And I think recognizing the reality of those deaths that we are having and the damage to our society and quantifying it would be a very good step to follow along. I look forward to continuing to work with you, and I appreciate the job you are doing and the testimony that you provided today, Mr. Patterson. Thank you, and I yield back.

Mr. ROTHFUS. The time of the gentleman has expired, and the chair recognizes the gentleman from Florida, Mr. Deutch, for 5 minutes.

Mr. DEUTCH. [inaudible].

Mr. GAETZ. Mr. Chairman, can I ask the gentleman to turn his microphone so I can hear him?

Mr. DEUTCH. I apologize. Thank you. Florida was the epicenter of the explosion of opioid abuse over a decade ago. In Florida, opioid addiction-related deaths increased 80 percent from 2003 to 2009. Addiction is cruel, ruthless, and unforgiving. Opioid pills prescribed after an injury or to treat chronic pain can too easily drag anyone in pain into the depths of addiction. The crackdown on pills has meant turning to street drugs for thousands of Floridians.

Mr. Chairman, we have used mandatory minimum sentences as 1951, and we boosted penalties through the last 3 decades of the twentieth century at the height of the war on drugs. But tough mandatory minimums for drug charges have not cut off access to drugs in the past, and they are not likely to stop the brutal tide of overdoses that we are facing today. I would like to share a story that I heard from Broward County public defender Howard Finkelstein, just to caution the work of this committee.

He told me about a 40-year-old woman in Broward County, Florida, who had no criminal record and was unable to work due to a disability. She was described by those who knew as a sweet lady. After being pursued multiple times by a confidential informant seeking pills, she gave in. She sold 35 Lorcet pills, a blend of Tylenol and hydrocodone, to the informant. After living 40 years without a criminal record, she was sentenced to a mandatory minimum sentence of 25 years in prison.

Does keeping this woman in prison until she is 65 do anything to help her, to help her family continue without their mom in the home, to help others who are addicted, to our society now paying for her incarceration? This committee needs to take a close look at the impact of our policing and prosecution policies around the country that do a lot to drive up the numbers of arrests, convictions, and fill our prisons, but may not be helping treat addiction or save lives.

Hyper-deadly drugs like fentanyl are finding a way into our communities. The rise of these synthetic opioids requires that we meet this challenge on its own terms. Their extreme potency makes it harder for law enforcement to stop them. With a few clicks on the internet, there is no longer a need for cartels or street dealers. Last year, Florida passed a law to impose mandatory minimum sentences for possession of fentanyl and other synthetic drugs, but evidence shows that boosting punishment is unlikely to stop the spread of these drugs.

This March, I held a roundtable on the opioid crisis with my colleague, Congresswoman Wasserman Schultz, in my district to talk with law enforcement, public health officials, and families about the response to the needs of our community. And what we heard was that, fundamentally, addiction is about mental health, and to save the lives of those in the grip of addiction, we need to get them help, not lock them up. Criminalizing addiction locks people out of our healthcare system and cuts off a real chance at recovery.

We need a comprehensive solution. I think we have delayed too long in getting a comprehensive response through the House to address this crisis. We need to focus on broadening access to addiction treatment that would truly save lives. Instead, just over a year ago, my Republican colleagues celebrated a vote to overturn Obamacare that would have taken comprehensive coverage from over 20 million people. Some Republican States, including my own State of Florida, have failed to expand access to care with Federal dollars by expanding Medicaid.

Expansion can allow more than 800,000 Floridians to gain access to comprehensive health coverage that includes mental health and substance abuse treatment as essential benefits. It is estimated that 300,000 of those 800,000 Floridians already need some level of care right now, and they are struggling to get it, but, apparently, my colleagues who voted for Trumpcare last year think that we should go the other direction, that we should end Medicaid expansion and fundamentally change the program structure.

It would replace guaranteed funding with a limited account for opioid treatment; to lock recovery clinic doors to those who desperately need help. It will undermine the emergency response needed to pull up the deep roots of Florida's addiction crisis. Twelve Floridians are lost every day to the scourge of addiction. It is a public health emergency, and treatment can help save the lives of our fellow Floridians.

Mr. Patterson, I would just ask you, given your experience, do you think a broader access to substance abuse and mental health coverage would help people struggling with addiction treatment stay in treatment?

Mr. PATTERSON. So, we are talking about addicted populations? You had a couple things combined in there.

Mr. DEUTCH. Okay.

Mr. PATTERSON. The sentencing issues put aside, I think for people that are not distributing drugs—and, obviously, DEA does not, you know, look at a certain level.

Mr. DEUTCH. I understand.

Mr. PATTERSON. The treatment availability should be there for those that are addicted to drugs. I think distribution is a different issue, though, than what you just talked about.

Mr. DEUTCH. Thank you very much. Thank you, Mr. Chairman.

Mr. ROTHFUS. The time of the gentleman is expired. The chair recognizes the gentleman from Florida, Mr. Gaetz, for 5 minutes.

Mr. GAETZ. Thank you, Mr. Chairman. Earlier in your testimony you said in response to a medical marijuana question, "We have a substance abuse problem, and we do not want to add to it." Is it the position of the DEA that democratizing access to medical marijuana will add to the substance abuse problem in this country?

Mr. PATTERSON. I think it is a conversation that we have to have. Again, when you say medical marijuana, is it a medicine that has been made from marijuana, or the current standard of the State has now said that marijuana is medicine?

Mr. GAETZ. Well, in either of those circumstances. But let's just take the circumstance where a State is said marijuana is medicine. Is it your view that that adds to the substance abuse problem?

Mr. PATTERSON. It is.

Mr. GAETZ. Opioids are prescribed principally as a chronic pain solution, right?

Mr. PATTERSON. Correct.

Mr. GAETZ. The National Academy of Sciences issued a report in 2017 entitled The Health Effects of Cannabis and Cannabinoids. Are you familiar with that work product?

Mr. PATTERSON. No, sir.

Mr. GAETZ. I will quote from it. It says, "There is conclusive or substantial evidence that cannabis or cannabinoids are effective for treatment of chronic pain in adults." Do you have any basis, scientifically or from any evidentiary standpoint, to disagree with that conclusion?

Mr. PATTERSON. Again, this is why I think we always talk about the research of the benefits of marijuana.

Mr. GAETZ. So, you support research into medical marijuana?

Mr. PATTERSON. We have said that all along, that we support the research of marijuana.

Mr. GAETZ. And after you implemented a rule in August of 2016 pushing the Department of Justice to create more research-based cannabis, they have not issued any more of those permits, have they? Or have not granted any.

Mr. PATTERSON. So, they have not been granted, but I think there is an important distinction that has to be understood. So, when we put that rule out it was in the efforts to help the research community.

Mr. GAETZ. But if none of the research permits have been granted, how has it helped them?

Mr. PATTERSON. Because there is an issue with how we put that solicitation out of that rule out, and that has to do with the single treaty, which I know, you know—I had to get up to speed on it. I did not understand it at first when I was told. But the reality is that the department has worked through this; once they have made their ruling, DEA will figure out how this looks moving forward.

Mr. GAETZ. But you have taken the position that medical cannabis—in response to my questions—adds to the problem. So, you have also agreed that opioids are prescribed for chronic pain, so I want to use my remaining time to delve into the extent to which medical cannabis in some places has been used as an appropriate substitute.

The Minnesota Department of Health had a research project with over 2,000 patients who had intractable pain that used medical cannabis. And those patients saw opioids prescribed at a rate 38 percent less than people who were not using medical cannabis. Do you have any basis with which to disagree with that finding that those patients saw a reduction in the need for opioids when they had access to medical cannabis?

Mr. PATTERSON. So, I am not familiar with that study. I think there are a number of studies out there that talk when people are presented, whether—I guess it would be with medical marijuana or with Tylenol or others—that there are many alternatives to opioids.

Mr. GAETZ. So, do you acknowledge, then, that medical marijuana is an alternative to opioids?

Mr. PATTERSON. No, I am saying I do not know that study. So, I mean—

Mr. GAETZ. What studies show that medical marijuana would increase the use of opioids? Are there any?

Mr. PATTERSON. I do not know.

Mr. GAETZ. So, you are the acting administrator of the DEA; you cannot cite a single study that indicates that medical marijuana creates a greater challenge with opioids. And you are unaware of the studies, including studies from the National Academy of Sciences, that demonstrate that medical marijuana can be an acceptable alternative to opioids. Is that what I am understanding?

Mr. PATTERSON. Yes.

Mr. GAETZ. The American Geriatric Society surveyed patients, and they found a 68 percent reduction in opioid use. Are you familiar with that?

Mr. PATTERSON. No, sir.

Mr. GAETZ. In New Mexico, medical cannabis patients saw a 70 percent reduction not only in opioids but in all scheduled drugs. Is that something you are familiar with?

Mr. PATTERSON. No, sir.

Mr. GAETZ. So, the sum of evidence from the States that have democratized access to medical cannabis—have you analyzed any data that looks at opioid death rates in medical cannabis States versus nonmedical cannabis States?

Mr. PATTERSON. No, sir.

Mr. GAETZ. You indicated earlier, and I am grateful for it, that that is an appropriate conversation to have. I wanted to take my last few moments to thank Chairman Goodlatte; he has signed on as a cosponsor to the Medical Cannabis Research Act, which I think builds on the work of DEA to push the Department of Justice to stop their obstruction when it comes to researching medical cannabis. Can we count on the DEA to be a partner in pushing for more research so that we can either validate or dismiss this information we are receiving from States?

Mr. PATTERSON. And I think we have been consistent in that message for the last number of years.

Mr. GAETZ. Thank you, Mr. Chairman.

Mr. ROTHFUS. The time of the gentleman has expired. The chair recognizes the gentlewoman from Washington, Ms. Jayapal, for 5 minutes.

Ms. JAYAPAL. Thank you, Mr. Chairman, and thank you, Administrator Patterson for being here and for your work. I am unfortunately going to miss the second panel, and so I did want to just raise something before turning to my questions for you that I was going to say in the second panel.

And that is in my hometown of Seattle we recognized early on that we cannot arrest our way out of the situation, not just for opioids but on other low-level crimes as well, and in 2011 we launched the Law Enforcement Assisted Diversion program, the LEAD program. It was the first known prebooking diversion program for people arrested on narcotics and prostitution charges in the United States, and it is a very, very unique collaboration between local law enforcement, prosecutors, treatment services, the Department of Corrections, public defenders, and the ACLU and others.

And actually, among LEAD participants, 60 percent are less likely to be arrested; 89 percent more likely to have a place to live; 46 percent more likely to have a job in the 6 months following enrollment.

Mr. Chairman, I seek unanimous consent to enter into the record an article on LEAD, as well as a University of Washington study on the efficacy of LEAD.

Mr. ROTHFUS. Without objection.

Ms. JAYAPAL. Thank you. And I want to thank Mr. Sensenbrenner, Mr. Johnson, and a number of Republicans that helped me to get some funds into the last budget omnibus spending bill that expands the LEAD program across the country into some of these critical areas that are dealing with opioids.

So, Mr. Patterson, according to a 24-page report that was prepared by the DEA last May, drugs frequently do not enter through land routes. The report provided numerous examples of this, noting, for instance, that the majority of heroin found in New Jersey is primarily smuggled into the United States by Colombian and Dominican groups via human couriers on commercial flights to the Newark International Airport.

You have been quoted previously saying, and this is your quote, “This is not an easy thing to fix. If there were two or three answers to solve this problem, then I should be fired. There are thousands of things that need to be addressed.”

And I wanted to bring up the fact that there have been many attempts to assert, by the White House and by Republican colleagues on the other side, that building a border wall is somehow going to solve the problem of the flow of illegal drugs into the United States. Did your intel report recommend building a border wall as a solution to the flow of drugs into the United States?

Mr. PATTERSON. That report—I do not recall specifically what its recommendations were—I will simply sum it up this way: Our current ports of entry are access points into this country where there is staffing. Now, I am not a border security person; I think we need secure borders, and ultimately, what that looks like I am not the right person to answer. If there is additional security on the border that allows additional CBP assets or others to work those points of entry, that is a critical piece.

Ms. JAYAPAL. Thank you, Mr. Patterson. I do have the report, and I can tell you it does not say anything about a border wall as a solution to the problem. In fact, does your own report not detail that, as you just said, drugs are entering the country not on the backs of human smugglers but actually in small quantities? Even if they are crossing the southern border, they are in the backs of legal vehicles; they are hidden away in little pieces; they are in tractor-trailers.

They are not being transported by individuals across the border, and a border wall that stops people from coming in is not the issue. It is these legal ports of entry that people are manipulating to get those drugs across. Is that correct?

Mr. PATTERSON. I do not discount that you do have people that smuggle smaller quantities across the border, you know, whether it is through their person or other means. I think the bulk that is coming out of Mexico is coming through the points of entry, or, as you brought up, other routes that we see: The Dominican Republic; directly out of China; you know, those types of events.

Ms. JAYAPAL. Thank you. So, would you support increased funding, for example, for the Coast Guard, something that the President had initially recommended decreasing funding? But the Coast Guard is actually responsible for the interdiction of drugs within our waters, for example.

Mr. PATTERSON. The Coast Guard is one of our most important assets when it comes to the control of especially cocaine coming out of South America, and I believe they could use more resources.

Ms. JAYAPAL. So, let me reiterate that a border wall does not solve the problems of drugs across into the United States. You have mentioned many times during your comments, and I have read some comments you have made before, that addressing demand is absolutely critical here. Can you comment on—and you only have 10 seconds—but the one or two most important things to address demand?

Mr. PATTERSON. So, demand, I think, comes through education, and the other piece is the conversations about prevention before it starts. I mean, I think a lot of the issues that come out in this is that once substance abuse starts, treatment is hard. Not necessarily in all drugs, but in most drugs, it is.

Ms. JAYAPAL. Thank you Mr. Patterson. I yield.

Mr. ROTHFUS. The time of the gentlewoman is expired. The chair recognizes the gentleman from Rhode Island, Mr. Cicilline, for 5 minutes.

Mr. CICILLINE. Thank you, Mr. Chairman. Thank you, Mr. Patterson. First, I want to thank the chairman and the ranking member for calling this hearing. And it is important to remember that drug overdose is the leading cause of injury deaths in the United States; 115 Americans die every day due to opioid overdose. In my home state of Rhode Island, last year we lost almost one Rhode Islander per day to this disease, and nearly half of those overdose deaths involve a prescription opioid.

And so, my first question is, my understanding is that there is a discrepancy between the Comprehensive Addiction Recovery Act, CARA, and the current DEA regulations on providing for a partial fill of a prescription. In the past partial fills could be made at the pharmacy when a pharmacy did not physically have enough quantity on hand. Under CARA, a partial fill can be made under several circumstances, including when a State has acted to limit prescriptions of opioids or a patient or prescriber requests an initial fill of an opioid prescription for a shorter time period.

This sort of discrepancy between the law that is CARA and DEA regulations is problematic for pharmacists. Can you tell me what steps the DEA is taking to bring its regulations into alignment with CARA and when we might expect those regulations to be promulgated and updated?

Mr. PATTERSON. I appreciate the question, sir, and it goes back to something I started off with, which is States in a lot of cases have already taken this on their own backs of fixing the, you know, State laws for much smaller initial prescriptions. And this is something that we obviously still owe related to our regulations in this space. It is critically important; we need to get it done. And it also, then, impacts the additional issues of quota and other type——

Mr. CICILLINE. It is on your agenda. Thank you. The Responsible Drug Disposal Act of 2010 gave authority to DEA to enable pharmacies and other entities who are licensed to handle controlled substances to collect unused medication from the public and destroy it. However, the Government Accountability Office found very low participation among pharmacies.

I am just wondering if you have a sense of why that is. Do you think it would be beneficial if more pharmacies participated, and what can we do to accelerate that participation?

Mr. PATTERSON. So, we have seen an uptick in the collection. I think it poses a number of challenges that—you know, distribution points, pharmacies, others—whether it is safeguarding or other issues that surround that. But I think this is a place where, again, our educational presence and us talking to people about getting these medications brought back in is absolutely critical, because we see so much diversion happening in that space still.

Mr. CICILLINE. And if you think there are things we can do to further enhance that, I trust you will let us know. Mr. Patterson, does the DEA offer any ongoing medical education or training to prescribers on the dispensing or prescribing of opioids? And if not, do you think your agency, if charged with that, has the ability to provide that kind of medical training?

Mr. PATTERSON. So, we obviously provide information through our outreach to both prescribers and to pharmacies as well as distributors and manufacturers. We cannot mandate CME, but I think it is probably one of the most valuable things that can be done. So, we use our registration or distribution list of our registrants to send out information. Again, I cannot make it mandatory that they——

Mr. CICILLINE. But there is no question. You think it would be beneficial if people——

Mr. PATTERSON. Absolutely.

Mr. CICILLINE. Okay. And my final question, because I know I do not have a lot of time. You mentioned that the DEA could do better in terms of disrupting or taking note of these distributors who are distributing orders that deviate from the norm, or unusual frequency, unusual quantities, and that there is in place only a civil fine; DEA needs to do a better job of that. Are there things we can be doing in Congress to give you additional resources or authority?

It seems to me if, as you described, it is just a cost of doing business, then that is not a great disincentive to do it. If, in fact, loss of licensure, criminal penalties, or other things were in place—why is DEA not doing a better job in the current framework, and what can we do to strengthen your ability to try to interrupt or prevent these distributions which are clearly problematic?

Mr. PATTERSON. I think it is a valid question, and hopefully I did not misspeak. Obviously, we have criminal tools in this space as well. I think probably all too often, though, we end up at the point of having a civil fine. And some of those are important, because again, as we heard earlier from one of the members, the change of a distribution center has a ripple effect. We know that, and we are cognizant of that.

There are times, however, when we have egregious behavior that we have to deal with, and I think there is definitely a change in the philosophy in the prosecutor's offices and with DEA, that we need to hold people more accountable than just a civil fine.

Mr. CICILLINE. Thank you. I yield back, Mr. Chairman.

Mr. ROTHFUS. The gentleman yields back. The gentlewoman from Florida, Ms. Demings, is recognized for 5 minutes.

Ms. DEMINGS. Thank you so much, Mr. Chairman, and Mr. Patterson, thank you so much for the job that you do. It is a moving target. One day you are the answer, and the next day you are the problem. But I think that not only should DEA be held accountable, but all of the stakeholders, including Congress, should be held accountable for the job that we do.

You talked a little bit about that with my colleague from Rhode Island, about some of the things that DEA could do differently in terms of accountability. I heard what you said to him, but could you just kind of elaborate just a little bit more on that particular issue? And how can Congress, as we deal with this crisis throughout our country, be more accountable as well in terms of helping to find solutions and not creating more problems?

Mr. PATTERSON. Right. Let me start with the second piece first. So, in the legislation space that provides us great assistance, and I recognize that every piece of legislation sometimes has its unintended consequences. There are more than 60 pieces that are out there right now in this opioid space, and you all should be applauded for the efforts you have done.

And we all need to make sure that when we see those unintended consequences, as we have seen in the past, we have to be very vocal about it with you so you know what is going to happen. DEA and HHS debate all the time over research, and research is critically important in this space as well, and we have to find common ground to address these problems.

Going back to the things that DEA needs to continue to do better—and this is the piece—and I greatly appreciate this hearing, actually, today, because I feel like this is one of those good days as opposed to the day that we are the enemy. We have made tremendous strides, I think, in this space over the last handful of years. So, it is using our data; it is figuring out ways to share our data. Right?

We have all had these stovepipes of information that we, for whatever reason, either do not feel we can share or cannot. The law enforcement community is all pulled together behind this, and you do not see the badges anymore; what you see is a combined effort. And I feel this even across the industry. Right? I mean, it truly feels like the moment where people are understanding that this is a disaster, and it is not just a talking point for people. It is a true movement of what is said. So, as a 30-year veteran of drug law enforcement, it is nice to see that even though a decade ago we had 35,000 overdoses, for whatever reason, this has truly woken everyone up.

So, our participation with our State and local partners, all these other things—but DEA has to continue to be more aggressive in terms of what it does. And not aggressive in a reckless way, but again holding people accountable, making sure that we are outspoken on where we see issues, and, frankly, not being afraid to push into that space.

When we talk about quota, quota is a tricky space for us to deal with. And all of these are balancing acts that we are going to have to deal with, but we should not be embarrassed—we probably should be embarrassed—but the mistakes that we made the past we learn from, and we have to move forward on that. That is why I appreciate today to at least highlight some of those things in what we are doing.

We see that all the time with the States right now. There are best practices; you know, the LEAD program got talked about a little bit earlier, though we did not really get to talk about it. You see these all over the country right now, and some are very successful, and some are failures.

I was just out in California; one of the things I talked to them about is "You do not have to reinvent this wheel; we can tell you where the things are going to work and are not going to work." It does not mean that they do that for every community, but these are the things that we all need to come together and we work on.

Ms. DEMINGS. You talked about fines having little impact on, say, drug manufacturers. What else do you believe could be done to ensure greater compliance?

Mr. PATTERSON. I think at some point we are going to have to hold these companies criminally accountable for some of their activities. And again, that is a tough balance to try and come to the right point on. Some are innocent mistakes, and generally we would never use an ISO on an innocent mistake. We want to work with the industry; we want to correct their behavior. But you see, it is not just in the drug distribution. You see it in banking; you see it in other places where civil fines just do not seem to catch anyone's attention.

Ms. DEMINGS. And finally, with hiring and retention, any challenges in that particular area? I know you spoke earlier a little bit about it. But any particular challenges with hiring and retention?

Mr. PATTERSON. Yes. So, I think these are struggles that we have dealt with for a host of reasons in hiring and positions. Like I said, the good news is that we can lean heavily on our State and local partners as we try and catch up, but there is a lot of challenges in that space. Retention; people seem to still like coming to work for DEA, so we are doing a good job there.

Ms. DEMINGS. Thank you very much. Mr. Chairman, I yield back.

Mr. ROTHFUS. The gentlewoman yields back. We thank Director Patterson for his attendance at today's hearing. That concludes our first panel, and we are going to invite our second panel to come up.

I would like to welcome our distinguished witnesses for a second panel. If you would please rise, and I can begin by swearing you in.

Do you swear that the testimony you are about to give is the truth, the whole, truth and nothing but the truth, so help you God? Let the record show that the witnesses answered in the affirmative. Thank you.

I would like to introduce the panel. Dr. Tim Westlake is a full- time emergency physician and is the emergency department director at Oconomowoc Memorial Hospital in Wisconsin. Among his many collateral responsibilities, Dr. Westlake is the vice chairman of the Wisconsin State Medical Examining Board and executive committee member of the Wisconsin EPDMP design team and cochairman of the Wisconsin State Coalition for Prescription Drug Abuse and Reduction.

Mr. Spencer Morgan is a Commonwealth's attorney for Accomack County, Virginia. Mr. Morgan started his professional career as a staff assistant in the office of our former colleague, Mr. Randy Forbes. Later, Mr. Morgan was a legislative assistant for the House Judiciary Committee Subcommittee on Crime, Terrorism, and Homeland Security. Welcome back.

Ms. Kristen Holman is the older sister of Garrett Holman. Garrett lost his life earlier last year to addiction. Ms. Holman has witnessed firsthand the devastation wrought by a destructive combination of drugs, including marijuana, ADHD medication, and synthetic opioids.

I would like to recognize my colleague, Mr. Cicilline of Rhode Island, to introduce our final witness on this panel, Dr. Josiah Rich.

Mr. CICILLINE. Thank you, Mr. Chairman. I appreciate the courtesy. It is a great honor for me to welcome Dr. Rich to the House Judiciary Committee. Dr. Rich is a professor of medicine at the Warren Alpert School of Medicine at Brown University and a practicing infectious disease specialist since 1994 at the Miriam Hospital Immunology Center, providing clinical care for over 22 years, and at the Rhode Island Department of Corrections, caring for prisoners with HIV infection and working on it in the correctional setting, doing research.

He has spent nearly a quarter of a century in public health and has been an extraordinary partner with local, State, and Federal Government in helping to develop good public policy. I have worked with him, and he has had the misfortune of being represented by me for 24 years in public life. But he was recently appointed by our Governor of Rhode Island, Governor Gina Raimondo, to the Overdose Prevention and Intervention Task Force expert team selected to advise the task force and formulate a strategic plan to address addictions and stop overdose in Rhode Island.

He is a cofounder of the nationwide Centers for AIDS Research Collaboration in HIV in Corrections Initiative and has served as an expert for the National Academy of Sciences, the Institute of Medicine, and many others; a real expert in issues of public health and addiction and the development of good public policy. And someone I have relied on for guidance over many years and really delighted that he will share his wisdom with this committee. I welcome Dr. Rich and thank you and yield back.

Mr. ROTHFUS. Your written statements will be entered into the record in their entirety, and we ask that you summarize, each of you, your testimony in 5 minutes. To help you stay within that time, there was a timing light on your table. When the light switches from green to yellow you have 1 minute to conclude your testimony; when the light turns red it signals your 5 minutes have expired. Dr. Westlake, you may begin. And if you could press the button so that your mic is on, please.

Statements of Timothy Westlake, MD, Hartland, Wisconsin; J. Spencer Morgan III, Commonwealth's Attorney, Accomack County, Virginia; Kristen Holman, Lynchburg, Virginia; and Josiah Rich, MD, Providence, Rhode Island

Statement of Timothy Westlake

Dr. WESTLAKE. Thank you. Chairman Rothfus, committee members, I appreciate the opportunity to talk to you today and for your leadership in addressing this issue. In my role on the Wisconsin Medical Examining and Controlled Substance boards I became the physician architect of the State's prescription opioid reform strategy and an expert on opioid scheduling. As an emergency physician on the front lines of the opioid battle field for the past 20 years, I have witnessed more tragedy than I care to recall.

Like you, I am laser-focused on what can be done to stop this senseless loss of life. It is why I am grateful for the opportunity to talk with you today and share a legislative solution that is actually working in Wisconsin right now. But first, a brief story about a young man named Archie Badura.

Every Sunday, we sat next to Archie and his family in church, where he was an altar server alongside my daughters. Archie got hooked on marijuana first, then prescription opioids pills; heroin followed shortly, and eventually fentanyl, a tragically all-too-familiar slide. The last time I saw Archie alive he was my patient in the ER. I had to resuscitate him with Narcan after he overdosed on fentanyl. Before discharging him, we pulled out a body bag, unzipped it, and pretended to fit him for it. It was a wakeup call.

Archie became serious about getting clean and started following recovery principles. He told his family he was going to beat the odds and not end up in a body bag. He stayed drug-free for 6 months after this. Sadly, he eventually relapsed on fentanyl and died at age 19. His mom, my friend Lauri, vividly remembers Archie being zipped up into a body bag identical to the one she had seen me showing him months earlier. In his honor, Lauri founded SOFA, Saving Others for Archie, and now helps others who are desperately trying to save their loved ones.

It is incontrovertible that the increased availability of prescription opioids has fueled the opioid epidemic. As a medical regulator, I have spent countless hours working to identify and implement best practices. For starters, we need more judicious prescribing practices. We are doing that in Wisconsin, not with top-down mandates but through education and partnerships within the medical community. In my written testimony I provide more detail about the cutting-edge prescription drug monitoring program reforms and educational reforms that we have put into place.

The fact is that the lion's share of medical regulation does and should occur at the State medical licensing board and health system levels. Where Congress can and has and can continue to be helpful is in law enforcement and in providing flexible funding to the States themselves to invest in communities where the dollars are most needed. When government intervenes too much, for example, with the development of the pain scale and pain as the fifth vital sign, there is too much room for unintended consequences.

By far, the deadliest front in the opioid war is the danger posed by creation of fentanyl-related substances. These deaths now surpass heroin deaths. The lethal dose of fentanyl is two milligrams, which means that there could be enough fentanyl, if this box were filled with fentanyl, that it would kill 900,000 people, which would be more than the entire population of Washington, D.C.

Fentanyl variations and related substances are so deadly that they can be used and are actually classified as chemical weapons. They are not just drugs. They are actually considered weapons of mass destruction. The bad guys use loopholes in the existing scheduling laws to create new legal fentanyl variants. These untested chemicals are then produced mostly in China and introduced into the opioid supply.

As our prescription opioid reforms take effect and the medical community returns to more judicious decision prescribing practices, the market for counterfeit pills continues to explode. Most illicit opioid users have no idea what they are consuming. With the advent of counterfeit pill production, they believe they are ingesting a safe, trade-name manufactured pill, when actually it is a fentanyl-related counterfeit substance. These pills can be alarmingly more strong than what they are purported to be, up to hundreds of times stronger.

The singer Prince died from a counterfeit Vicodin pill ingestion that he thought it was Vicodin; it was actually Fentanyl. During 2016, in one weekend there were 12 deaths in Milwaukee from counterfeit pills that contain cyclopropyl fentanyl, which at that time was legal and was shipped in on the Internet.

We saw this coming in Wisconsin, years ago. We worked closely with the DEA to get ahead of it. We created an enacting, novel scheduling language now being modeled nationally, X60 or the SOFA Act, Stopping Overdose of Fentanyl Analogues in homage to Saving Others for Archie. It controls by structure all likely and possible bioactive chemical fentanyl modifications. The novel catchall legislative language allows us to schedule proactively and not wait for loved ones to die before we can schedule each new modified fentanyl variant. So, instead of playing whack-a-mole with the variants as people die and we discover them, it unplugs the entire fentanyl machine.

The week after Wisconsin enacted SOFA, DEA published the identical scheduling language in the Federal Register as the method of Federal temporary scheduling. Chemists around the world and in China must be paying attention, because since that announcement 6 months ago, there have been no new fentanyl variants found.

In the previous 2 years, there were 17 that were found and scheduled, which represented hundreds of deaths. But the language needs to be written into the U.S. code, as the DEA administrator said, for the best permanent scheduling solutions. Many thanks to Mr. Sensenbrenner and Senator Ron Johnson who have the Federal SOFA Act, and thank you for their leadership on that.

When asked how often I see fentanyl overdoses, the answer is tragically far too often. The last shift I worked was 2 days ago on Sunday, and I was preparing my testimony, and I was interrupted to go resuscitate a fentanyl overdose. It is for this reason that I urge you to pass the legislation and make it so. Thank you for your time and consideration, and I look forward to answering any questions.

Mr. ROTHFUS. Thank you, Dr. Westlake. Mr. Morgan, you are recognized for 5 minutes.

Statement of J. Spencer Morgan III

Mr. MORGAN. Thank you, Mr. Chairman, ranking member, and members of the committee: thank you for inviting me to testify on this important topic. I intend to address several issues concerning opioid addition and the increased amounts of heroin and fentanyl from the perspective of a local prosecutor. Simply put, in the words of the Worcester County drug task force coordinator—or the equivalent of the criminal enforcement team there—there has never been a more dangerous time to purchase illicit drugs.

Little bit about Accomack County, we are at the southern tip of the Delmarva Peninsula. Accomack is a unique mixture of agriculture, tourism, and aerospace in industry through Wallops Island space port. Current population is right around 32,000 people.

When I first arrived in Accomack County in the fall of 2011 after graduating law school and taking the bar, opioids and heroine had really yet to make a huge widespread public impact on the county. Arrests were generally low, and we were aware of prescription medication abuse. However, the full extent of the problem had not been revealed.

At the same time, I did learn Worcester County, Somerset County, they were beginning to experience significant amounts of heroine at that time. In Accomack, the harbinger of what was just below the surface really became the widespread abuse of buprenorphine, or Subutex as the brand name is.

The drug used in the treatment, generally where the addict is treated with, in conjunction with drug treatment and counseling, and then titrated off the drug, which helps them manage the symptoms of opioid addiction became a currency among addicts for maintaining their addiction and trading for more powerful narcotics.

Once we began to see this, it was not long before we were seeing the substance attempted to be smuggled into our jails. And then, prosecuting those offenses and ultimately, and ironically, I ended up prosecuting someone involved in such a scheme for cleaning up the scene of an overdose death, where her boyfriend was found unresponsive, and police responded, EMTs responded, and she went back in while they were trying to save his life and hid away, or secreted away the signs of the heroin abuse.

I will note, however, that recently with the advents of Suboxone, a substance which contains naloxone, the inhibitor to prevent opioid interaction. We have seen decreased abuse of Suboxone, but by then, we were learning that we had dealers at the northern end of our county, who when they would serve clients with cocaine, they were providing gratis a bag of heroin and suggesting that the addicts return back when they wanted more of that.

Some of the challenges we have seen, not the least of which are the deadly nature of this substance, the substance fentanyl and carfentanil substances, carfentanil, fentanyl, certainly are deadly.

And one of the most tragic things I have experienced is the death of defendants and witnesses beyond availability of those people before we have a chance to go to even trial, or offer any of them any programs through the justice system that we have in Virginia for those addicts.

Some of these substances are so deadly, as Dr. Westlake has testified, that we have stopped field testing narcotics in Accomack County for fear of officer safety. The problem with our field testing is that if an officer were to come into contact with those substances, they could potentially overdose on the scene.

My time is running low, but I will say that there has been substantial headway in Accomack County. We currently are enjoying a level of cooperation between the medical treatment providers, substance abuse counselors and law enforcement than I think has ever been seen before. We have produced informational packets, which we supply our officers who can give addicts, be it a defendant or a suspect, a witness or a victim to crime in order to help get as many people in to substance abuse treatment and recovery as possible. We see it as a public health threat, where law enforcement can certainly partner with treatment providers and I will yield back the rest of my time, and happy to answer any questions.

Mr. ROTHFUS. Thank you, Mr. Morgan. The chair recognizes Ms. Holman, for your opening statement. Five minutes.

Statement of Kristen Holman

Ms. HOLMAN. Thank you. February 17th, 1996 was one of the best days of my life. My parents brought home the baby brother I had been asking for since I was able to speak. My little brother Garret grew to be one huge hardy kid, who always had the room laughing. His smile was contagious, and he always demanded everyone's attention.

We grew up in Forest, Virginia, and we had the best childhood. We were always outside, making up games, riding four wheelers, and meeting with friends throughout our neighborhood. Garret cared so deeply for everyone he loved. My brother had a bigger personality than words can describe. My brother would be the first one to stick up for someone, and he would be the first to stand out in a crowd.

Garret was diagnosed with ADHD very early in life. He was a hyper kid. He consumed everyone's energy at all times. When he became of age to make the decision to get off his medications for ADHD, he began to self-medicate. It started with marijuana.

With marijuana, Garret was able to self-medicate his condition on his own terms. He was able to function without feeling like he was forced to take a prescription medicine. He realized that this alternative would not work when he went to get a job, and realized he would be drug tested for any job he applied to. This is when he turned to more dangerous alternatives that did not show up on a drug test at the time.

There was no explaining to him the dangers of quitting these prescription meds so abruptly, and there was nothing that we could say or do that he wanted to hear. We were just forced to watch him choose this path while hoping and praying he would see the light and reach out to accept our help.

I watched my brother change from an amazing heartfelt, selfless person to someone I did not recognize. There was a darkness in his eyes, and an overall loss of life and love. Not only did I watch my brother change, I watched my parents and then myself slowly fade into that same dark place. The inability to help him made us all feel like we were not doing enough, when in reality, we became so heavily involved in him that we all lost ourselves. We lived life never knowing where we would get that one phone call that no one wants to hear.

As a sibling, I played referee between my mom and my dad, my parents and my brother, while often being angry at one or all of them, just because none of us had the answer. Addiction is a subject that many feel ashamed to speak of, and because of this feeling, we were left to suffer alone. Close family and friends knew of Garret's addiction, but no one but the four of us knew the true extent of it. Small talk and even such that should be fine became hard, and having conversations with people to worry my brother what he was constantly doing, and if I would see him again became the only thing I truly cared about.

Living in fear of losing my brother every day played a major stress role in my life, and I constantly dropped everything to be wherever I needed to be for Garret and my family. I spent hours and hours trying to talk to him, and trying to let him see how much love we all had for him. Garret was angry with himself over his addiction. He wanted to be happy and he could not. He tried so hard, and when he lashed out at us, it made it that much more hard for him.

In December of 2016, I received the news that my brother had overdosed. My dad revived him, and he was sent to the hospital. I remember getting that news and dropping everything and rushing to the car. When he finally woke up and we told him how lucky he was that he was still alive, he did not even blink. He was not thankful. He was not relieved. And that was because he was already gone. My little brother was not the person looking back at me anymore, and I did not recognize this person. And I could not understand why he was not hugging us and crying tears of excitement over getting a second chance at life.

My family knew we needed to do something drastic. We needed outside help. Our normal interventions were no longer buying us time with my brother. We needed a solution and an action plan. My parents forced him into a mental health evaluation, which he was only required to stay at for 5 days. After the 5 days, he reluctantly went to a 30-day in-house treatment program.

One week after he was released, my dad found him overdosed again, and revived once more. My dad forced a second evaluation, but the judge released him on February 6th, 2017. I lost my little brother and only sibling on February 9th, 2017 to a synthetic opioid that was delivered straight to him in the mail from China.

I cannot explain why this happened to my brother, and I do not know how to fix it. And I do not know what my family could have done differently. What I do know is that the drug addiction did not just take the life of my brother, but it took a big piece of my family's life. There are empty silences in conversations where he should be present. And there is a fight in all of us that still does not want to give up, and I do not believe it ever will.

Garret was not just a good person, he was a great person who fell into a terrible trap that none of us could get him out of. But we tried and tried and tried. My family feels that we failed Garret, but the truth is, this is something that millions and millions of families are dealing with. And people feel ashamed. And they do not want to speak out about what is going on. And that just leads people to suffer in silence.

Although it is too late for Garret, he is in my heart and head every day, and it only feels right for him to reach people at a national level. I cannot be any more inspired at this point to do whatever I can to reach out to families like mine. Thank you.

Mr. ROTHFUS. That was incredibly courageous. Garret would be proud of you. Thank you. The chair recognizes Dr. Rich for 5 minutes for his opening statement.

Statement of Josiah Rich

Dr. RICH. Thank you. It is a tremendous honor to be here and I want to thank Ms. Holman for such a courageous testimony. I have spent 25 years caring for people both in the community and behind bars. And, when I first went behind bars, it was to take care of people with HIV. And now, I found myself mostly taking of people with opiate use disorder. This rapidly evolving deadly epidemic demands a sustained public health approach, similar to the Ryan White CARE Act for the AIDS epidemic.

Opioid addiction is highly stigmatized, poorly understood by most people, and it is characterized by ongoing use despite negative consequences. Now, opiates are different than other addictive substances by two physiological properties, tolerance and withdrawal. Tolerance means you need an ever-increasing dose to get the same effect. And withdrawal is extremely painful when you abruptly stop opiates. You literally feel like you are dying.

So, this disease wraps around you like a boa constrictor. Every time you breathe out, it tightens, so when you try and breath in, you cannot. That results in changes in the brain chemistry and the brain pathways, and your response to stimuli. And it feels like you need opiates for your very survival. Just like you need to breath, you need to drink, you need to eat. So, people get desperate, because their ongoing use increases. They resort mostly to stealing, getting involved in the sec trade, getting involved in the drug trade.

So, what can we do about this? Our punitive approach has clearly failed. And, you would predict that from knowledge of the disease. So, treatment. Now, when we talk about treatment, you hear people talk about a treatment bed, a detox, and frankly, that does not work. That is an antiquated approach based on a drug-free model. And, 90 percent of the time, people relapse. And relapsing today, in the age of fentanyl contamination of our opiate supply is far more dangerous and results in death.

So, treatment that we have now that is effective, the best treatment we have is medications for addiction treatment, MAT. We have three FDA medications that when taken, they block the high of opiates and they block the withdrawal. And these are the two main drivers of ongoing use. They stabilize people lives, and allow them to work on their recovery.

In Baltimore, when they ramped up MAT, they drove overdose tests down 80 percent, similar results in France, and in Rhode Island, we rolled out MAT in our corrections department, our prison and jail, and we drove within year overdose deaths and people released from incarceration, we drove them down 60 percent. So, this is the proof of the concept, that MAT is what we need.

We also need for those who are unable or unwilling to get into MAT to outreach to them, to engage them, to give them the tools and the education they need to reduce their risks, including the lock zone and drug checking. There also have been many examples of public health and public safety collaborations, include Good Samaritan laws, offering the lock zone to first responders who, police and fire. We heard about a lead program in Rhode Island. We have safe stations, where the fire stations act to engage people and get them into care.

But, the punitive approach will disproportionally affect those most disadvantaged. And we hopefully have learned from our punitive approach to the crack epidemic, how it lead to mass incarceration of predominantly minority individuals.

So, the punitive approach will distract attention and resources away from what is clearly needed, which is a strong and sustained public health approach. Thank you.

Mr. ROTHFUS. Thank you, Dr. Rich. The chair recognizes the gentleman from Pennsylvania, Mr. Marino, for 5 minutes.

Mr. MARINO. Thank you, chairman. Appreciate it. Thank you for being here. I apologize for you having to be the second group that has to wait, but I want to pose a concept that I have had. I was a prosecutor for 18 years. I was a district attorney in Pennsylvania, and I was a US attorney with the Bush administration.

And, first of all, I will still stick to the fact that dealers, major dealers, need to be locked up. Period. People toting guns and shoving guns in people's side and drug deals need to be locked up. So, with that said, I have a concept, and I know that quite often, a person addicted to drugs will do some deliveries or dealing to get money to supply their habit. That is just all part of it. I do not necessarily, unless they are violent, want to see those people going to prison.

And, my concept is this opioid addiction is so much more worse than the cocaine and the crack cocaine, particularly because of the fentanyl. I want to see, and I tried to do this 2 years ago, and Karen Bass, a good friend of mine, on the other side, we are looking into this again. I want to see mandatory inpatient treatment. When a parent sees something going on with their child, or when a child sees something going on with their parent, we need a system, a central system where that person can call and ask for help, because it is the toughest thing to do. It is where do I go for help? So, we have to have some central location that can get those people, that person, or that family directly to someone who can help them in their area.

And, we have many hospitals across the country. We have good outpatient treatment facilities. But, to get off the opioids, to get off of heroin, that is going to take inpatient treatment, and it is going to take a long time. And what I think we should do is first of all make it into have that family member have the ability to go before the court and have an expert testify position that yes, this person is addicted to this. And this person needs inpatient treatment.

They cannot leave. It is going to be a lockdown situation. But in addition to the health needs, the mental health needs, we need to start working on the family as a whole, educating these people. Starting from pulling the bootstraps up. And then, the group will make a determination in that particular hospital as to when this person can have furlough, when they can get out, what we do when they get out. Just do not say, "You are out on the street now."

And, it is going to be, I think, one of the only ways in addition to going after the bad doctors, pharmacists, pharmaceutical companies and making them pay as well, one way, and/or another. So, what say you? So, you could start Dr. Rich, and go down the line.

Dr. RICH. Sure. Well, lot of material there to work. I agree with a number of things you said. I think the need for health and treatment and mental healthcare in addressing the family, and giving people real opportunities to get a better life, and that is really a big part of recovery.

You mentioned that we have treatment all over the country, and we have a need of inpatient. I would say we do not have treatment all over the country. We have a very fragmented system, and a lot of it is based on faulty thinking, the notion that you can get someone to a place, a bed, and that something magical is going to happen, and then they are going to come out. So, that does not work.

We do not require the inpatients most of the time. I would say that what we need to do is offer effective treatments that are proven. And most of the time that is not inpatient. Now, there are some cases where, you know, that is being explored in Massachusetts, for example they have—they are mandating people into treatment, exactly what you said. But instead of treatment programs, they have used an old jail. They have in jail cells.

Mr. MARINO. No, you see, mine, mine is——

Dr. RICH. And they are not getting medications.

Mr. MARINO. Mine is a hospital.

Dr. RICH. Right. Yep.

Mr. MARINO. With experts making that determination, and I see, and almost——

Dr. RICH. So, I think we can learn a lot from the Portuguese example, where that is exactly what they did. They did not mandate it. They made it available, made it realistic. That is how the rest of——

Mr. MARINO. But in my 18 years, I have never heard a person addicted to drugs not say to me, "I can get off any time I want." Dr. RICH. Well, they say different things to me.

Mr. ROTHFUS. The gentlemen's time has expired. The chair recognizes the gentleman from Rhode Island, Mr. Cicilline for 5 minutes.

Mr. CICILLINE. Thank you, and thank you to all of our witnesses, Ms. Holman. Thank you for being here. I know your brother is looking down on you very proudly for your courage. So, sadly, I have had many friends who have lost loved ones and children to this same disease. And, we all need to be reminded that is why we are here, and we need to come up with some answers.

Dr. Rich, I want to just focus a minute on what you just described. You know, I think a lot of folks, particularly families that are struggling with a loved one who has an addiction, the idea of getting them into a treatment facility, where they can have the peace of mind to know they are safe, seems like, sort of, you know, a natural inclination.

But it turns out, according to your testimony, that, while that may provide you peace of mind, it is actually not the best strategy in most cases for really addressing the addiction. And you, the work that you have done on what on the medically assisted treatment seems to be much more successful.

So, I am wondering if you could talk a little bit, in the face of that data, is it just old thinking? Why is that we continue to hear people talk about we need more beds, there has to be more placements. Is it just this reluctance on the using medicine, or what?

Dr. RICH. The medications are limited. You know, they are not perfect for everybody. They have a lot of side effects. They have a lot of problems. But they are the best thing we have.

The problem with the going to a detox is just as tolerance goes up very quickly, tolerance also goes down very quickly. And so, when you let people out of a detox, as we heard when Garret was released, he overdosed right away. Now, probably if he had been using up until that point that he took that dose, he would have had a much higher tolerance, and would not have overdosed right then and there.

So, we are setting people up for overdose by putting them through detox. And, they might not have detoxed 10 years ago, 5 years ago when we did not have fentanyl. But now we have fentanyl, and it is far too dangerous. So, you know, this is rapidly evolving. So, we really need to get with the times and get people on to these medications.

Now, there are some cases where, you know, maybe if the medication was tried and there is absolutely nothing else we can do, then maybe we need to be more of a big brother and be more controlling. But, we have already shown that by giving people access to, and continuing them on treatment, that they are going to reduce their overdose deaths. We need to roll that out right away.

Mr. CICILLINE. And that is the work that you have done in the prison with success. I think you said 61 percent success rate.

Dr. RICH. Sixty-one percent drop in overdose deaths within a year of starting that program, and people coming out of corrections. But, that does not have to be corrections. People should not have to go be incarceration——

Mr. CICILLINE. That was my impression.

Dr. RICH [continuing]. In order to get treatment. We can do that in pretrial arrest. We can do that in the hospitals, in the emergency rooms, in the clinics. We just need to roll it out. We need high quality programs that not only give the medications, we are really working on recovery work on the mental health work, all the other things that the congressman was talking about.

Mr. CICILLINE. And what do you think we can do? What can Congress do? I mean obviously, you know, providing resources so medically assistive treatment is available. Are there other things we can be doing in terms of closer regulation of prescriber activities? Better coordination through pharmacies? How much of that issue do you think is contributing to this real growth in opioid overdoses?

Dr. RICH. We have a whole population that is addicted now. And that started with the overprescribing. But they are there. And we can shut down the prescriptions. Some of them are going to say, "Oh, I guess I did not need that." But, most of them are going to go, at least for a time, and find out whatever they can find. So, that is very dangerous.

We also have people that have not started taking opiates. And we need to do whatever we can to prevent them from starting. And a big part of that is education, understanding what is going on.

Mr. CICILLINE. And finally, I know you have been part of the work that Governor Raimondo has been leading in Rhode Island that I think is really a model in terms of bringing all of the stakeholders and affected parties together to really develop a strategy and a plan. Maybe you could spend the last few minutes just talking about that.

Dr. RICH. Well, I was fortunate to be involved in that. The governor, instead of having a stakeholder process, had an expert driven process where they had experts making decisions rather than stakeholders saying, you know, fund my program. And that led to really looking at the evidence, getting a lot of information from the community and from the stakeholders, and developing a plan. We had a simple four-point plan expanding treatment, and 20,000 out of our population of a million were people that needed to be onto MAT.

And so, identifying where those people interact with systems and shutting them over into treatment. So, we have started to roll that out, and we think we can—we need to continue it, double down on that strategy.

Mr. CICILLINE. Thank you, Dr. Rich.

Mr. ROTHFUS. The gentleman's time has expired. The chair recognizes the gentleman from Louisiana, Mr. Johnson, for 3 minutes.

Mr. JOHNSON of Louisiana. Thank you, Mr. Chairman. We will be very brief. The bells mean that our votes have been called. So, we are all sort of, do not want to miss a vote. We are going to race out, so you will be just a few more minutes. I do not want there to be a perception today that what you have said here for the record is not important, just because we do not have a quorum. It is a busy day on the Hill. You know how this goes. But, your record is important to us. Everyone will review it. Your time is well spent here, and we greatly appreciate all of you, especially your personal tragedy. It makes a difference, it does.

Real quick practical question, and maybe this for Dr. Rich or Mr. Morgan. We referenced today buprenorphine, and I am just a constitutional law attorney. I do not know much about all this. But, my understanding is buprenorphine is one of the medications that is used to wean people off of opioids, is that right? It is not an opioid itself, right?

Dr. RICH. It is an opioid.

Mr. JOHNSON of Louisiana. Okay.

Dr. RICH. And it is what we called a mixed agonist. So, it partly turns on the receptor at low doses, and it also blocks you from getting high, and blocks you from going into withdraw.

Mr. JOHNSON of Louisiana. So, because of the blocking agent, it is one of the effective means to try to take people down off of their addiction?

Dr. RICH. Well, so, you know, a lot of people say, "Well, if I start on these medicines"—methadone, buprenorphine, commonly known as Suboxone, or deep on naltrexone, the vivitrol injection—"if I start this, how long do I have to stay on it?" And the answer is, for many people, a very long time. You need to stay on as long as you need to stay on. But, I think that the concept that somebody could be put on those medicines and weaned off in a short amount of time, and then they are going to be fine, this does not work that way.

Mr. JOHNSON of Louisiana. And so, what I am hearing, in my district back home, I have talked to a couple of pain management physicians. And they are feeling pressure from the insurance companies, because of perhaps what may be an overreaction to all this, to impose access limits or quantity limits on those who are appropriately using buprenorphine, or one of those derivatives. How do we separate those issues so that those patients are not adversely affected and caught up into the wave of those who have real addiction?

Dr. RICH. Buprenorphine, because of its properties, is the safest opioid to use. I find it is very effective for a lot of people with chronic pain. So, the insurance companies are reluctant to allow that, because there is a much bigger market of people with chronic pain. And it is an expensive medication. I routinely get letters saying, "Oh, well, have you tried oxytocin or, you know, oxycodone, or, others."

Mr. JOHNSON of Louisiana. I have people in my district, the insurance company said, "Why do you not go get on oxytocin?" Because they do not want to pay for buprenorphine anymore.

Dr. RICH. Exactly. But, we need to roll that out. There was mention of buprenorphine being a diverted substance. When we have studied people and asked them, "You know, have you gotten diverted buprenorphine?" They said, "Yes." And then we asked them, "Well, what did you use it for?" And they used it to treat these withdrawal symptoms. So, they are not using it to get high.

They are not going out to party with it. They are trying to treat themselves. They are using it as it is really indicated. But they cannot get access to it from their physicians, because there are not enough prescribers. So, they end up having to get it illicitly.

Mr. JOHNSON of Louisiana. I am way out of time, but I would love to talk with either or both of you later about mechanisms we can use for Congress to step in and help make that distinction for the people that really need it.

Dr. RICH. Sure.

Mr. JOHNSON of Louisiana. So, thanks for your time.

Mr. ROTHFUS. The chairman yields back. The chair recognizes himself for 3 minutes, if I can try to get a couple questions in before we have to run off for vote. So really, thank you everybody for participating in this very informative panel for us.

Mr. Morgan, your testimony referenced the synthetic drugs like fentanyl, especially their lethality. I especially represent a district in western Pennsylvania that has become an epicenter for synthetic opioid trafficking and usage.

One issue I hear about from other prosecutors are concerns dealing with forensic analysis, of blood toxicology and overdose death cases. Many times, the medical examiner reports list multiple controlled substances on the certificate's analysis, and this makes determining the precise cause of death difficult, as to which substance was responsible, or whether it was a combination of multiple substances. Have you encountered this problem regarding overdose cases in your jurisdiction?

Mr. MORGAN. We have not encountered that problem specifically. I am aware that it is a problem, when we get a certificate or a toxicology report from an ME's report that says there are these multiple amounts. The toxicologists in our certificate, as I understand it, will try and put that percentage by percentage into an equation or an amount in the blood, which is representative of the proportion of that sustenance.

Mr. ROTHFUS. Is proving causation a challenge in that context?

Mr. MORGAN. Yes. Proving causation, I imagine, would be a challenge. The quickest way I would combat that is I would get on the phone with my toxicologist within Virginia, the Department of Forensic Science, and speak with them. And look for an expert opinion to be tendered, ultimately a trial that says that this amount of fentanyl or this percent of fentanyl would be a cause of death or could be a cause of death.

But, in my experience, I think if I see fentanyl, it is going to be usually mixed with heroin. So, between fentanyl and heroin, I think I have good grounds to say beyond a reasonable doubt that this would be the cause of death. But I would need a toxicologist there, and that has presented problems in the past due to the volume of these types of cases around the State.

Mr. ROTHFUS. Dr. Westlake, you talked a little bit about some voluntary, as opposed to mandated—I think it is the context of prescription guidelines. I mean, part of the Comprehensive Addiction Recovery was to have Federal agencies take a look at this issue. I mean, can that help to establish some kind of standard of care, so that physicians at least can be aware of what would read a range of normal?

Dr. WESTLAKE. Yeah, I mean, I think that has already happened. I think with the release of the CDC guidelines, and then a lot of different States, in Wisconsin, for example, we had the State law passed that would promulgate guidelines from the medical examining board. And I think that is a key factor is that what I alluded to in my testimony was that we want the intervention into medicine to be from medicine itself and not from the legislature. I mean, if we look at the cause of the pain scale, pain crisis, opioid crisis to begin with, a lot of it came out the pain scale.

And so, I think we got to be really careful about interventions. But they are definitely necessary. And I think those educational interventions are already happening. And the CDC guidelines kind of lead the front of that. And I think education is happening. And we will see the results a couple years from now.

Mr. ROTHFUS. Ms. Holman, you know, what kind of options were presented for your brother when subjected to treatment?

Ms. HOLMAN. I mean, when we were seeking treatment?

Mr. ROTHFUS. Right.

Ms. HOLMAN. It was really hard to get anything, honestly. He got himself into trouble with law enforcement, so, he spent time in jail, and it seemed like it was easier to get him there than any kind of treatment.

Mr. ROTHFUS. You know, I really appreciate you being here. Your being here is going to help other families.

Ms. HOLMAN. I hope so.

Mr. ROTHFUS. So, I really encourage you to continue the work you are doing with your family.

Ms. HOLMAN. Thank you.

Mr. ROTHFUS. And know that you are not alone. And I think Dr. Rich talked about the stigma that has been out there, but I think your being here is going to help address that issue and help other folks find treatment. Dr. Rich, I appreciate where you are coming from, with respect to the punitive nature of what we have talked about, but do you draw any distinction at all between the user and the pusher?

Dr. RICH. Sure.

Mr. ROTHFUS. I look at this thing as a prevention enforcement treatment, prevention, enforcement, treatment. All three are important. And when you have people who come into or join this network of distribution, of this poison, that is responsible for the deaths of 10s of thousands of people in this country, you know, I want to go after those folks who are pushing this poison.

Dr. RICH. It is impossible to hear the tragedy that Ms. Holman described and not be angry about it. And, I share that anger. And people that are profiting from it, you know, it is a human response to want to punish them. We have tried that for 30 years, and the result is a disaster.

So, you know, I think we are going to get a much better result. Now, that does not mean I think we should legalize. I think we should try and clamp down as much as we can. But, if you have mandatory minimums, and you are sending 40-year-old mothers to——

Mr. ROTHFUS. I think you can look at things like that. But again, the premise being if you are pushing poison in our communities, you are going be held accountable with that. I am sorry, I have to go and vote. We are almost out of time. But I do want to thank everybody for coming in today.

This concludes today's hearing. Thank you to our distinguished witnesses for attending. Without objection, all members will have 5 legislative days to submit additional written questions for the witnesses or additional materials for the record. The hearing is adjourned.

[Whereupon, at 1:26 p.m., the hearing was adjourned.]

In: Battling the Opioid Epidemic
Editor: Vincent Hardy
ISBN: 978-1-53615-548-8

Chapter 2

THE DRUG ENFORCEMENT ADMINISTRATION'S ROLE IN COMBATING THE OPIOID EPIDEMIC*

The Subcommittee on Oversight and Investigations of the Committee on Energy and Commerce

Tuesday, March 20, 2018
House of Representatives, Subcommittee on Oversight and Investigations, Committee on Energy and Commerce,
Washington, DC.

The subcommittee met, pursuant to call, at 10:00 a.m., in room 2322 Rayburn House Office Building, Hon. Gregg Harper (chairman of the subcommittee) presiding.

Members present: Representatives Harper, Griffith, Burgess, Brooks, Collins, Barton, Walberg, Walters, Costello, Carter, Walden (ex officio), DeGette, Schakowsky, Castor, Tonko, Clarke, Ruiz, Peters, and Pallone (ex officio).

Also present: Representative McKinley.

Staff present: Jennifer Barblan, Chief Counsel, Oversight and Investigations; Mike Bloomquist, Staff Director; Ali Fulling, Legislative Clerk, Oversight and Investigations, Digital Commerce and Consumer Protection; Brittany Havens, Professional Staff, Oversight and Investigations; Christopher Santini, Counsel, Oversight and Investigations; Jennifer Sherman, Press Secretary; Alan Slobodin, Chief Investigative Counsel, Oversight and Investigations; Austin Stonebraker, Press Assistant; Hamlin Wade, Special Advisor, External Affairs; Christina Calce, Minority Counsel; Tiffany Guarascio,

* This is an edited, reformatted and augmented version of Hearing before the Subcommittee on Oversight and Investigations of the Committee on Energy and Commerce, House of Representatives, One Hundred Fifteenth Congress, Second Session, dated March 20, 2018.

Minority Deputy Staff Director and Chief Health Advisor; Chris Knauer, Minority Oversight Staff Director; Miles Lichtman, Minority Policy Analyst; Kevin McAloon, Minority Professional Staff Member; and C.J. Young, Minority Press Secretary.

Opening Statement of Hon. Gregg Harper, a Representative in Congress from the State of Mississippi

Mr. HARPER. We will call to order the hearing today on the Drug Enforcement Administration's role in combating the opioid epidemic.

Today, the Subcommittee on Oversight and Investigations convenes a hearing on the DEA's role in combating the opioid epidemic. This crisis is a top priority of the nation and certainly of this committee and subcommittee. Opioid-related overdoses killed more than 42,000 people in 2016. That's an average of 115 deaths each day. An estimated 2.1 million people have an opioid use disorder.

Since our earliest hearings in 2012, this subcommittee has been investigating various aspects of this epidemic. In May 2017, the Committee opened a bipartisan investigation into allegations of "opioid-dumping," a term to describe inordinate volumes of opioids shipped by wholesale drug distributors to pharmacies located in rural communities, such as those in West Virginia. From press reports and this investigation, we have learned of opioid shipments in West Virginia that shock the conscience.

Over 10 years, 20.8 million opioids were shipped to pharmacies in the town of Williamson, home to approximately 3,000 people.

Another 9 million opioids were distributed in just 2 years to a single pharmacy in Kermit, West Virginia, with a population of 406.

Between 2007 and 2012, drug distributors shipped more than 780 million hydrocodone and oxycodone pills in West Virginia.

These troubling examples raise serious questions about compliance with the Controlled Substances Act, administered by the DEA.

The CSA was enacted through this committee in 1970. This law established schedules of controlled substances and provided the authority for the DEA to register entities engaged in the manufacture, distribution, or dispensation of controlled substances. The CSA was designed to combat diversion by providing for a closed system of drug distribution in which all legitimate handlers of controlled substances must maintain a DEA registration, and as a condition of maintaining such registration must take reasonable steps to ensure their registration is not being used as a source of diversion. The DEA regulations specifically require all distributors to report suspicious orders of controlled substances in addition to the statutory responsibility to exercise due diligence to avoid filling suspicious orders.

This hearing has two goals. First, the subcommittee seeks to determine how the DEA could have done better to detect and investigate suspicious orders of opioids, such as the massive amounts shipped to West Virginia. The DEA has acknowledged to the committee that it could have done better in spotting and investigating suspicious opioid shipments. What were the deficiencies and has DEA addressed them? DEA has a comprehensive electronic database containing specific information at the pharmacy level. Could DEA use that database more effectively to investigate diversion and to facilitate compliance for the regulated industry?

The second goal is to find out whether the current DEA law enforcement approach is adequately protecting public safety. DEA statistics reveal a sharp decline since 2012 in certain DEA enforcement actions, immediate suspension orders, or ISOs, and orders to show cause. The number of ISOs issued by the DEA plummeted from 65 in 2011 to just six last year. Former DEA officials alleged in the Washington Post and on CBS' "60 Minutes" that the DEA's Office of Chief Counsel imposed evidentiary obstacles and delays for ISO and for orders to show cause submissions from the DEA field. The conflict between the DEA lawyers and the DEA investigators allegedly resulted in experienced DEA personnel leaving the agency and a loss of morale.

The goal of laws regulating controlled substances is to strike the right balance between the public interest in legitimate patients obtaining medications in a timely manner against another weighty public interest in preventing the illegal diversion of prescription drugs, particularly given the rampant and deadly opioid epidemic throughout the Nation. Our investigation is intended to assist the committee's continuing legislative effort to strike the right balance.

It is unfortunate that it's been a battle to get information out of the DEA. We have made recent progress with the DEA, but at this time our investigation still does not have the full picture. DEA has made some commitments that should hopefully help the committee gain the information it needs, and we expect the DEA to honor those commitments.

And I welcome today's witness, DEA Acting Administrator Robert Patterson. We have serious concerns about policy that we need to discuss today. But we are steadfast in our support and certainly want to salute the dedicated workforce at the DEA. We need an effective DEA in this crisis.

I want to thank the minority for their participation and hard work in this investigation, and I now yield to my friend, the ranking member, Ms. DeGette.

[The prepared statement of Mr. Harper follows:]

PREPARED STATEMENT OF HON. GREGG HARPER

Today the Subcommittee on Oversight and Investigations convenes a hearing on the Drug Enforcement Administration's (DEA) role in combating the opioid epidemic. The opioid crisis is a top priority of the nation and of this Committee. Opioid-related overdoses killed more than 42,000 people in 2016—115 deaths each day. An estimated 2.1 million people have an opioid use disorder.

Since our earliest hearings in 2012, this Subcommittee has been investigating various aspects of the opioid epidemic. In May 2017, the Committee opened a bipartisan investigation into allegations of "opioid-dumping," a term to describe inordinate volumes of opioids shipped by wholesale drug distributors to pharmacies located in rural communities, such as those in West Virginia. From press reports and this investigation, we have learned of opioid shipments in West Virginia that shock the conscience:

- Over 10 years, 20.8 million opioids were shipped to pharmacies in the town of Williamson, home to approximately 3,000 people.
- Another 9 million opioids were distributed in just 2 years to a single pharmacy in Kermit, West Virginia, population 406.
- Between 2007 and 2012, drug distributors shipped more than 780 million hydrocodone and oxycodone pills in West Virginia.

These troubling examples raise serious questions about compliance with the Controlled Substances Act, administered by the DEA.

The CSA was enacted through this Committee in 1970. This law established schedules of controlled substances and provided the authority for the DEA to register entities engaged in the manufacture, distribution, or dispensation of controlled substances. The CSA was designed to combat diversion by providing for a closed system of drug distribution, in which all legitimate handlers of controlled substances must obtain a DEA registration, and as a condition of maintaining such registration, must take reasonable steps to ensure their registration is not being used as a source of diversion. The DEA regulations specifically require all distributors to report suspicious orders of controlled substances, in addition to the statutory responsibility to exercise due diligence to avoid filling suspicious orders.

This hearing has two goals. First, the Subcommittee seeks to determine how the DEA could have done better to detect and investigate suspicious orders of opioids, such as massive amounts of opioids shipped to West Virginia. The DEA has acknowledged to the Committee that it could have done better in spotting and investigating suspicious opioid shipments. What were the deficiencies, and has DEA addressed them? DEA has a comprehensive electronic database containing specific information at the pharmacy level.

Could DEA use that database more effectively to investigate diversion and to facilitate compliance for the regulated industry?

The second goal is to find out whether the current DEA law enforcement approach is adequately protecting public safety. DEA statistics reveal a sharp decline since 2012 in certain DEA enforcement actions, Immediate Suspension Orders (ISOs) and Orders to Show Cause (OTSCs). The number of ISOs issued by the DEA plummeted, from 65 in 2011 to just six last year. Former DEA officials alleged in the Washington Post and on CBS "60 Minutes," that the DEA's Office of Chief Counsel imposed evidentiary obstacles and delays for ISO and OTSC submissions from the DEA field. The conflict between the DEA lawyers and the DEA investigators allegedly resulted in experienced DEA personnel leaving the agency and a loss of morale.

The goal of laws regulating controlled substances is to strike the right balance between the public interest in legitimate patients obtaining medications in a timely manner against another weighty public interest in preventing the illegal diversion of prescription drugs, particularly given the rampant and deadly opioid epidemic throughout the nation. Our investigation is intended to assist the Committee's continuing legislative effort to strike the right balance.

It is unfortunate that it's been a battle to get information out of the DEA. We have made recent progress with the DEA, but at this time our investigation still does not have the full picture. DEA has made some commitments that should hopefully help the Committee gain the information it needs, and we expect the DEA to honor these commitments.

I welcome today's witness, DEA Acting Administrator Robert Patterson. We have serious concerns about policy to discuss, but we are steadfast in our support and salute the dedicated workforce at the DEA. We need an effective DEA in this crisis.

I also want to thank the Minority for their partnership and hard work in this investigation. I now yield to my friend, the Ranking Member, Ms. DeGette.

Ms. DEGETTE. Thank you so much, Mr. Chairman.

And I am happy to kick off the whole series of hearings with the Energy and Commerce Committee this week with this Oversight and Investigations hearing.

Opioid overdose is now the number-one cause of unintentional death in the United States. Every day we hear reports of Americans dying and leaving loved ones, often children, to pick up the pieces, and these reports are heartbreaking.

The crisis has also had an economic toll. Estimates are that it's cost this country a trillion dollars since 2001, and here's the point at my opening statement where I show that Congress can still be bipartisan because today I want to talk, as the chairman did, about our committee investigation, examining exactly how the opioid epidemic developed.

Our investigation, as the chairman said, focused on West Virginia, which has the highest opioid death toll in the Nation. The numbers that we are seeing coming out are simply shocking. A major 2016 news investigation, for example, reported that distributors shipped 780 million opioids to this state between 2007 and 2012. Again, in 5 years, they shipped 780 million opioids to this small State of West Virginia. Now, we focus on West Virginia but I am hoping that the lessons we learned will apply nationwide, including in my home State of Colorado.

Administrator Patterson, I join the Chairman in welcoming you here. We have a lot of questions and we'd like to know what you think failed us in West Virginia and, more importantly, what we can do to avoid this again. We know something had to have gone wrong. For example, in DEA's own court filings, in 2008 the distributor shipped one pharmacy in West Virginia 22,500 hydrocodone pills per month. But our investigation also found that a number of pharmacies were sent even many times more that amount. For example, the Chairman talked about Kermit, West Virginia. We looked at one pharmacy in Kermit, which has a few hundred people. Drug distributors supplied this pharmacy with more than 4.3 million doses of opioids, more than 350,000 per month in a single year, and then the next year 4 million doses of opioids.

What on earth were people thinking? Now, when the DEA finally shut down this pharmacy and took its owner to court, the owner admitted at its height the pharmacy filled one prescription per minute. Who could think that this was a legitimate use?

News reports from the time describe pharmacy workers throwing bags of opioids "over a divider and onto a counter to keep pace." One law enforcement agent noticed a cash drawer "so full the clerk could not get it to close properly." And this was not the only pharmacy to receive such massive quantities of opioids. In another example, between 2006 and 2016, distributors shipped over 20 million doses of opioids to two pharmacies in one town of 3,000 people.

I want to know if the DEA thinks that this amount of pills sent to these pharmacies was excessive. In addition, the Controlled Substances Act and applicable regulations required the distributor to tell DEA how many pills that distributor sold and to what pharmacies. DEA compiles this information into a database called the Automation of Reports and Consolidated Orders System. It's called ARCOS.

I want to know how the DEA made use of ARCOS data from 2006 on and whether it relied on that data to monitor the number of pills that distributors sent to West Virginia. Did the DEA perform analytic assessments of the pills the pharmacies received? Did it look at how many pills distributors sent to a town or region as a whole? And if so, I want to know why the DEA didn't act to stop these shipments.

I want to know whether the distributors themselves exercised appropriate due diligence before sending millions of pills to pharmacies. For example, in a letter sent to all drug distributors in 2006 and 2007, the DEA gave them a list of circumstances that might be indicative of diversion, all of which plainly require distributors to know their customers before shipping them any opioids at all. I want to know if the drug distributors met this standard when they shipped those pills to tiny West Virginia and, similarly, did the distributors comply with their obligations. And I want to know also what the DEA is doing right now to stop painkillers from flooding our communities today.

We have had a lot of hearings on this, Mr. Chairman, but this is the first one to look in a hard way at this crisis developed. We spend countless hours of law enforcement time trying to stop illegal drugs from coming into this country and here we are, sending millions of doses of opioids to tiny little towns in West Virginia, all of this supposedly legally.

I think I can speak for the whole committee to say this needs to stop, it needs to stop now, and we need to figure out how we are going to protect our constituents and our citizens.

I yield back.

Mr. HARPER. The gentlewoman yields back.

The chair will now recognize the chairman of the full committee,

Chairman Walden, for purposes of an opening statement.

OPENING STATEMENT OF HON. GREG WALDEN, A REPRESENTATIVE IN CONGRESS FROM THE STATE OF OREGON

Mr. WALDEN. Thank you, Mr. Chairman, and thank you for your leadership on this very important issue to the people we represent.

For nearly a year, this committee has been investigating how inordinate numbers of pills were shipped to pharmacies in rural West Virginia. The numbers that we have seen thus far, as you've heard, Mr. Patterson, are nothing short of staggering—more than 20 million prescription opioids shipped to a West Virginia town with a population of fewer than 3,000 people. Another West Virginia pharmacy, in a town with a population of fewer than 2,000 people, received an average of 5,600 prescription opioids a day during a single year.

As part of our investigation, we have also looked at the Sav-Rite pharmacies in Kermit, West Virginia, a town with a population of about 400.

During last October's full committee hearing, I asked your colleague at the DEA a very straightforward question: which companies provided the Sav-Rite No. 1 pharmacy with so many opioids that it ranked 22nd in the entire United States of America for the number of hydrocodone pills received in 2006?

After an extended and unnecessary delay, we finally received the DEA data and now know the answer to that question. But this isn't the end of the matter, however.

We have learned that in 2008, a second Sav-Rite location opened just 2 miles away from the original pharmacy. However, the second Sav-Rite was forced to close and surrender its DEA registration after it was raided by federal agents in March 2009. Now, in most instances, this would be a success story. But in this case, the original Sav-Rite pharmacy—the one that had received 9 million pills in just 2 years—stayed open for another two years, and in those 2 years, Sav-Rite No. 1 dispensed about 1.5 million pills into the community. So the question is, how did that happen? How is it possible?

The raid on Sav-Rite 2 was based on observations made during undercover investigations conducted at both Sav-Rite locations as well as a pill mill medical practice. As part of the undercover operation, Federal investigators saw pharmacy customers sharing drugs with one another in the parking lot, and as you've heard, a cash drawer so full the clerk could not close it, and learned that the owner of the Sav-Rite pharmacies apparently developed a "getrich-quick scheme" with a pill mill medical practice. This scheme may have filled their cash drawers, but it was devastating to the community.

It doesn't make any sense as to why the DEA did not shut down both pharmacies at the same time. They were owned by the same person. They were part of the same criminal scheme. DEA has acknowledged that breakdowns occurred and lessons were learned, in this case and in others. We need to make sure DEA has fixed its own problems so that an effective DEA is part of the many solutions needed to combat the opioid crisis.

As you know, people are dying. Lives are being ruined. We must be united in our efforts to end this horrible epidemic. That is why myself and this entire committee have been so frustrated that it has taken so long to obtain DEA's full cooperation in this investigation.

And while progress is being made in DEA's efforts—and I appreciated our meeting on Friday—we still have plenty of unanswered questions coming in to today's hearing. So I am hopeful we can learn the answers to those questions today and I am also pleased with the commitments DEA has made to fulfill our remaining requests in this investigation. And I expect those commitments to be honored, period. If they are not, we'll be back talking again soon.

Our most pressing questions are intended to get DEA on a better path. Every one of us on this dais and in this room supports a strong and effective DEA. We know you have an enormous and important job to do with dedicated agents and we are grateful to all those in law enforcement personnel at your agency. Quite simply, we want you to have the tools and the resources you need to help us combat this epidemic, among the other many duties you have at DEA.

So I want to thank you for again being with us today, Acting Administrator Patterson, and we look forward to your candor.

And I would like to yield the balance of my time to the gentleman from Virginia, Mr. Griffith. Before I do that, I would remind the committee we will have two full days of hearings starting tomorrow and Thursday reviewing 25 pieces of legislation on the opioids epidemic, and we hope and expect everyone on the committee to attend those hearings. With that, I yield to the gentleman from Virginia. [The prepared statement of Mr. Walden follows:]

PREPARED STATEMENT OF HON. GREG WALDEN

Thank you, Mr. Chairman, for holding this hearing on DEA's role in combating the opioid epidemic, a top priority of this committee.

For nearly a year, this committee has been investigating how inordinate numbers of pills were shipped to pharmacies in rural West Virginia. The numbers that we have seen thus far are nothing short of staggering—more than 20 million prescription opioids shipped to a West Virginia town with a population of fewer than 3,000 people. Another West Virginia pharmacy, in a town with a population of fewer than 2,000 people, received an average of more than 5,600 prescription opioids a day during a single year.

As part of our investigation, we have also looked at the Sav-Rite pharmacies in Kermit, West Virginia, a town with a population of approximately 400 people.

During last October's full committee hearing, I asked your colleague at the DEA a very straightforward question: Which companies provided the Sav-Rite #1 pharmacy with so many opioids that it ranked 22nd in the entire country for the number of hydrocodone pills received in 2006?

After extended delay, we received the DEA data and now know the answer to that question. This is not the end of the matter, however.

We have learned that in 2008, a second Sav-Rite location opened, just two miles away from the original pharmacy. However, the second Sav-Rite was forced to close and surrender its DEA registration after it was raided by federal agents in March 2009. In most instances, this would be a success story. But in this case, the original Sav-Rite pharmacy-the one that received 9 million pills in just 2 years-stayed open for more than two years. In those two years, Sav-Rite #1 dispensed about 1.5 million pills into the community. How is this possible? The raid on Sav-Rite 2 was based on observations made during undercover investigations conducted at both Sav-Rite locations as well as a pill mill medical practice. As part of the undercover operation, federal investigators saw pharmacy customers sharing drugs with one another in the parking lot, a cash drawer so full that the clerk could not close it, and learned that the owner of the Sav-Rite pharmacies apparently developed a "get-rich quick scheme" with a pill mill medical practice. This scheme may have filled their cash drawers, but it was devastating the community. It doesn't make any sense as to why the DEA did not shut down both pharmacies at the same time—they were owned by the same person and were part of the same criminal scheme. DEA has acknowledged that breakdowns occurred, and lessons were learned-in this case and others. We need to make sure DEA has fixed its own problems so that an effective DEA is part of the many solutions needed to combat the opioid crisis. People are dying. Lives are being ruined. We must be united in our efforts to end this horrible epidemic. That is why myself and this entire committee have been so frustrated that it has taken this long to obtain DEA's full cooperation in this investigation.

And while progress is being made in DEA's efforts, we still have plenty of unanswered questions coming into today's hearing. I am hopeful that we can learn the answers to those questions today. I am also pleased with the commitments DEA has made to fulfill our remaining requests in this investigation. I expect those commitments to be honored. If they are not, we'll be back here again soon.

Our most pressing questions are intended to get DEA on a better path. Every one of us on this dais, and in this room, supports a strong and effective DEA. We know you have an enormous job to do and we are grateful to all of the dedicated law enforcement personnel at the agency. Quite simply, we want you to have the tools and the resources you need to combat this epidemic, among the other many duties of the DEA.

So thank you again for being here with us today, Acting Administrator Patterson. We look forward to your candor, and I would like to yield the balance of my time to the gentleman from Virginia, Mr. Griffith.

Mr. GRIFFITH. Thank you, Mr. Chairman.

We have an implied constitutional responsibility to conduct oversight and ensure that the Controlled Substances Act strikes the correct balance between the public interest in legitimate patients obtaining medications against the weighty public interest in preventing the illegal diversion of prescription drugs.

A key issue is whether the DEA is adequately protecting public safety. DEA statistics reveal a sharp decline and immediate suspension orders—ISOs—since 2012. ISOs are a DEA administrative tool not to punish but to protect the public from rogue doctors or pharmacists who would continue to provide opioids to drug abusers unless their registration was immediately suspended.

Former DEA officials alleged in the Washington Post and on CBS "60 Minutes" that the DEA's office of chief counsel, starting around 2013, changed its evidentiary requirements for ISO submissions from the DEA field. DEA documents provided to the Committee seem to substantiate this allegation.

Now, ISOs remind me of DUI cases in Virginia. When a police officer gets a driver off the road who's been drinking, their license to drive is administratively suspended in order to protect the public.

Trial on the merits is delayed, but not public safety. It's a similar principle here. Immediately suspend the rogue operator and protect the public.

I yield back.

Mr. HARPER. The gentleman yields back.

The chair will now recognize the ranking member of the full committee, Mr. Pallone, for five minutes.

Opening Statement of Hon. Frank Pallone, Jr., a Representative in Congress from the State of New Jersey

Mr. PALLONE. Thank you, Mr. Chairman.

The opioid epidemic continues to devastate communities and families in every part of America, and every day 115 Americans lose their lives in an opioid overdose.

We must do more to help those struggling with addiction, and I am committed to working with all of my colleagues to advance meaningful legislation and resources to help combat this crisis. Families all across this nation are looking to us for help, and it is my hope that DEA will work cooperatively with us on this effort.

In addition to advancing efforts to respond to this crisis, Congress also has a responsibility to figure out what went wrong and how it went wrong and how to make sure something like this never happens again. And that is why this committee has been engaged in a bipartisan investigation into the role both DEA and drug distributors have in addressing the ongoing opioid crisis and what systems failed to protect the communities that have been so overwhelmed by this epidemic.

So I hope that the lessons we learn will help us address this urgent problem throughout the country, from New Jersey to West Virginia and beyond.

Clearly, something went wrong. The safeguards designed to prevent opioids from being diverted into the wrong hands simply did not work and our committee's investigation has found that drug distributors shipped millions of pills to multiple small-town pharmacies in West Virginia every year. For example, a pharmacy in a town of 2,000 people received 16.5 million doses of opioids over a 10-year period and there were other pharmacies in that area as well.

There is simply no way that there was an actual medical need for this incredible volume of opioids in this rural sparsely-populated area and I would hope that DEA can tell us what broke down in the safeguards that should have protected communities from these abusive practices. These include failures by both the distributors and the DEA.

For example, I have questions about the data that DEA collects and why they did not use it more aggressively to prevent the oversupply of opioids in certain—in certain cases. We know that distributors are required to tell DEA how many pills they ship each month and where those pills go. It is not clear, however, that DEA has used this data in the past, and if DEA is using this data now to help it curtail excessive pill distribution.

Distributors are also required to alert DEA when a pharmacy places an order for what appears to be a suspiciously large quantity of pills. It appears that distributors have not always alerted DEA of those suspicious orders and may not even have had adequate systems in place to identify inappropriately large orders. But at the same time, it is also not clear that DEA has always done enough with the suspicious orders they receive from distributors to alert the agency to possible anomalous shipments, and I hope we can get answers to both of these questions.

And when multiple distributors ship to a single pharmacy, possibly causing an oversupply, it is not clear that DEA has had an adequate system to identify and flag to the distributors that an oversupply problem may be unfolding. Unlike DEA, who has access to comprehensive distribution data, distributors can only see what they supply to an individual pharmacy. Yet, if DEA is not flagging when multiple distributors are at risk of collectively oversupplying a pharmacy, then the result is another example of a system failure that can lead to diversion.

So it seems likely that failing to report suspicious orders by distributors has hurt DEA's ability to monitor the distribution of controlled substances and I hope that we will hear that this is no longer an issue today, and if it is, I'd like to know what tools DEA needs to help it to enforce this requirement. At the same time, I do hope that DEA is making full use of suspicious orders when they are reported to their field offices.

Finally, Mr. Chairman, while our investigation has focused on what went wrong in West Virginia, I also want to know how DEA is monitoring distributors across the country now. Addictive drugs are still abundant in our communities and now new opioids are also being introduced to the market.

So I hope that DEA is actively or proactively analyzing shipments of these pills and, where appropriate, stepping in and stopping the over-distribution of these drugs.

So I just want to thank Administrator Patterson for appearing before us. This issue is extraordinarily important and no entity can address it alone. DEA and Congress must be allies in combating the opioid crisis and only by understanding what went wrong can we fix this system for the future.

So just, again, I know you're in the hot seat today but this is something that we need to work on together.

Thank you, Mr. Chairman.

[The prepared statement of Mr. Pallone follows:]

PREPARED STATEMENT OF HON. FRANK PALLONE, JR.

Thank you, Mr. Chairman. The opioid epidemic continues to devastate communities and families in every part of America. Every day, 115 Americans lose their lives to an opioid overdose.

We must do more to help those struggling with addiction, and I am committed to working with my colleagues to advance meaningful legislation and resources to help combat this crisis. Families all across this nation are looking to us for help, and it is my hope that DEA will work cooperatively with us on this effort.

In addition to advancing efforts to respond to this crisis, Congress also has a responsibility to figure out what went wrong, how it went wrong, and how to make sure something like this never happens again. That is why this Committee has been engaged in a bipartisan investigation into the role both DEA and drug distributors have in addressing the ongoing opioid crisis, and what systems failed to protect the communities that have been so overwhelmed by this epidemic.

I hope that the lessons we learn will help us address this urgent problem throughout the country, from New Jersey to West Virginia and beyond.

Clearly, something went wrong. The safeguards designed to prevent opioids from being diverted into the wrong hands simply did not work.

Our Committee's investigation has found that drug distributors shipped millions of pills to multiple small-town pharmacies in West Virginia every year. For example, a pharmacy in a town of 2-thousand people received 16.5 million doses of opioids over a 10-year period. And there were other pharmacies in that area.

There is simply no way that there was an actual medical need for this incredible volume of opioids in this rural, sparsely populated area. I would hope that DEA can tell us what broke down in the safeguards that should have protected communities from these abusive practices. These include failures by both the distributors and DEA.

For example, I have questions about the data that DEA collects, and why they did not use it more aggressively prevent the oversupply of opioids in certain cases. We know that distributors are required to tell DEA how many pills they ship each month, and where those pills go. It is not clear, however, how DEA has used this data in the past, and if DEA is using this data now to help it curtail excessive pill distribution.

Distributors are also required to alert DEA when a pharmacy places an order for what appears to be a suspiciously large quantity of pills. It appears that distributors have not always alerted DEA of these suspicious orders, and may not even have had adequate systems in place to identify inappropriately large orders. But at the same time, it is also not clear that DEA has always done enough with the suspicious orders they receive from distributors to alert the agency to possibly anomalous shipments. I hope we can get answers to both of these questions.

And when multiple distributors ship to a single pharmacy, possibly causing an oversupply, it is not clear that DEA has had an adequate system to identify and flag to the distributors that an oversupply problem may be unfolding. Unlike DEA who has access to comprehensive distribution data, distributors can only see what they supply to an individual pharmacy. Yet, if DEA is not flagging when multiple distributors are at risk of collectively oversupplying a pharmacy, then the result is another example of a system failure that can lead to diversion.

It seems likely that failing to report suspicious orders by distributors has hurt DEA's ability to monitor the distribution of controlled substances. I hope that we will hear that this is no longer an issue today, and if it is I'd like to know what tools DEA needs to help it enforce this requirement. But at the same time, I do hope that DEA is making full use of suspicious orders when they are reported to their field offices.

Finally, while our investigation has focused on what went wrong in West Virginia, I also want to know how DEA is monitoring distributors across the country now. Addictive drugs are still abundant in our communities, and now new opioids are also being introduced to the market.

I hope that DEA is acting proactively to analyze shipments of these pills and, where appropriate, stepping in and stopping the over-distribution of these drugs. I want to thank Administrator Patterson for appearing before us today. This issue is extraordinarily important, and no entity can address it alone. DEA and Congress must be allies in combatting the opioid crisis, and only by understanding what went wrong can we fix this system for the future.

Thank you.

Mr. HARPER. The gentleman yields back.

I ask unanimous consent that the members' written opening statements be made part of the record. Without objection, it will be entered into the record.

Additionally, I ask unanimous consent that Energy and Commerce members not on the Subcommittee on Oversight and Investigations be permitted to participate in today's hearing.

Without objection, so ordered.

I would now like to introduce our witness for today's hearing. Today, we have Mr. Robert Patterson, the Acting Administrator for the Drug Enforcement Administration. We appreciate you being here with us today, Mr. Patterson, and you are aware that the committee is holding an investigative hearing and when so doing it has been our practice of taking testimony under oath.

Do you have any objection to testifying under oath?

Mr. PATTERSON. I do not.

Mr. HARPER. Witness response is no.

The chair then advises you that under the rules of the House and the rules of the committee, you're entitled to be accompanied by counsel. Do you desire to be accompanied by counsel during your testimony today?

Mr. PATTERSON. I do not.

Mr. HARPER. Responds that he does not. In that case, I would ask that you rise and please raise your right hand and I will swear you in.

[Witness sworn.]

You are now under oath and subject to the penalties set forth in Title 18 Section 1001 of the United States Code. You may now give a 5-minute summary of your written statement. You can hit the button on the mic and you have 5 minutes to summarize your testimony. Thank you again for being here, Mr. Patterson.

TESTIMONY OF ROBERT W. PATTERSON, ACTING ADMINISTRATOR, DRUG ENFORCEMENT ADMINISTRATION

Mr. PATTERSON. Thank you, and good morning.

Committee Chairman Walden, Subcommittee Chairman Harper, Ranking Members Pallone and DeGette, and distinguished members of the subcommittee, thank you for the opportunity to be here today to discuss the opioid epidemic and DEA's role in combating this crisis.

Over the past 15 years, our nation has been increasingly devastated by opioid abuse, an epidemic fueled for a significant period of time by the overprescribing of potent prescription opioids for acute and chronic pain. This indiscriminate practice created a generation of opioid abusers, presently estimated at more than 3 million Americans.

Over the past few years, we have begun to see a dramatic and disturbing shift. As a result of the increased awareness of the opioid epidemic, prescriptions for opioids have started to decline — obviously, somewhat a success. But organizations, in particular the well-positioned—in particular, the well-positioned Mexican drug cartels have filled this void by producing and distributing cheap powdered heroin, often mixed with illicit fentanyl and other fentanyl-related substances and selling it to users in both traditional powder form and, in some cases, pressed into counterfeit pills made to resemble illicit pharmaceuticals.

There are two central elements DEA is addressing as part of this administration's collective efforts to turn this tide, with a third piece that must also be addressed. First and foremost is enforcement. Based on our investigations, actions are undertaken every day using our criminal, civil, or administrative tools to attack the traffic in illicit drugs and the diversion of the licit supply.

Second is education. I strongly believe there is a real value and a natural fit for the DEA in this space and look whenever possible to partner with leaders in prevention and education.

The third element is treatment. The DEA is committed to doing what we can to improve access to drug treatment and recovery services, working alongside our partners at the Department of Health and Human Services, to utilize evidence-based strategies that minimize the risk of diversion during this public health emergency.

Ultimately, the only way to fundamentally change this epidemic is to decrease demand for these substances and address the global licit and illicit supply concerns through the efforts of DEA and all of its partners. The action of DEA's Diversion Control Division are critical with respect to addressing the licit supply. Diversion of prescription opioids by a few has a disproportionate impact on the availability of prescription opioids. The fact remains that a majority of new heroin users stated that they started their cycle of addiction on prescription opioids. As a result, we are constantly evaluating ways to improve our effectiveness to ensure that our more than 1.7 million registrants comply with the law.

Our use of administrative tools and legislation that changed our authorities in this area has been the subject of numerous media reports. Let me address that issue up front. DEA has continued to revoke approximately 1,000 registrations each year through administrative tools such as orders to show cause, immediate suspension orders, and surrenders for cause. We have and will continue to use all of these tools to protect the public from the very small percentage of registrants who exploit human frailty for profit. Where a licensed revocation is not necessary we have aggressively pursued civil actions and MOUs designed to ensure compliance.

Over the last decade, DEA has levied fines totaling nearly $390 million against opioid distributors nationwide and entered into MOUs with each. DEA has also reprioritized a portion of its criminal investigators and embedded them in with diversion investigators and enforcement groups, referred to as tactical diversion squads. We currently have 77 of these groups nationwide who are solely dedicated to investigating, disrupting, and dismantling individuals and organizations involved in diversion schemes.

DEA's Diversion Control Division has simultaneously worked to improve communication and cooperation with the registrant community. As an example of this outreach, DEA offers year-round training free of charge to pharmacists, distributors, importers, and manufacturers. DEA just completed training more than 13,000 pharmacists and pharmacy technicians on the important role they play in ensuring they only fill valid prescriptions.

In May, DEA will initiate a similar nationwide effort to provide training on the vital role that prescribers play in curbing this epidemic. This effort will start with specific focus on States where we have seen little decrease or, in some increases, an increase in opioid prescribing rates.

Administrative action, civil fines, and criminal cases are all important steps. Where we have fallen short in the past it is by not proactively leveraging the data that has been available to us.

Although I am happy to discuss what happened in the past, I focus my time on moving our agency forward and appreciate the opportunity to update you on where we are today and where we intend to go. For example, in January we utilized ARCOS data overlaid with data from HHS and, when available, state PMP programs. The result was approximately 400 targeted leads that DEA was able to send to its 22 field divisions nationwide for further investigation.

We are working all the Federal agencies in the space while we continue to work well with our colleagues at ONDCP, CCD, NIDA. The mutual issues that we face today have created stronger and critical partnerships with FDA and HHS.

I'll finish up by saying I'd like to recognize the Health Subcommittee's efforts to hold a legislative hearing starting tomorrow on more than 25 pieces of legislation. That effort not only underscores the unprecedented nature and complexity of the opioid crisis but also demonstrates that we must all take action to address this threat together.

Thank you for this opportunity and I look forward to your questions.

[The prepared testimony of Mr. Patterson follows:]

STATEMENT OF ROBERT W. PATTERSON, ACTING ADMINISTRATOR, DRUG ENFORCEMENT ADMINISTRATION, BEFORE THE SUBCOMMITTEE ON OVERSIGHT AND INVESTIGATIONS, COMMITTEE ON ENERGY AND COMMERCE, U.S. HOUSE OF REPRESENTATIVES, MARCH 20, 2018

Chairman Walden, Ranking Member Pallone, and Members of the Committee: on behalf of the approximately 9,000 employees of the Drug Enforcement Administration (DEA), thank you for the opportunity to discuss the threat posed by the opioid epidemic. The misuse of controlled prescription drugs (CPDs) is inextricably linked with the threat the United States faces from the trafficking of heroin, illicit fentanyl, and fentanyl analogues.

Drug overdoses, suffered by family, friends, neighbors, and colleagues, are now the leading cause of injury-related death in the United States, eclipsing deaths from motor vehicle crashes or firearms.[1] According to the Centers for Disease Control and Prevention (CDC), there were nearly 64,000 overdose deaths in 2016, or approximately 174 per day. Over 42,249 (66 percent) of these deaths involved opioids. The sharp increase in drug overdose deaths between 2015 to 2016 was fueled by a surge in fentanyl and fentanyl analogue (synthetic opioids) involved overdoses.[2]

The misuse of CPDs and the growing use of heroin, fentanyl, and fentanyl analogues are being reported in the United States in unprecedented numbers. According to the Substance Abuse and Mental Health Services Administration (SAMHSA) 2016 National Survey on Drug Use and Health (NSDUH), 6.2 million people over the age of 12 misused psychotherapeutic drugs (e.g., pain relievers, tranquilizers, stimulants, and sedatives) during the past month.[3] This represents 22 percent of the 28.6 million current illicit drug

---

[1] Rose A. Rudd, Noah Aleshire, Jon E. Zibbell, & R. Matthew Gladden. Increases in Drug and Opioid Overdose Deaths – United States, *2000-2014 Morbidity and Mortality Weekly Report*, 2016;64:1378-1382.

[2] CDC WONDER data, retrieved from the *National Institute of Health* website; http://www.drugabuse.gov as reported on NIDA's website.

[3] Substance Abuse and Mental Health Services Administration. (2017). Key substance use and mental health indicators in the United States: Results from the 2016 National Survey on Drug Use and Health (HHS Publication No. SMA 17-5044, NSDUH Series H-52). Rockville, MD: *Center for Behavioral Health Statistics and Quality, Substance Abuse and Mental Health Services Administration*. Retrieved from https://www.samhsa.gov/data/.

users and is second only to marijuana (24 million users) in terms of usage.[4] There are more current misusers of psychotherapeutic drugs than current users of cocaine, heroin, and hallucinogens combined.[5]

The increase in the number of people using heroin in recent years – from 373,000 past year users in 2007 to 948,000 in 2016 – is troubling.[6] More alarming is the proliferation of illicit fentanyl and its analogues. DEA investigations reveal that fentanyl and its analogues are increasingly being added to heroin and frequently pressed into counterfeit tablets resembling CPDs. Because of its high potency, the more illicit fentanyl and related analogues are introduced to the 11.5 million people that misused a pain reliever in the previous year, the more likely that drug overdoses will continue to climb.[7]

Controlled Prescription Drugs

In 2016, almost 3.4 million Americans age 12 or older reported misusing prescription pain relievers within the past month.[8] This makes prescription opioid misuse more common than use of any category of illicit drug in the United States except for marijuana. Whereas the vast majority of individuals misusing opioid CPDs do not go on to use heroin, this information provides valuable insight into the role that CPDs play in the opioid epidemic and underscores the need for a robust regulatory program that seeks to stop diversion of CPDs.

Black-market sales for opioid CPDs are typically five to ten times their retail value. DEA intelligence reveals the "street" cost of prescription opioids steadily increases with the relative strength of the drug. For example, hydrocodone combination products (a Schedule II prescription drug and also the most prescribed CPD in the country)[9] can

---

[4] Substance Abuse and Mental Health Services Administration. (2017). Key substance use and mental health indicators in the United States: Results from the 2016 National Survey on Drug Use and Health (HHS Publication No. SMA 17-5044, NSDUH Series H-52). Rockville, MD: *Center for Behavioral Health Statistics and Quality, Substance Abuse and Mental Health Services Administration*. Retrieved from https://www.samhsa.gov/data/.

[5] Substance Abuse and Mental Health Services Administration. (20 17). Key substance use and mental health indicators in the United States Results from the 2016 National Survey on Drug Use and Health {HHS Publication No. SMA 17-5044, NSDUH Series H·52). Rockville, MD: *Center for Behavioral Health Statistics and Quality, Substance Abuse and Mental Health Services Administration.* Retrieved from https://www.samhsagov/data/.

[6] Center for Behavioral Health Statistics and Quality. (2017). *2016 National Survey on Drug Use and Health: Detailed Tables.* Substance Abuse and Mental Health Services Administration, Rockville, MD.

[7] Ibid.

[8] Substance Abuse and Mental Health Services Administration. (2017). Key substance use and mental health indicators in the United States: Results from the 2016 National Survey on Drug Use and Health (HHS Publication No. SMA 17-5044, NSDUH Series H-52). Rockville, MD: *Center for Behavioral Health Statistics and Quality, Substance Abuse and Mental Health Services Administration*. Retrieved from https://www.samhsa.gov/data/.

[9] On October 6, 2014, DEA published a final rule in the *Federal Register* to move hydrocodone combination products from Schedule III to Schedule II, as recommended by the Assistant Secretary for Health of the U.S. Department of Health and Human Services.

generally be purchased for $5 to $7 per tablet on the street. Slightly stronger drugs like oxycodone combined with acetaminophen (e.g., Percocet) can be purchased for $7 to $10 per tablet on the street. Even stronger prescription drugs are sold for as much as $1 per milligram (mg). For example, 30 mg oxycodone (immediate release) and 30 mg oxymorphone (extended release) cost $30 to $40 per tablet on the street. The costs that ensue with greater tolerance make it difficult to purchase these drugs in order to support a developing substance use disorder, particularly when many first obtain these drugs for free from the family medicine cabinet or from friends.[10]

Heroin

The vast majority of heroin consumed in the United States is produced by powerful Mexico-based transnational criminal organizations (TCOs), such as the Sinaloa Cartel and New Generation Jalisco Cartel, and transported to the United States across the Southwest Border. These TCOs are extremely dangerous, violent, and will continue to leverage established transportation and distribution networks within the United States.

Not surprisingly, some people who misuse prescription opioids turn to heroin. Heroin traffickers produce high purity white powder heroin that costs approximately $10 per bag, and usually contains approximately 0.30 grams per bag. This makes heroin significantly less expensive than CPDs. Heroin produces a "high" similar to CPDs and can keep some individuals who are dependent on opioids from experiencing painful withdrawal symptoms. For some time now, law enforcement agencies across the country have been specifically reporting an increase in heroin use by those who began misusing prescription opioids.[11]

According to reporting by treatment providers, many individuals with serious opioid use disorders will use whichever drug is cheaper and/or available to them at the time.[12] Heroin purity and dosage amounts vary, and heroin is often adulterated with other substances (e.g., fentanyl and fentanyl analogues). This means that heroin users are at higher risk of unintentional overdose because they cannot predict the dosage of opioid in the product they purchase on the street as heroin.[13] Additionally, varying concentrations

---

[10] Substance Abuse and Mental Health Services Administration. (2017). Key substance use and mental health indicators in the United States: Results from the 2016 National Survey on Drug Use and Health (HHS Publication No. SMA 17-5044, NSDUH Series H-52). Rockville, MD: Center for Behavioral Health Statistics and Quality, Substance Abuse and Mental Health Services Administration. Retrieved from https·//www. samhsa.gov/datal.

[11] U.S. Department of Justice, Drug Enforcement Administration, *2016 National Heroin Threat Assessment Summary, DEA Intelligence Report*, April, 2016, available at: https://www.dea.gov/divisions/hq/2016/ hq062716_attach.pdf.

[12] U.S. Department of Justice, Drug Enforcement Administration, *2014 National Drug Threat Assessment Summary*, November, 2014.

[13] Stephen E. Lankenau, Michelle Teti, Karol Silva, Jennifer Jackson Bloom, Alex Harocopos, and Meghan Treese, Initiation into Prescription Opioid Misuse Among Young Injection Drug Users, *Int J Drug Policy*, Author

found in diverted or counterfeit prescription opioids purchased on the street have led to increased unintentional drug overdose deaths.

A report published by SAMHSA analyzing data through 2011 found that four out of five recent new heroin users had previously misused prescription pain relievers.[14] The reasons an individual may shift from one opioid to another vary, but today's heroin is high in purity, less expensive and often easier to obtain than illegal CPDs.

Overdose deaths involving heroin are increasing at an alarming rate, having increased more than five-fold since 2010.[15] Today's heroin at the retail level costs less and is more potent than the heroin that DEA encountered two decades ago. It is also not uncommon for heroin users to seek out heroin that dealers claim is "hot," meaning that it is likely cut with fentanyl or its analogues. Users seeking "hot" heroin is an indicator that as higher opioid tolerance levels develop among users, they will continue to seek out more potent forms of opioids.

Fentanyl and Fentanyl Analogues

Fentanyl is a Schedule II controlled substance produced in the United States and widely used in medicine. It is an extremely potent analgesic used for anesthesia and pain control in people with serious pain problems and in such cases, it is indicated only for use in individuals who have high opioid tolerance.

Illicit fentanyl, fentanyl analogues, and their immediate precursors are often produced in China. From China, these substances are shipped through private couriers or mail carriers directly to the United States or alternatively shipped directly to TCOs in Mexico, Canada, or the Caribbean. Once in the Western Hemisphere, fentanyl or its analogues are prepared to be mixed into the U.S. heroin supply domestically, or pressed into a pill form, and then moved to the illicit U.S. market where demand for prescription opioids and heroin remain at epidemic proportions.

In some cases, traffickers have industrial pill presses shipped into the United States directly from China and operate fentanyl pill press mills domestically. Mexican TCOs have seized upon this business opportunity because of the profit potential of synthetic opioids, and have invested in growing their share of this market. Because of its low

manuscript; available in PMC 2013 Jan 1, Published in final edited form as: *Int J Drug* Policy, 2012 Jan; 23(1): 37-44. Published online 2011 Jun 20. doi: 1016/j.drugpo.2011.05.014. and; Mars SG, Bourgois P, Karandinos G, Montero F, Ciccarone D., "Every 'Never' I Ever Said Came True": Transitions From Opioid Pills to Heroin Injecting, *Int J Drug Policy*, 2014 Mar;25(2):257-66. doi: 10.1016/j.drugpo.2013.10.004. Epub 2013 Oct 19.

[14] Substance Abuse and Mental Health Services Administration, *Associations of Nonmedical Pain Reliever Use and Initiation of Heroin Use in the United States*, Department of Health and Human Services, August 2013, *available at*: https://www.samhsa.gov/data/sites/default/files/DR006/DR006/nonmedical-pain-reliever-use-2013.htm.

[15] CDC WONDER data accessed on 10/15/17, as reported at *NIDA's* website: 3,036 heroin overdoses in 2010; 15,446 overdoses in 2016. https://www.drugabuse.gov/related-topics/trends-statistics/overdose-death-rates.

dosage range and potency, one kilogram of fentanyl purchased in China for $3,000 $5,000 can generate upwards of $1.5 million in revenue on the illicit market.

According to the DEA National Forensic Laboratory Information System (NFLIS), from January 2013 through December 2016, over 58,000 fentanyl exhibits were identified by federal, state, and local forensic laboratories.[16] During 2016, there were 36,061 fentanyl reports compared to 1,042 reports in 2013,[17] an exponential increase over the past four years. The consequences of fentanyl misuse are often fatal and occur amongst a diverse user base. According to a December 2017 CDC Data Brief, from 2015 to 2016, the death rate from synthetic opioids other than methadone, a category that includes fentanyl, doubled from 9,580 (age adjusted rate 3.1) to 19,413 (the age-adjusted rate of drug overdose deaths involving synthetic opioids other than methadone (drugs such as fentanyl, fentanyl analogs, and tramadol) doubled between 2015 and 2016, from 3.1 to 66.2 per 100,000).[18]

Florida's Pill Mills – Start of the Proliferation of CPDs

Between 2005 and 2009, Florida was the epicenter of many illegal operations whereby hundreds of millions of dosage units of controlled substances were diverted into United States illicit markets. During this time, the diversion of millions of dosage units of hydrocodone products was facilitated by rogue internet pharmacies and unscrupulous prescribers who provided prescriptions to drug seekers utilizing internet sites.[19] The *Ryan Haight Online Pharmacy Consumer Protection Act* (P.L. 110-425) took effect in April of 2009, combined with intensified law enforcement and regulatory actions, virtually eliminated the threat posed by domestic rogue internet pharmacies.

As the number of domestic internet-based pharmacies began to decline in 2008, law enforcement observed a significant rise in the number of rogue pain clinics or "pill mills," particularly in Florida.[20] In 2009, there was a high concentration of pain clinics located in the tri-county area of South Florida (comprised of Broward, Miami-Dade, and Palm Beach Counties). According to data provided by the State of Florida, by 2010, Broward County alone was home to approximately 142 rogue pain clinics. Federal, state, and local law enforcement investigations identified thousands of drug seekers that routinely traveled to Florida-based rogue pain clinics to obtain pharmaceutical controlled

[16] U.S. Department of Justice, DEA, NFLIS, actual data queried on October 13, 2017.

[17] U.S. Department of Justice, DEA, NFLIS, actual data queried on October 13, 2017.

[18] Rose A. Rudd, Noah Aleshire, Jon E. Zibbell, & R. Matthew Gladden Hedegaard, H., Margaret Warner, and Arialdi M. Miniño. Drug Overdose Deaths in the United States, 1999–2016 Increases in Drug and Opioid Overdose Deaths – United States, 2000-2014 Morbidity and Mortality Weekly Report, *NCHS Data Brief*, 2016;64:1378-1382No. 294, Dec 2017. https://www.cdc.gov/nchs/data/databriefs/db294.pdf.

[19] The final rule rescheduling hydrocodone combination products from schedule III to schedule II of the Controlled Substances Act was published in the Federal Register on August 22, 2014, and became effective on October 6, 2014. 79 FR 49661.

[20] It addition, the amount of heroin seized at the South West border increased over 300 percent from 2008 to 2013.

and non-controlled substances, such as oxycodone, hydromorphone, methadone, tramadol, alprazolam, clonazepam, and carisoprodol.

After obtaining controlled prescription drugs, these individuals would travel back to their home states and illegally distribute the drugs that ultimately flooded the illicit market in states along the entire East Coast and Midwest.

West Virginia

During this same timeframe, some DEA-registered practitioners in West Virginia turned their practices into pill mill operations, indiscriminately writing prescriptions for opioids. One pill mill operation in Kermit, West Virginia, was highlighted in a 2016 article published by the *Charleston Gazette-Mail* in which roughly nine million opioid pills were sent over the course of two years to a town with a population of 392 people.[21] DEA, along with its Federal, State, local, and tribal partners, identified the individuals involved in violations of the Controlled Substances Act (CSA) and worked with the U.S. Attorney's Office for the Southern District of West Virginia to arrest several individuals, all of whom were sent to jail for their crimes. Stemming from the same operation, DEA and its State and local counterparts took action taken against the Sav-Rite Pharmacy in Kermit, including the arrest of the owner and forfeiture of more than $400,000.

Unfortunately, West Virginia continues to be the State with the highest rate of death due to drug overdoses with 52 overdose deaths per 100,000 population in 2016.[22] Consequently, DEA has devoted additional resources to West Virginia by increasing its presence in the State. In 2016, DEA established an Assistant Special Agent in Charge position in Charleston, West Virginia. A senior level manager now oversees the entire State from the State's capital, rather than Washington, DC. Additionally, in 2016 DEA added a second Tactical Diversion Squad (TDS) in Clarksburg and in 2017 DEA headquarters deployed one of its two "mobile" TDS groups to West Virginia. These groups pursue criminal investigations against those who traffic CPDs. In 2018, DEA is deploying six new heroin enforcement teams focused on combatting the flow of heroin and illicit fentanyl. The enforcement teams will be based in communities facing significant challenges with opioids, including Charleston, West Virginia, and five additional locations.

DEA has also established a new Field Division in Louisville. This office covers Kentucky, Tennessee, and West Virginia and will enhance DEA enforcement efforts within the Appalachian mountain region and unify drug trafficking investigations under a

---

[21] https://www.wvgazettemail.com/news/cops_and_courts/drug-firms-poured-m-painkillers-into-wv-amid-rise-of/article_99026dad-8ed5-5075-90fa-adb906a36214.html, retrieved March 7, 2018.

[22] Hedegaard H, Warner M, Minino AM. Drug overdose deaths in the United States, 1999 – 2016. *NCHS Data Brief*, no 294. Hyattsville, MD: National Center for Health Statistics. 2017/CDC.

single Special Agent in Charge. DEA anticipates that this change will produce more effective investigations on heroin, fentanyl, and prescription opioid trafficking, all of which have a significant impact on the region. The division will also better align DEA with the U.S. Attorney's Office districts in those areas, similar to current Bureau of Alcohol, Tobacco, Firearms and Explosives (ATF) and Federal Bureau of Investigation (FBI) offices, and also with the Appalachia High Intensity Drug Trafficking Areas Program. Funded by the White House Office of National Drug Control Policy (ONDCP).

DEA Lessons Learned and Response to the Proliferation of CPDs

Effective Registrant Outreach

Due to the complexity of DEA's regulatory program, the Diversion Control Division has worked aggressively to improve its communication and cooperation with its more than 1.7 million registrants, who represent medical professionals, pharmaceutical drug manufacturers, and those in the drug supply chain. DEA works with its registrant population by: (1) hosting Pharmacy Diversion Awareness Conferences (PDACs) throughout the country; (2) administering the Distributor Initiative Program with a goal of educating distributors on how to detect and guard against diversion activities; and (3) maintaining an open dialogue with various national associations such as the National Association of Boards of Pharmacy (NABP), American Medical Association (AMA), Federation of State Medical Boards A, and other groups to address diversion problems and educate the medical community on improving prescribing practices.[23]

By the end of 2017, DEA had hosted 100 PDACs in 50 states (as well as the District of Columbia and Puerto Rico) training more than 13,100 pharmacists, pharmacy technicians, and others on the important role they play in ensuring that valid prescriptions for controlled substances are filled. In May 2018, DEA will initiate a nationwide program to offer similar training to individual practitioners.

In addition to the training opportunities offered to registrants, DEA has also begun a program to proactively send targeted email messages to various segments of its registrant population on matters of mutual interest. For example, in February 2018, DEA sent correspondence to 1.3 million doctors nationwide alerting them of the CDC's recommendations for opioid prescribing for acute pain and alerted practitioners of a free training webinar available from CDC. DEA is working on similar correspondence alerting these same practitioners about resources available from SAMHSA on locating a substance abuse treatment provider in their state. We have also sent targeted messages to DEA's Schedule I researcher population on enhancements made to streamline the registration process for them, as well as to the manufacturer and distributor populations

---

[23] In FY2017 alone, Diversion has participated in 1,407 outreach efforts.

on new enhancements aimed at assisting them with fulfilling their regulatory responsibilities to identify and report suspicious orders. In the coming months, DEA will send targeted messages on certain practitioners on how they may utilize telemedicine to treat opioid use disorder.

Prescription Drug Monitoring Programs

Prescription drug monitoring programs (PDMPs) are state-run electronic database systems used by practitioners, pharmacists, medical and pharmacy boards, and law enforcement, but access varies according to state law. These programs are established through state legislation and are tailored to the specific needs of each state. DEA strongly champions robust PDMPs and encourages medical professionals to use this important tool to detect and prevent doctor shopping and other forms of diversion. Currently, 49 states have an operational PDMP. Missouri will become the 50th, pursuant to the Governor's Executive Order in July 2017. As of January 2018, 40 of these states require controlled substance prescribers to use the state's PDMP prior to prescribing a controlled substance, in certain circumstances, as mandated by each state's legislation.[24]

While PDMPs are valuable tools for prescribers, pharmacists, and law enforcement agencies to identify, detect, and prevent nonmedical prescription drug use and diversion, PDMPs do have some limits in their use for detecting diversion at the retail level. For example, drug traffickers and drug seekers willingly travel hundreds of miles to gain easy access to pain clinics and physicians that are operating unscrupulously and outside of the law, making interconnectivity between PDMPs vital. As a result, ONDCP and the Bureau of Justice Assistance (BJA) currently offer assistance for interstate and state-tribal PDMP linkages. CDC supports states to advance interventions for preventing prescription drug overdoses, through its *Prevention for States* program, which could include activities focused on improving interoperability between PDMPs and Electronic Health Record (EHR) technology and provide real-time provider access. The Indian Health Service (IHS) developed a policy that requires federal IHS facilities to report all controlled substance prescriptions to their respective State PDMPs and requires federal prescribers to check State PDMPs prior to prescribing opioids for a period longer than seven days. Forty-four states[25] are currently able to exchange prescription data between certain states. In some instances, data sharing may be limited to a single neighboring state. In other instances, data sharing may span states within a specific region. There are currently two interstate data sharing hubs in operation: RxCheck, BJA's open standards solution

---

[24] *PDMP Center of Excellence*, Brandeis University. http://www.pdmpassist.org/pdf/Mandatory_Query_Conditions_20180102.pdf retrieved March 6, 2018.

[25] States with the capacity to participate in interstate data sharing include Alabama, Alaska, Arizona, Arkansas, Colorado, Connecticut, Delaware, District of Columbia, Florida, Georgia, Idaho, Iowa, Illinois, Indiana, Kansas, Kentucky, Louisiana, Maryland, Maine, Massachusetts, Michigan, Minnesota, Mississippi, Montana, Nebraska, New Hampshire, New Mexico, New York, North Dakota, New Jersey, Nevada, Ohio, Oklahoma, Pennsylvania, Rhode Island, South Carolina, South Dakota, Tennessee, Texas, Utah, Vermont, Virginia, Wisconsin, West Virginia.

developed and operated in partnership by the IJIS Institute (IJIS) with funding from BJA; and PMP Interconnect (PMPi), a proprietary solution operated by NABP. As of August 2017, nine states are live or are implementing interstate data sharing using both hubs, 36 states are live or are implementing interstate data sharing using the PMPi hub only, and 4 states are live or are implementing interstate data sharing using the RxCheck hub only.

Federal partners are working to address the interoperability. Brandeis University's PDMP Training and Technical Center, funded by BJA, has assisted the IHS to improve interoperability between IHS, its pharmacies and PDMPs. The BJA currently provides funding to 30 states through the *Harold Rogers PDMP program* for PDMP implementation or enhancements or enhanced data sharing, including interstate data sharing. CDC supports work in states to enhance and maximize PDMPs as a public health and clinical tool.

Law enforcement access to request, view, and utilize PDMP data in support of ongoing investigations in a manner that protects personally identifiable information is vital. Access to information in support of active State and Federal investigations varies widely from state to state, with some states requiring a court order in order for law enforcement to obtain data.

Medication Disposal

On September 9, 2014, DEA issued a final rule, titled "Disposal of Controlled Substances." These regulations implement the Secure and Responsible Drug Disposal Act of 2010 (P.L. 111-273) and expand upon the previous methods of disposal by including disposal at drop-boxes in pharmacies and law enforcement agencies, mail back programs and drug deactivation systems if they render the product irretrievable. Through these regulations, DEA continues to focus its national attention on the issue of the misuse of prescription drugs and related substance use disorders, and promotes awareness that one source of these drugs is often the household medicine cabinet, as 53% of persons aged 12 or older who misused pain relievers in the past year bought or took the pain relievers from a friend or relative, or that friend or relative gave it to the user for free.[26] These regulations provide a safe and legal method for the public to dispose of unused or expired CPDs. As of March 2018, 3,812 DEA registrants have become "authorized collectors."

Since 2010, DEA has held its National Drug "Take Back" Initiative (NTBI) to provide a convenient and safe option to dispose of unused, expired and/or unwanted prescription drugs. DEA's most recent NTBI was held on October 25, 2017. As a result of all fourteen National Take Back Days, DEA, in conjunction with its State, local, and

---

[26] Substance Abuse and Mental Health Services Administration. (2017). Key substance use and mental health indicators in the United States: Results from the 2016 National Survey on Drug Use and Health (HHS Publication No. SMA 17-5044, NSDUH Series H-52). Rockville, MD: *Center for Behavioral Health Statistics and Quality, Substance Abuse and Mental Health Services Administration.* Retrieved from https://www.samhsa.gov/data/.

tribal law enforcement partners, has removed a total of 9.02 million pounds (4,508 tons) of medications from circulation. The DEA's next National Take Back Day is scheduled for April 28, 2018.

Automated Reporting and Consolidated Orders System (ARCOS) Data

ARCOS reporting is required by 21 U.S.C. §827(d)(1) and applicable DEA regulations. Manufacturers and distributors of schedule I, II, or III narcotic controlled substances (and GHB) must report the manufacture, sale, purchase, loss, or other disposition of these controlled substances (e.g., a manufacturer's sales to distributors; a distributor's sales to pharmacies, hospitals/clinics, and doctors). DEA's Diversion Control Division has taken numerous steps to examine sales and monitoring processes in ARCOS. For example, Diversion Control utilizes various reports and records to monitor trends or determine anomalous transactions, which can then be developed into investigative leads. A unit within the Diversion Control's Pharmaceutical Investigations Section uses aggregated ARCOS data to identify patterns and trends in the flow of narcotic controlled substances through the closed system of drug distribution. This unit prepares regular threat assessment reports for each of DEA's 22 Field Divisions to prioritize DEA resources in furtherance of criminal, civil, and regulatory investigations. Additionally, DEA is working on enhancements to the ARCOS system, which will require those entities submitting data to ARCOS to fix any transaction errors in order for the report to be accepted. This will help the ARCOS system to capture more accurate data and provide a more "real time" snapshot of the flow of controlled substances within the drug supply chain. Finally, DEA is working collaboratively with a coalition of 41 States Attorneys General and a second coalition of 7 States Attorneys General to provide non-public, law enforcement sensitive ARCOS data to support their active investigations against certain manufacturers and distributors.

Suspicious Order Reports (SORs)

Since the enactment of the CSA in 1970, all DEA registrants who distribute controlled substances have a statutory duty to "maintain effective controls against diversion" of controlled substances into other than legitimate medical, scientific, and industrial channels. The first regulations implementing the CSA in 1971 contained a provision regarding "suspicious orders of controlled substances." This provision, which has remained essentially unchanged since 1971, currently appears in 21 CFR § 1301.74(b) and reads as follows: "The registrant shall design and operate a system to disclose to the registrant suspicious orders of controlled substances. The registrant shall inform the Field Division Office of the Administration in his area of suspicious orders when discovered by the registrant. Suspicious orders include orders of unusual size, orders deviating substantially from a normal pattern, and orders of unusual frequency."

These reports are currently fielded and verified by DEA personnel and can be used as a tool to identify and pinpoint vulnerabilities throughout the closed system of drug distribution. Since 2010, DEA has found that certain distributors were not adequately following their internal controls or not reporting suspicious orders. Through negotiated settlements involving civil penalties and compliance agreements and other means, DEA has worked with DEA-registered manufacturers and distributors to strengthen suspicious order monitoring and reporting. DEA is also exploring ways to ensure that suspicious orders would be submitted to a central database. Centralized reporting would provide for a more efficient review, dissemination, and investigation of suspicious activity.

In addition, we have launched a new tool within the ARCOS system to assist drug manufacturers and distributors with their regulatory obligations under the CSA. The tool will allow a distributor (or manufacturer) to enter the DEA registration number of a prospective purchaser (pharmacy, hospital, doctor, etc.) as well as a drug code for the controlled substance the buyer wishes to purchase and the ARCOS application will return a count of the number of registrants who have sold that particular controlled substance to that prospective purchaser in the last 6 months. This new query application will help distributors identify red flags indicative of suspicious orders.

Finally, DEA Diversion Control urges DEA registrants and the public at large to "submit a tip" regarding possible CSA violations, including: illicit drug distribution or trafficking; suspicious online pharmacies selling controlled substances over the internet; and the illegal sale and distribution of a prescription drug by individuals, including doctors and pharmacists. These tips are submitted to a DEA Field Divisions for prompt action by either a DEA Special Agent or a professional staff member. These tips are submitted through DEA's Diversion Control website (https://www.deadiversion.usdoj.gov/tips_online.htm). DEA also maintains a telephone hotline (877-RxABUSE) for the community to submit tips which may establish leads relating to the potential diversion of controlled substances.

Tactical Diversion Squads

DEA Tactical Diversion Squads investigate suspected violations of the CSA and other federal and state statutes pertaining to the diversion of controlled substance pharmaceuticals and listed chemicals. These unique groups combine the skill sets of Special Agents, Diversion Investigators, and a variety of state and local law enforcement agencies. They are dedicated solely towards investigating, disrupting, and dismantling those individuals or organizations involved in diversion schemes (e.g., "doctor shoppers," prescription forgery rings, and DEA registrants who knowingly divert controlled substance pharmaceuticals). Between March 2011 and present, DEA increased the number of operational TDSs from 37 to 77. In addition, DEA established two mobile TDS that can deploy quickly to "hot spots" around the country in furtherance of the Diversion Control Division's mission.

Production Quotas for Schedule II Opioids

The Diversion Control Division is responsible for setting Aggregate Production Quotas (APQs) every year. These APQs are the "total quantity of each basic class of controlled substance listed in Schedule I or II necessary to be manufactured during the following calendar year to provide for the estimated medical, scientific, research, and industrial needs of the United States, for lawful export requirements, and for the establishment and maintenance of reserve stocks."[27] Since 2014, DEA has observed a decline in prescriptions written for certain Schedule II opioids. These declines have led to overall reductions in licit demand which in turn, have directly impacted the factors DEA considers when establishing the APQs for Schedule II opioids. In October 2016, DEA announced a 25 percent reduction (or more) in the 2017 APQs for many prescription opioids, including oxycodone, hydrocodone, fentanyl, hydromorphone, and morphine. Hydrocodone was reduced to 66 percent of the previous years' (2016) level. In late 2017, DEA announced a nearly 20 percent reduction in the 2018 APQs (from the 2017 levels) for controlled substances, and these reductions included the aforementioned opioids as well as oxymorphone, codeine, and meperidine. These decreases can be attributed to combined local, state, and federal activities and interventions, including creating new partnerships, enforcing current regulations, and dissemination of provider education and guidance documents, including the CDC *Guideline for Prescribing Opioids for Chronic Pain* released in March 2016. In addition, we are encouraged that more states have enacted and enforced laws mandating the use of PDMPs by medical providers and pharmacists which provides prescribers with valuable information to guide their medical decisions.

DEA's 360 Strategy

To counter the opioid crisis, DEA initiated and continues to expand upon its 360 Strategy. The strategy leverages existing Federal, State, local, and tribal partnerships to address the problem on three different fronts: law enforcement, diversion control, and demand reduction. Our enforcement activities are directed at the violent cartels and drug trafficking gangs responsible for feeding the heroin and prescription drug epidemic in our communities. We are also enhancing our diversion control efforts and working with community partners for them to implement evidence-based programs and efforts designed to reduce demand and to prevent the same problems from resurfacing.

As part of the 360 Strategy, DEA recently partnered with Discovery Education, a division of Discovery Communications, to develop and distribute a prescription opioid and heroin education curriculum to middle and high school students, their teachers, and parents. We are calling it *Operation Prevention* and have started nationwide deployment of this program. Our goal is to educate children about the science of addiction and the

[27] 21 CFR 1303.11(a).

true danger of prescription opioids and heroin, and to "kick start" life-saving conversations in the home and classroom.

This award-winning program is available at no cost to schools nationwide and includes resources such as standards-aligned lesson plans, interactive student activities, parent resources and more – all available through an online portal. Operation Prevention launched in October 2016 with a virtual field trip, viewed live by more than 200,000 students, in all 50 States and in seven foreign countries. This program will run for at least three consecutive school years (through spring 2019) and is free for all law enforcement, prevention, treatment, and community groups to use and distribute. As of February 2018, the program has reached more than 2.1 million students.

Since its implementation in 2016, the 360 Strategy has been implemented in eight cities– Louisville, Kentucky; St. Louis, Missouri; Pittsburgh, Pennsylvania; Milwaukee, Wisconsin; Dayton, Ohio; Albuquerque, New Mexico; Charleston, West Virginia; and Manchester, New Hampshire. DEA is expanding this program to additional locations including Salt Lake City, Utah and New Jersey in 2018. Our enforcement efforts will continue across the United States with our law enforcement and community partners.

Conclusion

The United States continues to be affected by a national opioid epidemic, which has been spurred, in part, by the rise of misuse of prescription opioids. DEA can and must do better and will continue to use all criminal, civil, and regulatory tools possible to identify, target, disrupt, and dismantle individuals and organizations responsible for the illicit distribution of pharmaceutical controlled substances in violation of the CSA. DEA expects that demand for opioids will continue to be met in part by Mexican-based TCOs that produce high purity heroin, which is being laced with fentanyl, fentanyl analogues, and other synthetic opioids, and then pressed into counterfeit pills. DEA will continue to address this threat by pursuing these TCOs, which have brought tremendous harm to our communities. Working with DOJ and our interagency partners, DEA will continue to engage our international counterparts, especially China. We look forward to continuing to work with Congress to find solutions necessary to address the threats posed by controlled prescription drugs, heroin, fentanyl, and other synthetic opioids.

***

Mr. HARPER. Thank you, Mr. Patterson. It'll now be the opportunity for members to ask you questions regarding your statement and look for solutions to the problems that we have and I will begin by recognizing myself for 5 minutes for questioning.

Over the past year, this committee has been investigating opioid dumping and as part of this probe the Committee found some disturbing examples, and I will share a couple of these, some that we have touched on. A single pharmacy in Mount Gay-Shamrock, West Virginia, population 1,779, received over 16.5 million hydrocodone and oxycodone pills between 2006 and 2016. Distributors sent 20.8 million opioid pills to Williamson, West Virginia, population 2,900, during the same period, and in 2006 a pharmacy located in Kermit, West Virginia, population 406, ranked 22nd in the entire country in the overall number of hydrocodone pills it received with a single distributor supplying 76 percent of hydrocodone pills that year.

Would you agree that, on its face, these distribution figures represent inordinate amounts of opioids shipped to such rural markets?

Mr. PATTERSON. I would.

Mr. HARPER. Distributors are required to file reports of shipment amounts on certain controlled substances to the DEA database called the Automated Reports and Consolidated Ordering System, or ARCOS. These reports are filed monthly. Is that correct?

Mr. PATTERSON. Sir, either monthly or quarterly.

Mr. HARPER. What's the distinction between when one is done quarterly or monthly? Who makes that determination?

Mr. PATTERSON. It is done by a distributor or a manufacturer.

Mr. HARPER. OK. Ten years ago, would the ARCOS database have been able to flag DEA diversion investigators about unusual patterns such as the stunning monthly increases of shipment amounts or disproportionate volume of controlled substance sales at a pharmacy?

Mr. PATTERSON. Ten years ago, I think that would be doubtful.

Mr. HARPER. OK. Did the DEA attempt to leverage the data in ARCOS to help support DEA investigations of opioid diversion in West Virginia?

Mr. PATTERSON. Back at that time frame?

Mr. HARPER. Just tell me when. When did they start utilizing that?

Mr. PATTERSON. Sir, so ARCOS data I think pre probably 2010 was an extremely manual process. As that system has gotten more robust and, certainly, through the last handful of years we've used that in a much more proactive manner.

Mr. HARPER. Would the DEA ARCOS database be able to flag such signals of opioid diversion today? Your answer is, obviously, a yes.

In 2006 and 2007, DEA sent at least three letters to wholesale drug distributors regarding their compliance obligations under the Controlled Substances Act. The letters reminded the companies of their duties to monitor and report suspicious orders of opioids. Yet, during this time, according to DEA enforcement actions, drug distributors failed to maintain effective controls against diversion.

Why did the DEA communications with industry fail to prevent the kinds of major breakdowns apparent in West Virginia?

Mr. PATTERSON. I think when you go back to that timeframe on the suspicious orders reports, there were two major failures. One was either a lack of information contained therein or not filing them in this instance that they had. I think that started the problem, quite frankly and a lot of the frustration came from chasing down the registrants and ultimately reminding them of their responsibility in this regulated area.

Mr. HARPER. Over the last 10 years, the DEA reached settlements with drug distributors for failing to maintain effective controls against diversion of opioids or failing to report suspicious orders. Yet, after these settlements, drug distributors continued to fail to comply with the regulatory requirements. Why were these initial settlements not effective in achieving compliance from these distributors?

Mr. PATTERSON. And again, this goes back to the frustration of the day, and I know that the folks that were in diversion back in 2010 and 2012 struggled with the fact that these MOUs or MOAs have been put in place with these companies and they blatantly violated them again.

Mr. HARPER. So how is DEA utilizing ARCOS today? Is it effective today?

Mr. PATTERSON. So, sir, ARCOS as a stand-alone database is a good pointer. I think, as I said in my opening statement, ARCOS data and what we have learned, combined with state PMP HHS data, gives you a much better outlier problem.

In some of the cases that we have looked at, depending on the situation, ARCOS data would not have found those particular issues, right. If it's a smaller level or a single place. So the reality is is what we need is all of these data sets essentially working in conjunction with each other.

Mr. HARPER. Are there movements to improve ARCOS? Is that constantly monitored and updated and refined?

Mr. PATTERSON. So we are constantly working with this data now in a very proactive way. We've joined with two state coalitions of states' attorneys-general to work with data sharing in this space, especially with the PMP data as well as our counterparts at HHS.

Mr. HARPER. Thank you, Mr. Patterson.

The Chair now recognizes the ranking member, Ms. DeGette from Colorado, for 5 minutes.

Ms. DEGETTE. Thank you so much, Mr. Chairman, and I agree, Mr. Patterson, that we do need to look forward how we can improve things. But I don't think we can do it without examining the past, and this ARCOS system is the perfect example.

I want to spend a few minutes following up on what the chairman was asking you, my understanding is ARCOS was in place during this whole time period, 2006 to 2016, correct?

Mr. PATTERSON. That's correct, ma'am.

Ms. DEGETTE. And so what was happening the data was just being reported in but nothing was really being done with it. Isn't that correct?

Mr. PATTERSON. I would say it was used in a very reactive way.

Ms. DEGETTE. Right. So you said that a lot of times you wouldn't have been able to tell this from ARCOS.

I am going to assume, though, if we had been analyzing this data we would have found the 184,000 pills per month that McKesson was sending to Kermit if someone had looked at it. Wouldn't you think so?

Mr. PATTERSON. I do agree with that.

Ms. DEGETTE. Yes. And wouldn't you agree that in Kermit—I think you said yes when the chairman said this—it was 2.2 million pills in a year in Kermit.

All you'd have to do is look at that raw data and see that, wouldn't you?

Mr. PATTERSON. That's correct.

Ms. DEGETTE. And so really the fact—well, let me—let me ask you another question. The Controlled Substances Act and the applicable regulations require the distributors to know their customer.

So distributors are supposed to report orders of unusual size, orders deviating substantially from a normal pattern, and orders of unusual frequency to the DEA.

Isn't that correct?

Mr. PATTERSON. It is, ma'am.

Ms. DEGETTE. So it's not just the DEA that has a burden to analyze the ARCOS data and to identify problems. But even before that, the distributors have a burden, right?

Mr. PATTERSON. The key burden is actually on the distributor.

Ms. DEGETTE. Right. Exactly. So do you think that if you were McKesson Corporation and you were looking at all these prescriptions in Kermit, would you think they knew those customers?

Mr. PATTERSON. Well, one, the obligation was there to know their customers.

Ms. DEGETTE. Right. Do you think that you possibly could know the customers when you're sending that many prescriptions in there?

Mr. PATTERSON. I think McKesson's answer would be that they did their part on this.

Ms. DEGETTE. Well, what's your answer?

Mr. PATTERSON. Obviously, I think they should have done more.

Ms. DEGETTE. Well, I would think so. Do you think that orders of this magnitude—2.2 million doses of hydrocodone to one Sav-Rite pharmacy—do you think that that's an order of an unusual size?

Mr. PATTERSON. I do, ma'am.

Ms. DEGETTE. And do you think that it deviates from a normal pattern?

Mr. PATTERSON. I do.

Ms. DEGETTE. OK. Let me ask you another question.

Now, looking back on this case, do you think that the distributors in all of these situations that the Chairman and I have been talking about—do you think that they failed to adequately exercise good due diligence over what they were doing?

Mr. PATTERSON. Certainly, on the appearance of it. I can't tell you what their due diligence was. But——

Ms. DEGETTE. Oh, we are going to ask them that. Don't worry.

You're not here to represent them.

Now, in December, the Washington Post and "60 Minutes" reported that McKesson distributed large volumes of opioids from its Aurora, Colorado distribution facility in 2012. One pharmacy that received these shipments reportedly sold as many as 2,000 opioids per day. Have you retroactively applied ARCOS data to the Colorado situation to see if there were distribution patterns similar to what we saw in Kermit, West Virginia?

Mr. PATTERSON. I believe that's the case, ma'am, that ultimately the DEA litigated and received a settlement. I don't know if we went back currently and have looked at that same number.

Ms. DEGETTE. And what was the settlement? Mr. PATTERSON. It was $150 million.

Ms. DEGETTE. From McKesson to—— Mr. PATTERSON. The U.S. government.

Ms. DEGETTE. The U.S. government. As a result of McKesson's failure to adequately follow the law on distributing those opioids. Is that right?

Mr. PATTERSON. That's correct.

Ms. DEGETTE. And so what do you think Congress can do so that we don't have a total slip-up like we did in all of these cases in West Virginia and around the country, really?

Mr. PATTERSON. Well, look, the fundamental change that we have already made is our recognition of how we can use the various data sets and paying attention to what we are doing.

The outreach to industry—and I think this is a topic that I assume will come up at some point—we have to work with the industry and the industry, obviously, has their responsibility.

But we have 1,500 people to monitor 1.73 million registrants.

Ms. DEGETTE. So, really, you think the initial burden to assess this is on the industry. But then the DEA has an important enforcement?

Mr. PATTERSON. Oversight.

Ms. DEGETTE. Yes, thank you.

Thank you, Mr. Chairman.

Mr. HARPER. Gentlewoman yields back.

The chair will now recognize the chairman of the full committee, Mr. Walden, for 5 minutes for questions.

Mr. WALDEN. Thank you, Mr. Chairman.

Mr. Patterson, we need to find out whether DEA is really addressing the lessons you say DEA has learned.

Case in point is the one I raised, the questionable enforcement approach regarding the two Sav-Rite pharmacies in Kermit, West Virginia that I mentioned in my opening statement.

Sav-Rite No. 2 was shut down in April of 2009, correct?

Mr. PATTERSON. I don't know the specific dates. I know there were two pharmacies. One was shut down and one wanted criminal——

Mr. WALDEN. Yes, our data show April of 2009 Sav-Rite 2 was shut down. Sav-Rite 1 was not shut down until over 2 years later when the owner of the pharmacy entered a guilty plea to charges that he illegally issued prescriptions, correct?

Mr. PATTERSON. That's correct.

Mr. WALDEN. And in April 1st of 2009, an article in the local Herald Dispatch reported that the two Sav-Rite pharmacies and a local pain clinic were under federal investigation for operating a drug operation. The article reported an affidavit from Federal investigators who stated there were two overdose deaths linked to this network.

So my question is why did DEA shut down Sav-Rite No. 2 but not Sav-Rite No. 1 in April of 2009 if both pharmacies were part of a network linked to deaths?

Mr. PATTERSON. Sir, I would have to get back to you on that one particular issue and I will you the reason why. It's my understanding it was part of the criminal process in that case and I don't know the answer for why that was. But I would be happy to get that back to you.

Mr. WALDEN. Thank you.

So why would the DEA even consider such an arrangement when it knew the owner operated the pharmacies 2 miles apart, one of which the DEA claimed to be the prime reception location for the flood of pills—that's a direct quote—being sent to the area and linked to overdose deaths? Same owner, same operator, 2 miles apart?

Mr. PATTERSON. I agree with you, and it's something I will get back to you on.

Mr. WALDEN. During the time the DEA allowed Sav-Rite No. 1 to remain in operation, this pharmacy received somewhere between 1 and 2 million hydrocodone and oxycodone pills. Allowing Sav-Rite 1 to continue to dispense such a volume of opioids posed a continuing risk to public health and safety. Isn't that right?

Mr. PATTERSON. I would agree.

Mr. WALDEN. So, Mr. Patterson, what's the biggest priority? Protecting public safety or deferring to an ongoing criminal investigation?

Mr. PATTERSON. It should have been to protect public safety.

Mr. WALDEN. So in this case, the government originally entered a plea agreement with the pharmacy owner that didn't even call for any prison time. The lack of any prison time troubled the judge and eventually the defendant was sentenced to 6 months in prison.

What kinds of evidentiary challenges would have been involved in such a case and would putting an immediate suspension order on hold really help solve these challenges?

Mr. PATTERSON. So putting an immediate suspension order on hold, again, I don't know the particular facts of that criminal case and I would be happy to get back to you.

I will tell you that I have a very strong opinion and this has been relayed throughout our agency that whether it's an immediate suspension or whether a surrender for cause, that if we are having harm issues that that suspension needs to occur even in lieu of a criminal prosecution.

Mr. WALDEN. And have you gone back and looked? Are there any records in your possession that would speak to this issue of why that decision was made?

Mr. PATTERSON. I would be happy to go back and look, sir.

Mr. WALDEN. And will you provide those to us unredacted?

Mr. PATTERSON. I would be happy to take that back and take a look at it for you.

Mr. WALDEN. That wasn't the answer I was looking for.

Mr. PATTERSON. I don't want to commit to the department's files. But I would be happy to take that back and I will take your concern back about getting them unredacted.

Mr. WALDEN. Yes. We've had this discussion in private. We'll have it in public. We'll have it in private.

The long and short of it is we just want to find out what was going on, what was the thinking, why the change in operation. People died and things were not—we don't want to see your agency repeat that.

We are beholden to the constituents we represent and I think the public has a right to know, don't you?

Mr. PATTERSON. I fully understand your concern and I agree with you.

Mr. WALDEN. Would this happen again today?

Mr. PATTERSON. Certainly, I think with our mentality, the answer would be no. Like I said, what we wish to do, sir, is stop public harm. I've had this conversation with U.S. attorneys' population, states' attorneys' population.

I see in too many instances on ISOs, current ones that I sign off on, where there has been a delay that I don't find appropriate.

Mr. WALDEN. So how do you weigh when to proceed with an ISO versus a criminal case?

Mr. PATTERSON. I would take it, quite frankly, no different than what we would do in a criminal case in the field, and in this case, I find that we have the ability.

So we have certain protocols where we evaluate risk of ongoing criminal activity in traditional criminal cases. In this case, because the person has a registration, we can immediately stop that harm.

Mr. WALDEN. And what's immediate? Is that 90 days? Twenty-five days? Tomorrow?

Mr. PATTERSON. I think the frustration in this is it takes time to build even that ISO charge, which is the reason why, in a lot of cases, we've gone to surrenders for cause or a voluntary surrender in which we go in and try and remove that registration.

Mr. WALDEN. So how long are we talking about to build that case?

Mr. PATTERSON. I think probably, in an efficient manner, 45 to 90 days.

Mr. WALDEN. So during that period, they can continue to dispense these drugs?

Mr. PATTERSON. The same way an illicit person would be out on the street as we gather the evidence we needed to present the charge.

That's why, sir, I go back to my point on surrender for cause, or a voluntary surrender. If I can walk in and lay out to that person why they need to surrender that and I can do it in a day and that's the method that we have actually been using much more aggressively than the ISO process, then we are going to do that.

Mr. WALDEN. What's the average time to go to a voluntary surrender?

Mr. PATTERSON. It depends. With very aggressive people it happens relatively quickly. There's always a quick balance with a criminal case and then evidence that they need to look at for that.

And, like I said, again, our conversations with prosecutors in the field have been that decision has to get made quickly.

Mr. WALDEN. All right. I know my time has expired.

I would imagine Mr. Griffith is going to have a comment or two on this as well.

With that, Mr. Chairman, I yield back, and thank you again.

Mr. HARPER. Thank you, Mr. Chairman.

The chair now recognizes the ranking member of the full committee, Mr. Pallone, for 5 minutes.

Mr. PALLONE. Thank you, Mr. Chairman.

Mr. Patterson, I want to ask you about another pharmacy in West Virginia so I can better understand why DEA was not able to stop the distributors from oversupplying certain pharmacies.

This one is the Family Discount Pharmacy in Mount Gay-Sham-rock, West Virginia. Mount Gay-Shamrock has a population of just under 2,000. DEA's data shows that distributors shipped 16.5 million opioid pills to this pharmacy between 2006 and 2016, including 2 million pills in three consecutive years. By contrast, the Rite-Aid Pharmacy down the street received a total of about 2 million pills during this entire 11-year period.

So do you agree that over 16 million pills is an excessive amount of opioids for Family Discount Pharmacy to have received relative to the size of the town it served?

Mr. PATTERSON. Especially when you compare it to the other pharmacy. Correct.

Mr. PALLONE. I thank you.

One distributor has provided evidence suggesting that between May 2008 and May 2009 they sent DEA 105 suspicious order reports stating that this pharmacy regularly ordered high volumes of pills.

For example, this distributor apparently told DEA that Family Discount ordered 25 500-count hydrocodone bottles on June 16th, 2008, and that's 12,500 pills just in the one day. On October 10th, Family Discount ordered 32 500-count hydrocodone bottles, or 16,000 pills in a single day, again, for a town of only 2,000 people.

Now, merely reporting these suspicious orders does not absolve the distributor of its additional responsibilities. Is that correct?

Mr. PATTERSON. That's correct.

Mr. PALLONE. So distributors still have to actually refuse shipments to suspicious pharmacies?

Mr. PATTERSON. They can, yes.

Mr. PALLONE. Additionally, it appears that distributors continue to ship this pharmacy over a million opioid pills each year in the 5 years after these reports were made and even the distributor who told us they reported the pharmacy to DEA continued to supply them after submitting those reports.

So, Mr. Patterson, it would appear that, again, something broke down to allow so many opioids to be shipped to this pharmacy. Just tell us what happened here. Why are so many opioids sent to this pharmacy at the same time that DEA has received a number of suspicious order reports? What do you think happened?

Mr. PATTERSON. Sir, so, again, on any of these individualized cases I am going to have to go back and take a look at the specific instances of what happened.

I will give you, I think, the concern I have with the ARCOS— not just ARCOS data but the suspicious orders, which is that was a decentralized function. It would go out to our division—those reports.

We are now bringing those in as well to our headquarters for proper deconfliction and visibility of what we see. I will take on face value the facts that you just proffered to me and I would be happy to go back and take a look at the Family Discount scenario. As I sit here, I don't have the particulars on the case from that time.

Mr. PALLONE. Well, we appreciate your following up. That's obviously why we are asking the questions. I don't expect you to know everything right off the bat.

But let me just say this. Between 2006 and 2010, did the DEA have any data analysts assigned to scrutinize information from distributors about the amount of pills shipped to particular pharmacies? Did you have any kind of data analysts, in that respect?

Mr. PATTERSON. So my understanding of the people that were handling the ARCOS data it was a completely manual process, meaning everything was coming in on paper or tapes, which would have to be verified.

So you have this 1-month to 3-month delay to begin with. They would have to have errors in their report that would go back and forth. So what you found yourself with is a set of data that sometimes would take a year-plus to get correct, and then in that timeframe, sir, we are using it very much as a reactive tool. In other words, someone would come in and provide some piece of information on a pharmacy or a doctor or some other issue and then they would go and look at the ARCOS data. It was not done in a——

Mr. PALLONE. So does that mean then, if I understand you, that it would be too long a period of time before would they realize how excessive this was?

Mr. PATTERSON. Well, if it was still ongoing, obviously, it would be an ability to look at that current situation. In a lot of these cases you see where these problems occurred for either a year or two and then disappeared or they were ongoing. But——

Mr. PALLONE. And is that problem being corrected or what do you suggest we do?

Mr. PATTERSON. It has been corrected, sir. So, again, I think that for the Committee to understand is ARCOS is an extremely different tool in 2018 than it was even in 2010 or 2011.

Mr. PALLONE. So you feel that you already have the tools to correct it—you don't need anything else?

Mr. PATTERSON. I feel that tool, with other data, is an important way for us to look proactively at the very specific issues that we are talking about today.

Mr. PALLONE. All right. Thank you.

Mr. HARPER. The gentleman yields back.

The chair will now recognize the gentleman from Texas, Mr. Barton, for 5 minutes.

Mr. BARTON. Thank you, Mr. Chairman.

This is a difficult hearing because I think everybody has the same bottom line. But your agency doesn't appear to be willing to aggressively try to help us solve this or at least deal with this crisis.

According to the latest numbers that this committee staff has, 115 people a day are dying of opioid overdoses and two-thirds of those are legally prescribed drugs. So about 80 people a day are dying from taking legally-prescribed prescription drugs. Now, they may be getting that prescription in an illegal way—in other words, they don't really need it. You're the head of the agency that's supposed to do something about it.

Now, I don't know much about you but, apparently, your background has been on the illegal side of DEA. Is that correct?

Mr. PATTERSON. That is correct.

Mr. BARTON. OK. How long have you been in your current position?

Mr. PATTERSON. Since October of 2017.

Mr. BARTON. OK. And I doubt that you volunteered for the job.

We still don't have a Trump administration appointee who's been recommended to the Senate. So for the foreseeable future in terms of drug enforcement the buck stops with you, even though you're, as I understand it, a career civil servant. Is that correct?

Mr. PATTERSON. That's correct.

Mr. BARTON. OK. Are you familiar with the Washington Post articles that have been running the last 3 to 4 months? One of them talks about the tension between the field enforcement offices and the Washington administrative officials.

Mr. PATTERSON. I have.

Mr. BARTON. OK. Do you agree or disagree with the basic thrust of those articles—that the enforcement people were very enthusiastic and willing to really go after the distribution centers and the drug manufacturers and the pharmacies and the Washington staff, for lack of a better term, stonewalled them or toned them down?

Mr. PATTERSON. So I believe that's an overstatement. I think you have a number of issues that, quite frankly, play out in this space, some of which have to do with personalities. But I don't find that the folks in the field, for the most part, had this belief that they were shut down. I do think there were people that felt that way at headquarters but not necessarily in the field.

Mr. BARTON. Are you familiar with a gentleman named Clifford Lee Reeves, II?

Mr. PATTERSON. I am.

Mr. BARTON. You don't think he stonewalled them or toned them down?

Mr. PATTERSON. Sir, as I've talked about with everybody I've met on this situation, I will simply explain this. I could put three people in a room and talk about probable cause and they could all have different opinions on——

Mr. BARTON. Well, let me put it this way. You and your associates in Washington have stonewalled this committee for the last 6 or 7 months.

It took a threat of Chairman Walden to subpoena the attorney general of the United States to finally break loose some documents.

We didn't get those documents, I understand, until yesterday. Now, that's not the Washington Post, sir. That's your people in Washington interacting with Energy and Commerce Committee staff on a bipartisan basis. That's not hypothetical. That's real.

Now, we are as much a part of the problem as anybody because the Congress has not aggressively addressed it. But we are beginning to, and as long as you're the head of the DEA, I personally, as Vice Chairman of this committee, expect you to work with us and to tell your people to work with the committee staff. Can you do that?

Mr. PATTERSON. Sir, I took over this job in October. I met with——

Mr. BARTON. OK. I want to know will you do what I just asked you to do? Yes or no. Will you tell your people to work with committee staff to help address this problem?

Mr. PATTERSON. Of course, and I have since November and we've been turning documents over since that time.

Mr. BARTON. Well, you didn't turn them over until yesterday, sir, and some of the documents you turned over were so redacted that it just looked like black marks on the pages.

Mr. PATTERSON. Sir, we've been turning documents over since November to the tune of more than 10,000 pages of documents that have come over here in the last month.

Mr. BARTON. Yes, and how many of those pages do you think are useable?

Mr. PATTERSON. Well, we sat down yesterday with staff to go—— Mr. BARTON. Because this hearing was today.

Mr. PATTERSON [continuing]. The concerns. Sir, I would respectfully disagree with that.

Mr. BARTON. Well, at least you're respectfully disagreeing and I appreciate that.

Mr. PATTERSON. I am fully committed, sir, to working with this committee and being as transparent as I can be.

Mr. BARTON. Well, you just remember, 80 people a day are dying because of legal prescription drugs that are probably being illegally prescribed. Remember that.

I yield back.

Mr. HARPER. Gentleman yields back.

The chair will now recognize the gentlewoman from Florida, Ms. Castor, for 5 minutes.

Ms. CASTOR. Thank you, Chairman Harper.

Administrator Patterson, I am sure you know about the multi-district opioid litigation in the Northern District of Ohio, which consolidates over 400 lawsuits brought by cities and counties and other states' communities against the drug distributors, manufacturers, and pharmacy chains. The most important source of information in that major lawsuit is going to be most likely the ARCOS data, and I understand DEA initially resisted providing ARCOS data to the federal judge.

A DEA official testified in response to my question in the Health Subcommittee hearing last month that the resistance was based upon a need to protect proprietary information. But now the court in this case has recently entered a protective order describing how the parties should treat the confidential ARCOS data when DEA disclosed it.

It's apparent to me that the ARCOS data will be pivotal in appropriately resolving the case and assigning accountability. Do I understand now that DEA has agreed to provide 9 years of data on opioid sales including the identifies of manufacturers and distributors that sold 95 percent of opioids in every State from 2006 to 2014?

Mr. PATTERSON. That is correct, under the protective order.

Ms. CASTOR. Under the protective order. So this will not be the last major challenge to manufacturers and distributors and others that are responsible. Will DEA likely cooperate in those cases too?

Have you set up a standard—is this a decision, going forward, that other judges and litigants can count on?

Mr. PATTERSON. I would believe it's under the same circumstances and conditions that we would comply the same way with anyone else that came in under those same terms.

Ms. CASTOR. So when will that data be provided to the Federal court in the northern Ohio case?

Mr. PATTERSON. I can get back to you on the date. I think it's very short term.

Ms. CASTOR. OK. The Committee's analysis of ARCOS data has been very concerning. The trends in West Virginia—we've just really skimmed the surface, I think.

My colleagues have outlined some of these. I am concerned that there are other regions all across the country where distributors may have supplied pharmacies with excessive quantities of opioid pills and that that information may be overlooked.

How is DEA currently using the older ARCOS data, say, from 2006 to the present to go back and look at past crimes, and if you could explain what you're doing now.

Mr. PATTERSON. No, I appreciate the question and I think it's an important issue.

So the 400 packages that we just put out are current-day packages that we want to investigate—in other words, where harm is continuing. I shouldn't say where harm is definitely continuing but where those outliers are that we want to go back and take a look at, why is that occurring, right?

Some of these actually end up being reasonable issues. There's an oncology department there. There's some reason why there's a higher level of that medication going to that area.

I think the key is is that once we get a handle on current issues that we are dealing with we want to roll backwards and look at 2012, 2013, 2014, and 2015 where we still have the ability to take a look at that data and make it make sense.

I can tell you that there's a number of cases ongoing in DEA without going into detail on them, looking at just that issue right now with manufacturers and——

Ms. CASTOR. And what is the statute of limitations? If you go back and the Committee has seen some of this in graphical forms where 2006 it ramped up and then because now the spotlight is being shined on it that the excessive distribution has scaled down.

Do you have the ability to go back and hold them accountable for that peak dangerous distribution of opioids?

Mr. PATTERSON. So on the criminal side, I believe it would be 5 years. On civil, I would have to find out. I am not sure how far back you can go civilly.

Ms. CASTOR. So you are——

Mr. PATTERSON. As long as it is an ongoing issue, then you fall into that timeframe.

Ms. CASTOR. And there was a lot of criticism by the Pulitzer Prize-winning Charleston Gazette Mail that the state didn't take advantage of data at their fingertips. How are you cooperating with states in providing that data so they can hold folks accountable?

Mr. PATTERSON. So this gets back to the issue, I think, with PMP which—and this is why these two data sets are so critical with each other.

We see the distribution to the pharmacy. PMP data in the states will then show you the distribution out of the pharmacy, right. So that whole connection, that's where those other outliers become very critical for us to take a look at.

Some states, and this is the issue that we have addressed throughout the members that we've met through and the states that we've talked to, some states share this data. Some states require a subpoena, which is also fine. Some states don't share. This is a problem that we have and, frankly, I think an issue that I would hope that someone looks at on a legislative fix, at a minimum to make the states cooperate with each other because you have bordering states, in some cases, that are still not participating and cooperating with each other, which is exactly how a lot of this diversion happens.

Ms. CASTOR. Thank you very much. I yield back.

Mr. HARPER. Gentlewoman yields back.

Before we proceed, I want to clarify for the record that the DEA has been producing documents and the vast majority of the roughly 9,700 pages we have received have come in during the last month.

Those documents had substantial redactions. Staff identified key documents for you and yesterday the DEA brought up some of those for us to view in camera. And I will note that those documents still contain some redactions.

So there's still much work to be done. I wanted to clarify that for the record, that the bulk of these came in after Chairman Walden's press conference and we'll continue to work with you in this effort.

Mr. PATTERSON. Thank you, sir.

Mr. HARPER. Now the chair will recognize the Vice Chairman of the Subcommittee, the gentleman from Virginia, Mr. Griffith, for 5 minutes.

Mr. GRIFFITH. Thank you, Mr. Chairman.

Mr. Patterson, I am going to need your assistance on some of this because what I am going to do is ask a series of questions which require a yes or no answer.

First, if you would take a look at the email before you dated 5/6/2011. I show it to you here, and I would ask unanimous consent to put that into the record.

Mr. HARPER. Without objection.

[The information appears at the conclusion of the hearing.]

Mr. GRIFFITH. And apparently, secret DEA official wrote, because his name is blacked out, our first and most prominent social responsibility as government officials in the DEA is to protect the public. I think that trumps all other activities. I think that's what Congress/citizens would expect us to do. You agree with that statement, don't you? Yes or no.

Mr. PATTERSON. Yes.

Mr. GRIFFITH. One of the key tools for DEA to fulfill this mission is through an immediate suspension order—I will henceforth refer to those as ISOs. This is an administrative tool used as an emergency intervention to stop a rogue doctor or pharmacist from continuing to prescribe or dispense opioids that would possibly kill drug seekers and/or put the public at risk.

You agree with that as well, don't you?

Mr. PATTERSON. I do.

Mr. GRIFFITH. An essential element for requesting the ISO is concern about imminent danger to public health or safety. A pharmacy in Oviedo, Florida received an increase of oxycodone of almost 2,500 percent compared to 1 year earlier. Local police arrested customers in the parking lot of this pharmacy for selling/trading pills.

Police officers were concerned customers were getting high in the parking lot and getting on the roads, endangering the public. The continued dispensing of opioids by this pharmacy with its parking lot of drug pushers and drug users who get high and then drive on the public roads would pose an imminent danger to the public, wouldn't you agree? Yes or no.

Mr. PATTERSON. Yes.

Mr. GRIFFITH. You would also agree, I assume, that speed is crucial in issuing imminent suspension orders to protect the public?

Yes or no.

Mr. PATTERSON. I would.

Mr. GRIFFITH. I will just tell you, 45 to 90 days that you told the Chairman of the Full Committee is not acceptable. Please refer to another email before you and I ask unanimous consent to put that in the record and this one is dated August 22nd—or 20th—there's two different dates on it.

Mr. HARPER. Without objection.

Mr. GRIFFITH. 2013.

All right. The email chain in August 2013 shows that DEA lawyers were requiring the DEA field to submit an expert witness report to describe the expert's assessment of data and documents prior to submitting either or both request for an immediate suspension order and orders to show cause.

Are you aware of this new requirement that was imposed in 2013? Yes or no.

Mr. PATTERSON. No.

Mr. GRIFFITH. And I expected that.

Regarding medical experts being required, DEA counsel Lee Reeves wrote, "To be clear, this is not a chief counsel office requirement policy. This is the requirement of the administrator and the courts."

Are you aware that the medical experts are required by the DEA administrator? Yes or no.

Mr. PATTERSON. No.

Mr. GRIFFITH. Mr. Reeves also wrote that as a general matter, these cases without expert testimony are the exception rather than the rule.

So, generally, DEA is requiring medical expert testimony before the field can submit an ISO to the chief counsel's office for review. Is this still the policy of the DEA? Yes or no.

Mr. PATTERSON. It is not a policy, no.

Mr. GRIFFITH. I appreciate that. Thank you.

Mr. Reeves cites the DEA administrator's decision in the Ruben case for requiring medical experts. However, the Ruben case is a show cause case, not an ISO.

This decision basically says that if a state doesn't provide guidance on certain medical standards, the DEA must use an expert to explain why the doctor's activities fell below the standard of care.

However, you would not need a medical expert if the state had a statute of regulations on prescribing standards. Yes or no, or I don't know?

Mr. PATTERSON. I don't know that.

Mr. GRIFFITH. All right. Fair enough.

Let's discuss this policy of requiring experts, and I know that you're trying to shift from some of that but let's discuss it.

It would take some time for the DEA field to find a medical expert, wouldn't you agree?

Mr. PATTERSON. I would.

Mr. GRIFFITH. And to obtain the services of a medical expert the DEA would have to issue a sole source contract and the agency and the expert would have to figure out and reach an agreement on fee and deliverables. Isn't that true?

Mr. PATTERSON. I don't necessarily know about the contract but it would require some type of compensation.

Mr. GRIFFITH. And after all of that, the medical expert would need to review prescription monitoring program, data patient files, and other information. It's going to take some time for the medical expert to review and render an opinion, isn't it?

Mr. PATTERSON. It would.

Mr. GRIFFITH. Yes. After the medical expert completes the review then the chief counsel's office would need additional time to review the field submission of the request for an immediate suspension order. Isn't that true?

Mr. PATTERSON. Yes.

Mr. GRIFFITH. This scenario assumes no delays along the way, and realistically this process, in many ISO cases, will take weeks, won't it?

Mr. PATTERSON. I would believe so.

Mr. GRIFFITH. And that's where you get your 45 to 90 days. If the DEA registrant sought a restraining order against the ISO, the delay in timing getting the medical expert and going through all the steps we just went through would in fact weaken the DEA's case in court for immediacy, wouldn't it?

Mr. PATTERSON. I would believe so.

Mr. GRIFFITH. Yes, it would.

And so in fact, insisting on an expert medical testimony for the ISO—I get the trial in cheap, the merits. But to protect the public, insistent on a medical expert in advance is endangering the public and endangering your case on the ISO because it takes away the immediacy factor. Wouldn't you agree?

Mr. PATTERSON. Yes, and I——

Mr. GRIFFITH. OK. I got to keep moving because I am already out of time.

All right. Maybe I can get some more opportunity later. Thank you, Mr. Chairman. I yield back.

Mr. HARPER. Gentleman yields back. The chair will now recognize the gentleman from California, Mr. Ruiz, for 5 minutes.

Mr. RUIZ. Mr. Patterson, thank you for coming. I am a board-certified emergency physician and I can't tell you how personally I take it whenever a patient comes in overdosed, not breathing, and blue.

It's not uncommon to see a blue-colored patient being strolled in in an emergency situation, having been dumped from a car from friends who found this person overdosed, not breathing. And as emergency physicians we cut to the chase and we start resuscitating the patient. We know exactly what to do no matter if it's from overdose of opiates or any other reason why a patient is comatose. Whether we start the ABCs—airway breathing circulations— and we bring them back, as much as possible.

So I am going to cut to the chase here and ask you to be very frank and direct.

You screwed up. The DEA knew that there was a lot of opioids being shipped, an extraordinary amount and not outliers, and when you said earlier that there's two things that you were going to do from now on it's very concerning that those two things were to recognize how to use the data, and two, pay more attention to what you're doing. That leads me to believe that you were collecting data that you did not know how to use, and two, you weren't paying attention to your job within the DEA.

So I am going to be very straightforward. What are you doing different now that you're going to recognize how to use the data?

Mr. PATTERSON. Sir, I appreciate the concern and I think what I've tried to explain is the data—when we are talking about a lot of these cases that you have brought up we are talking about a time period in which this data was——

Mr. RUIZ. OK. Be specific on what are the changes you're going to do now. Not giving me the reasons why or an excuse. Tell me what are you going to do now that's different.

Mr. PATTERSON. So let me give you a handful of the differences.

Mr. RUIZ. Yes.

Mr. PATTERSON. On the suspicious orders, we have regulations that are in the final stretch to deal with that. We have a website that's now been built for the distributors to understand their customers better where they can go in and see partial information on other people that distributed to that particular pharmacy for the past 6 months.

We are working with all of our other partners both in the Health and Human Services side and the states to try and combine all this data, to look at it in a very proactive manner.

Mr. RUIZ. What are your flags? What numerical equations have you used to flag something for the pharmacies and for the distributors?

Mr. PATTERSON. I would have to get you what the specific flags are for them. I mean, they——

Mr. RUIZ. Are they new flags or are they old flags, like——

Mr. PATTERSON. No, they're our baselines for any given area as to traditional, what the prescribing rates have been in those particular areas and anything that's an anomaly to that is a flag.

All right. So when we've talked about these issues before we have a——

Mr. RUIZ. And who's looking at those flags? Who's the one in your department who's actually putting their eyes on this computer and reporting these?

Mr. PATTERSON. A unit within the diversion.

Mr. RUIZ. OK. And how many people are in that unit?

Mr. PATTERSON. I would have to get that number for you.

Mr. RUIZ. OK, because you have——

Mr. PATTERSON. Again, most of it's generated by computer.

Mr. RUIZ. OK.

Mr. PATTERSON. So it's not necessarily a manpower-intensive endeavor to do.

Mr. RUIZ. OK. And so when you said that now you're going to start paying attention to what you're doing, tell me about that. What are the organizational changes that you have made to start paying attention to doing your job?

Mr. PATTERSON. I don't think I said now that we are doing it. I think we've been doing it for a period of time.

Mr. RUIZ. Well, you said moving forward that now, what you have to do is to pay attention to what you're doing. That means to imply that there was some kind of slip-up before.

So what exactly are you doing? What are the changes? I want to practice my ABCs for a patient who's coming in. I want to know what you're doing exactly that you're going to make sure that this doesn't happen again.

Mr. PATTERSON. Again, that's some of the issues I just talked to you about and how we use data, or not community outreach. Well, community outreach with the prescribing——

Mr. RUIZ. Have you changed any organizational structure? Is there any accountability metrics that you have included in your department? Have you increased the staffing in certain areas?

What are you doing to pay better attention to your job?

Mr. PATTERSON. Over the past few years, we've increased staffing and diversion. We have a new head of diversion control coming in.

He and I have sat down and spent time on this particular issue as to other proactive ways we can look at it. I met with the U.S. attorney and states' attorneys to talk about these issues of working criminal cases or civil cases and how they impact our administrative issues for the criminal prosecutions.

They want to continue to gather evidence. If we have some harm that's being done and we can stop it, then we have to start to balance this out in a better and more proactive way. So there are dozens of things we are doing differently. This is not just a one issue fix.

Mr. RUIZ. Well, those are the things that I am particularly concerned and want to know more about because that's what's going to create the change is by making changes in your department in order to use your data more efficiently and also to start paying attention whether it's through computers or personnel, because a computer can flag all it wants to flag but if a human is not taking those warnings and having action based on what your computer is flagging then it's just going to be a flashing flagging computer.

Mr. PATTERSON. Understood.

Mr. HARPER. Gentleman yields back.

The chair will now recognize the gentleman from Texas, Dr. Burgess, for 5 minutes.

Mr. BURGESS. Thank you, Mr. Chairman.

And Mr. Patterson, I want to acknowledge that I asked for you to come to my office and you complied with that, and for that I am deeply appreciative with the information that you shared with me.

Obviously, this is something about which many of us feel very, very strongly. Clearly, we want to get some answers.

The subcommittee has interest in knowing about differences between voluntary suspension orders and immediate suspension orders. I will stipulate that both exist and that we could argue which is a more propitious path to follow. Are there other tools you have in your tool box in addition to immediate suspension order and the voluntary suspension order?

Mr. PATTERSON. Sure. There's a whole range. There's letters of admonition, orders to show cause. There's a host of administrative tools that we have that we can use in this space, and depending on—and to go back to an issue that Mr. Griffith had brought up, depending on, quite frankly, whether it's a doctor or a pharmacy may be a very different reaction than what we would do or evidence we would gather against maybe a distributor.

Mr. BURGESS. Let me ask you a question, because I can't take credit for it—my staff did this—but went to your Diversion Control Division and pulled down a document that's called "Cases Against Doctors" and this is produced by the U.S. Department of Justice and Drug Enforcement Administration.

I presume it's your product. It's about a hundred pages long. It goes back, basically, to 2002 through October 12th of 2017. It's a hundred pages or about three cases per page, so that's 300 cases against doctors in the last 15 years. Does that sound about right?

Mr. PATTERSON. Sir, I don't know. That's a complete list of all doctors that cases have been worked or is it a guide to help people and where people have gotten into trouble?

Mr. BURGESS. Well, I will tell you what concerns me as I look through this is that most of the dates are pre-2009. So I guess my question would be where is the data from 2010 onward and perhaps that's something we can follow up with together because I do share the provider's perspective on this. We want to be able to provide pain relief when it's required of us and it's appropriate.

At the same time, we obviously do not want to be jeopardizing public safety and the integrity of society the way the opiate crisis is endangering us currently. But I think this could be very important information. You referenced, at the start of your testimony, that over-prescribing is perhaps one of the number-one problems.

Well, if that's the case, then it's this sort of information that is, I think, going to be very helpful to us as policy makers how do we develop the correct policy.

Let me just ask you, did I understand this figure correctly? You referenced $309 million in fines at the DEA level. Is that correct?

Mr. PATTERSON. In civil fines, $390 million or $309 million. Mr. BURGESS. So OK, that ballpark—$300 to $400 million.

We'd appropriated a billion dollars in cures for treatment of this problem. We are looking at another $6 billion in the appropriations bills that are coming through right now. So you see the disparity there.

Someone, whether it be suppliers, prescribers is causing a problem to exist. You're finding them but it's only minuscule compared with the amount that it's actually costing society in trying to save people, salvage people, get people back to productivity.

That doesn't even address the fact that, again, people are taken out of being productive citizens when they enter into this type of behavior. Is that correct?

Mr. PATTERSON. I agree, sir. And may I just add? So these fines come as, again, and some of the members have already mentioned this balance, right, of ensuring pain medicines for people.

So I think the fines generally come with, quite frankly, the heavier piece of that is the memoranda of understanding or memoranda of agreement of how they'll behave, moving forward.

Mr. BURGESS. Correct. I get that.

Let me just ask you this, because I think it was Mr. Barton referenced 80 people a day who were dying—115 was the total number but 80 per day are dying because of what you described as over-prescribing. And then we've got these lists that in my observation are not up to date. Do we know how many people were dying a day from over-prescribing in 2007, 2008, 2009 in that timeframe?

Do you have a figure?

Mr. PATTERSON. I don't have it here. I would be happy to get that stat for you. It still was an alarming number, even back in that time period, sir.

Mr. BURGESS. And then that begs the question. And again, I appreciate the effort that you're putting into it now. But it's been right there in front of us for well over a decade, decade and a half and, clearly, it requires all hands on deck in our approach. And, again, I appreciate your being very forthcoming with my office and I appreciate that.

Mr. Chairman, I will yield back.

Mr. HARPER. Gentleman yields back.

The chair will now recognize the gentlewoman from New York, Ms. Clarke, for 5 minutes.

Ms. CLARKE. I thank you, Mr. Chairman, and I thank our ranking member.

Mr. Patterson, it's clear in many cases certain drug distributors supply very large volumes of opioids to some pharmacies in West Virginia. But we've also seen from DEA's data that many of these pharmacies were buying from multiple distributors. For example, in 2009, the West Virginia pharmacy, Hurley Drug, received over 2 million opioid pills from six different distributors, including over 300,000 from one distributor, over 600,000 from a second distributor, and over 900,000 from a third.

So it's bad enough if one distributor over-supplies a pharmacy.

But when you look at the total shipments that Hurley Drug received from all distributors, it was about 2 million pills, which is over seven times what a similar pharmacy will be expected to receive, according to DEA's own data.

So DEA is the only entity that can see the volumes that multiple distributors are simultaneously sending to a single pharmacy. Is that correct?

Mr. PATTERSON. From the distributor level, yes, ma'am.

Ms. CLARKE. So, Mr. Patterson, was DEA performing analytics a decade ago to identify these kinds of patterns at individual pharmacies?

Mr. PATTERSON. Again, ma'am, in a reactive manner at that time.

Ms. CLARKE. OK. So I would like to look at DEA's data on another pharmacy in West Virginia—Sav-Rite Pharmacy in the small town of Kermit received hydrocodone from five different distributors in 2008. A few distributors provided relatively normal amounts that don't seem to raise alarms. However, one distributor shipped 1.2 million pills and another shipped nearly 2 million. All told this pharmacy got nearly 4 million pills that year, which is nearly 15 times what a similar pharmacy would be expected to receive, according to DEA's data.

Mr. Patterson, if you rely on distributors to report suspicious orders from pharmacies, how do you flag pharmacies trying to stay under the radar by buying from multiple distributors?

Mr. PATTERSON. So, ma'am, this is where, again, the data that we use today—not the data, I shouldn't say the data—but how we use the data is very different today, and this is also where the critical nature comes into us working with the states.

Those same pharmacies, that PMP data which show that amount of distribution from those pharmacies, so we have that distributor in and then the pharmacy out, depending on the PMP program.

So the key is for us to work together on that and, again, I can say repeatedly in 2008, 2009, and 2010 we did not use this data in the way that we are now using it and I think that's the key.

I get that we have this issue from a decade ago, that we have to resolve in terms of how we used it. And, again, where we fell short in that we'll take responsibility for it. I think the system is much more robust and used in a much different way in——

Ms. CLARKE. So can you give us a little bit more insight into how you're proactively analyzing the data to ensure that pharmacies are not being over supplied by multiple distributors? That has not come across clearly to us this morning. How are you actually doing that disruption?

Mr. PATTERSON. Again, so as we talked about in the opening, we are proactively looking at data not just across DEA and that ARCOS database that we've talked about but HHS, PMP programs where we are sharing that information and looking to proactively target outliers.

Ms. CLARKE. So what happens once you're flagged in this regard?

Mr. PATTERSON. So we——

Ms. CLARKE. What exactly happens?

Mr. PATTERSON. We send that information out to the field for investigators—those TDS groups or diversion groups, depending on how they're being used to go out and work those cases to find out is it a legitimate amount of prescriptions that are going there or is there illegitimate diversion occurring in those areas.

Ms. CLARKE. And has that worked thus far? Because, you said this was over a decade ago. I am assuming that you have already begun sort of this new protocol. What are your findings?

Mr. PATTERSON. Yes, ma'am. So the interesting thing is of those 400 packages that went out, a good majority of what we saw in that data and the outliers and what they identified were ongoing cases that we already had, which shows that that data set works to develop and target those areas where we have problems.

To the extent that we didn't have cases on those other ones and they were warranted, we've opened cases on those facilities or doctors or distributors to take a look at that behavior.

Ms. CLARKE. Mr. Patterson, I just want to share with you that this is an ongoing crisis. Once we are able to disrupt this supply chain, we know that these supply chains become supplanted by more nefarious actors.

And so, I really want to impress upon you and your agency to be as forward leaning in this regard as possible because once those pills are cut off, we know that that's when the illicit trade picks up in velocity.

Mr. PATTERSON. Yes, ma'am. And as we've talked about, again, in the opening, I think that shift has already occurred.

Ms. CLARKE. Thank you. I yield back, Mr. Chairman.

Mr. HARPER. Gentlewoman yields back. The chair will now recognize the gentleman from New York, Mr. Collins, for 5 minutes.

Mr. COLLINS. Thank you, Mr. Chairman, and thank you, Mr. Patterson for being here.

I think you can tell and your get out of jail free card today, you have been in this particular job 5 months. I would hope 5 months from now you would not be giving many of the same answers.

Following up on what Mr. Ruiz said, I think we are just all frustrated. There seems to be the bureaucracy mindset in the DEA today, much like we've seen in the VA. And we are finally seeing heads rolling in the VA. Not as fast as we want. I am just curious, because there's no doubt there was an abject failure of the DEA, going back the last 10 years.

Have a lot of heads been chopped off? Have you got a new team in place?

Mr. PATTERSON. Sir, so as I said, we have a new head of Diversion Control. I think the last two people that have done that job have done and both successful in turning around that program.

Mr. COLLINS. Well, not to interrupt but to interrupt, I think the right people can turn this around in 48 hours. I am a turn around guy. That's what I've spent my whole life doing.

You bring a new team in and people get called in the office every day and they walk out saying, somebody just hit me up the side of the head with a baseball bat. I am either going to get my act together or I am going to get out of Dodge.

This isn't a time to be polite or nice or let's do better tomorrow.

No, this is an abject failure, and if I am sitting in that seat and McKesson processed 1.6 million orders and only 16 were deemed suspicious, that's absurd. I don't know what kind of computers you have but that's absurd. It means no one was watching.

And you can say well, that was being done in the district level. But it's indefensible. When we look in West Virginia and two suspicious orders so, let's maybe jump ahead, and in 2008, Cardinal Health was fined $34 million for not reporting suspicious orders.

All right. So let's go forward 8 years later. They're still not doing it. Two guesses. First—second one doesn't count. How much do you think you fined them 8 years later for the same problem? Thirty-four million dollars, the same amount. In most places the second offense—all right, first offense $34 million, eight years later the same problem, the same fine? Should have been tenfold. Should have been $340 million dollars.

What did your agency do? And this was a year and a half ago. You guys don't get it and if you're not—this committee agrees on a lot. I don't think we've ever agreed across the board on an issue as much as we are agreeing your agency needs to be turned upside down, not just a little shakeup here and there but turned upside down. It starts with you. If you can't do it, you ought to get out.

So when I look at some of the things—so we have distributors. We have pharmacies. We have doctors. Well, I happen to live next door—literally, next door to one of the doctors, Dr. Gosy, in Clarence, New York, and I saw his six sports cars parked out there with all new—his name in the community was Dr. Pain. And this wasn't something new.

When I look back, it took the DEA a good 7 years to come after my next door neighbor. By the way, he doesn't live there anymore. But he had set up a script line in 2012 where people could call in and fill scripts with PAs under basically no supervision.

So at what point—how could you allow a single physician—my next door neighbor, literally, in Clarence, New York—to write more prescriptions for opioids, millions of them, than any other doctor or in fact any other hospital in the State of New York?

There's 20 million people in New York. My particular town of Clarence has about 50,000 people, and one doctor in the town of Clarence was writing more prescriptions than any doctor in the State of 20 million people or any hospital including New York City.

Took you guys 5 years to figure out there might be something suspicious? Would you agree that's unacceptable?

Mr. PATTERSON. Sir, so I wouldn't have any data on a particular prescriber. DEA doesn't hold that set of data.

Mr. COLLINS. Well, he's now been indicted. They've seized his cars. They've seized his bank accounts.

Mr. PATTERSON. So at some point, whether that was a DEA case or a state local case, I don't know what it was that investigated him and——

Mr. COLLINS. It was a federal case.

Mr. PATTERSON. OK. So at some point we learned of that and then there was——

Mr. COLLINS. Yes, but what's going on with your computer systems and other things? It takes you 4 or 5 years. I know how computers work, pretty much. I don't know how old yours are. Maybe they're XT tabletops. I am not sure.

But this kind of data should be instantaneously available.

Mr. PATTERSON. And, sir, I go back to the states control prescription monitoring program, not DEA. We control into a pharmacy. The doctor——

Mr. COLLINS. Well, maybe you should be kicking some butt going down the chain. I mean, if I was sitting in your job and you're on the hot seat right now, and you're telling me now, I mean, placing the blame on the states, that doesn't cut it in our world here. We are not looking to place blame. We are looking for solutions.

My time has expired. We look forward to you coming back in another 4 or 5 months and having a different set of answers.

Thank you, sir.

Mr. HARPER. Gentleman yields back.

The chair will now recognize the gentleman from New York, Mr. Tonko, for 5 minutes.

Mr. TONKO. Thank you, Mr. Chair.

I want to find out if DEA uses data gathered through its ARCOS system to game disability into how many opioid pill distributors send to a town or region as a whole, even if the distributions are spread out over multiple pharmacies.

Administrator Patterson, one town examined by the committee was Williamson, West Virginia, population 3,000. Our committee's investigation focused on two pharmacies in Williamson. The first is Tug Valley Pharmacy.

Mr. Chair, could I ask that we please show minority exhibit three on the screen?

OK. We have here the Tug Valley Pharmacy. According to DEA's ARCOS data, between 2006 and 2016, Tug Valley Pharmacy received over 10 million doses of opioids from 13 different distributors. This includes over 3 million pills just in 2009. So Administrator Patterson, this is an unbelievable quantity of opioids for a pharmacy this size in a town of 3,000. Does DEA believe the amount of opioids this pharmacy received was excessive?

Mr. PATTERSON. In 2009 I would say so, sir.

Mr. TONKO. And, again, Mr. Chair, if we could please put minority exhibit four up on the screen. This is the second pharmacy in Williamson—Hurley Drug—that we see on the screen here.

ARCOS data show that Hurley received over 10.5 million doses of opioids from 11 different distributors between 2006 and 2016.

This includes over 2 million doses in both 2008 and in 2009. Mr. Patterson, again, this strikes me as an excessive amount of opioids for a pharmacy in a town of 3,000 to receive.

Do you agree that this is unreasonable?

Mr. PATTERSON. I would agree.

Mr. TONKO. I've mentioned that both of these pharmacies are located in Williamson and, incidentally, both of them are still in operation today.

I want to show you where they are located. So if we could please post minority exhibit five on the screen, and combined distributor shipped over 20.8 million doses of opioids to these two pharmacies, which you can see on our screen, are located only blocks apart and they did that 20.8 million doses of opioids between 2006 and 2016.

Mr. Patterson, between 2006 and 2016, what kind of ARCOS data analyses did DEA do to alert it when distributors shipped an unwarranted amount of opioids into a town or region so that it could stop these excessive distributions?

Mr. PATTERSON. Again, sir, I would have to go back and look at that specific example and look at the data set in terms of where those periods of time were.

As I already testified previously, we use the data in a very different way today than we did then. But I would want to go back and specifically look at the time frame and what was going on and I can get back to you on that.

Mr. TONKO. If the data were used today, as you use it today would it have avoided something like this?

Mr. PATTERSON. I would hope so.

Mr. TONKO. Well, can we have a little more of an answer? I am hoping is good, but——

Mr. PATTERSON. I would like to—part of the important issue that we are talking about today is to go back and look at these specific examples.

Like I said, I have seen examples where on ARCOS data we actually can't see some of these anomalies. So I think, in taking these examples back and looking at them and we are using a time frame of 2006 to 2016, I can't tell you for the last couple of years what that ARCOS data has been, as I sit here.

Traditionally, what we've seen is very high levels of distribution into those places between 2008 to 2010 or 2011 when we started to look at this data in different ways.

Still not nearly as proactively as we do today. But that's why I would like to take this example back and look and get back to you on essentially what's happened with that.

Mr. TONKO. Thank you.

I have been dealing with this issue a great deal in my district and when I hear of opioids being the gateway to the illness of addiction, it's very disturbing, and the heartache and the pain and, unfortunately, the death associated with that illness is a crisis and we need to do something very valuable here and I would implore that the folks at DEA be smarter in their approach.

And with that, I yield back, Mr. Chair.

Mr. HARPER. Gentleman yields back.

The chair now recognizes the gentleman from Pennsylvania, Mr. Costello, for 5 minutes.

Mr. COSTELLO. Thank you, Mr. Chairman.

Are you aware that the DEA's chief ALJ authored quarterly reports describing DEA's declining use of ISOs and noted in June 2014, "an alarming low rate of agency diversion enforcement activity" on a national level?

Mr. PATTERSON. I have read those, yes.

Mr. COSTELLO. For the last several years, the chief ALJ has reported declining number of ISOs to the DEA administrator on a quarterly basis. This issue had also been raised in the committee's investigation.

Why has the number of DEA ISOs declined significantly over the past few years?

Mr. PATTERSON. I think there's two things when you look at those statistics.

I think that, although warranted, the statistics were very high in 2010 and 2011 because of the issue that we were dealing with in Florida and how those ISOs were being used. I think during this latter part we have gotten to a point of in trying to expedite the surrender of registrations we have much more gone into a posture of trying to get voluntary or surrender for cause orders.

Mr. COSTELLO. Is there still a need today, as there was in 2011, for the DEA enforcement tool of ISOs?

Mr. PATTERSON. Yes.

Mr. COSTELLO. A 2013 report by the chief ALJ stated the DEA's chief counsel had "instituted a new vetting QA initiative" that could be slowing the progress of diversion cases.

What was this initiative?

Mr. PATTERSON. I don't know if it was initiative or if it was guidance. I think the——

Mr. COSTELLO. What was the guidance? Yes.

Mr. PATTERSON. I think the issue at play here was directed towards distributors, not necessarily directed at doctors and pharmacies.

Mr. COSTELLO. Have you provided that guidance in full to this committee?

Mr. PATTERSON. We have not.

Mr. COSTELLO. Will you?

Mr. PATTERSON. That's a conversation that we've had with Mr. Walden and we'll continue to work forward on that——

Mr. COSTELLO. When a state revokes the medical license of a doctor, that doctor is no longer eligible to have a DEA registration associated with that medical license, correct?

Mr. PATTERSON. That's correct.

Mr. COSTELLO. When the doctor no longer has state authority to prescribe does the DEA have to conduct any further investigation or can DEA execute revocation of DEA registration by just obtaining the certificate of the medical license revocation?

Mr. PATTERSON. We can do an order to show cause.

Mr. COSTELLO. No investigation is needed?

Mr. PATTERSON. That's correct, because they've lost state authority.

Mr. COSTELLO. After a state revocation of the doctor's medical license, how quickly is DEA notified about the revocation and how long does it take for DEA to revoke the doctor's DEA registration?

Mr. PATTERSON. That's where we need to be working with the state medical boards to learn of that information. Our field division offices are responsible for that.

Mr. COSTELLO. Are the vast majority of DEA enforcement actions in diversion litigation cases comprised of these no state authority cases that do not involve DEA investigation?

Mr. PATTERSON. In terms of the orders to show cause?

Mr. COSTELLO. That's correct.

Mr. PATTERSON. That's correct.

Mr. COSTELLO. Yes?

Mr. PATTERSON. Yes.

Mr. COSTELLO. Is it estimated to be about 80 percent of their actions?

Mr. PATTERSON. I would believe that's probably a fair number.

Mr. COSTELLO. Mr. Chair, I would like to yield the balance of my time to you, Mr. Griffith.

Mr. GRIFFITH. Thank you very much.

When I was asking you questions earlier, we talked about the ISOs and the apparent requirement—I know you didn't do it but the apparent requirement for a medical expert in advance of issuing an ISO and the fact that that would take a number of weeks and you said 45 to 90 days. I went through all the different steps that might actually lead to that.

So you agree that it's the DEA's mission to protect the public safety and we agree that there's a tremendous amount of delay and part of that delay in no small measure is the requirement that before you get that administrative tool of the ISO you have to get a medical expert.

So can you, as acting administrator, agree with me today that you would be willing to reexamine the medical expert requirement?

Mr. PATTERSON. Absolutely.

Mr. GRIFFITH. And I appreciate that.

Mr. PATTERSON. And again, we are using the word requirement.

I think these documents are in reference to distributors and not doctors and pharmacies. But I would be happy to go back and look into that further.

Mr. GRIFFITH. Yes, it was actually reference to doctors and pharmacies. But that's OK. As long as we are working it out, that's where we want to go. We want to make things better.

And one of the reasons that I get so passionate about this is you saw Mr. Tonko's minority slide of Hurley Drug earlier. Well, Hurley, Virginia, is 33 miles from Williamson, West Virginia, where that drug store is located. And anybody with any sense knows that a big bunch of those pills were coming into my district.

Likewise, I had some additional questions that dealt with the fact that we have problems with red flags being raised that apparently takes a while to be picked up on.

So we had a doctor in Giles County who was sending his patients over to West Virginia to get drugs. We have a situation in Martinsville where they have, according to the CDC, they prescribe more opioid pain killers than anywhere else in the U.S. per capita and where another doctor was prescribing opioids for patients in North Carolina.

So I look forward to working with you to solve these problems.

But these are real world problems, real world people, and real word deaths.

Mr. PATTERSON. I agree with you.

Mr. GRIFFITH. I yield back. I now recognize Congresswoman Walters for five minutes.

Mrs. WALTERS. Thank you, Mr. Chairman.

Mr. Patterson, it's my understanding that the DEA often uses tips and information it receives from state and local law enforcement to develop cases against entities or individuals suspected of engaging in or facilitating illicit drug diversion. Is that correct?

Mr. PATTERSON. Correct.

Mrs. WALTERS. According to the DEA, the Automated Reports and Consolidated Ordering System, or ARCOS, provides the agency with retail level data regarding controlled substance transactions.

Does this mean, for example, ARCOS can show many doses of hydrocodone or oxycodone an individual pharmacy received in a given year?

Mr. PATTERSON. Yes.

Mrs. WALTERS. In fact, as part of its investigation, the Committee has obtained and analyzed ARCOS data for parts of West Virginia to great effect. So we recognize how important a tool it can be.

In February of this year, DEA announced that it was adding a feature to ARCOS that will allow manufacturers and distributors to view the number of companies that have sold a particular controlled substance to a prospective customer in the preceding 6 months.

Mr. Paterson, does this policy enable companies to see the amount of controlled substances its current customers are receiving from other suppliers?

Mr. PATTERSON. Yes. Part of the suspicious orders is them knowing their customers to know when to file these concerns.

Mrs. WALTERS. Does the newly added features in ARCOS provide state and local law enforcement with greater access to the system's retail level data?

Mr. PATTERSON. I would have to find out if it provides at the state level. When we work investigations with the state level—the state and local level, obviously, we can share that data as part of an investigation.

This is also part of the issue that we are dealing with the states' attorneys general on as to how to share these data sets to be more proactive.

Mrs. WALTERS. OK. According to a letter the DEA sent to the committee in November of last year, DEA will share ARCOS data with law enforcement on a need to know basis and when they are operating in coordination with the DEA for investigative purposes.

So is it fair to say that the state and local law enforcement entities do not have access to DEA ARCOS data on a real-time basis?

Mr. PATTERSON. If we are working an investigation we'll share that data in real time with them.

Mrs. WALTERS. OK. Is DEA developing any proposals that will enhance state and local law enforcement's ability to access and utilize ARCOS data?

Mr. PATTERSON. Again, we are working jointly with them and this also goes back to the effort with our states attorneys general.

Mrs. WALTERS. OK. In order to effectively combat the opioid epidemic we need an all hands on deck approach. The DEA has data that could assist state and local law enforcement to identify potential sources of illicit drugs in their communities and I think the agency should be exploring every avenue to provide this data to law enforcement as quickly as possible.

It seems to me that providing state and local police with access to ARCOS data would be beneficial to the DEA as well, effectively providing the agency with additional eyes and ears on the ground, likely resulting in additional leads being produced to the agency.

Mr. Patterson, will you commit to examine ways to improve state and local law enforcement's access to ARCOS data so that bad actors might be able to be identified with greater frequency and effectiveness?

Mr. PATTERSON. Yes, ma'am.

Mrs. WALTERS. Thank you, and I yield back the balance of my time.

Mr. HARPER. I now recognize the gentlelady from Indiana, Mrs. Brooks.

Mrs. BROOKS. Thank you, Mr. Chairman.

Hello, Mr. Patterson. Since 2011, the number of immediate suspension orders issued by the DEA, as you have even noted, declined significantly from a high of 65 in 2011 down to a low of 6 in 2017. So I want to talk about that a little bit.

Are there instances in which the DEA pursues an immediate suspension order, the ISO, in parallel with related potential criminal investigation?

Mr. PATTERSON. So, ma'am, since October, so the administrator's position signs the ISOs when they're issued. What I have traditionally seen is because of the process of where a criminal case is being investigated there's been a delay in the ISO process as they're gathering evidence.

One of the concerns I have, and it goes back to, again, what Mr. Griffith said, is that cuts against the very argument that we have an imminent problem that we are trying to deal with.

So, again, my conversations that I've had with both U.S. and states attorneys are is that we have to act much faster in these cases in terms of if we have ongoing harm and we have the ability to stop that harm, even at the peril of a criminal case, then that's what we should be doing.

Mrs. BROOKS. And let's be clear. The U.S. doesn't do the immediate suspension orders. Those are done by the DEA.

Mr. PATTERSON. The DEA. It's an administrative action.

Mrs. BROOKS. And are you saying that the U.S. attorneys were asking—as a former U.S. attorney are you saying the U.S. attorneys were asking or telling DEA not to issue ISOs?

Mr. PATTERSON. In trying to gather evidence in their criminal case.

Mrs. BROOKS. I understand, but that can take months if not years sometimes in criminal cases. Do you believe that's what happened prior to you coming in October of 2017—that delays happened?

Mr. PATTERSON. I think that's been an ongoing theme of what some of these delays are caused by.

Mrs. BROOKS. And why would the DEA delay that type of administrative action in pursuit of a criminal investigation? Why?

Mr. PATTERSON. Because people believe that the criminal investigation is an important endeavor towards whether it's that doctor or that pharmacy.

Mrs. BROOKS. Well, it is very important, no doubt, because that person is, obviously, distributing—or the belief is distributing illicitly. But why would an immediate suspension—is that so that undercover operations can happen with the physician?

Mr. PATTERSON. Yes, ma'am.

Mrs. BROOKS. And the prescriber?

Mr. PATTERSON. The gathering of evidence.

Mrs. BROOKS. And what is the new guidance, and I appreciate the importance of gathering of evidence, but what is the new guidance relative to ISOs and criminal investigations that you are contemplating or that are in place now, and is that guidance in writing?

Mr. PATTERSON. So it is not formalized. This is conversations that I've been having with the AGAC, the, you know, advisory—— Mrs. BROOKS. I served on the attorney general's advisory counsel. Mr. PATTERSON. And to the extent that I've been meeting with states' attorneys to try and talk to them about the same issues.

So I think we have to, again, a lot of this is striking a balance.

I, frankly, feel that a lot of these cases can be worked backward on the criminal aspect.

I understand that their desire in a lot of these cases is to be able to get contemporaneous evidence, use undercover, right, as opposed to having to use witnesses that have come in that maybe not have the best of backgrounds.

So I understand that balance. The concern I have, like I said, if we are using an ISO, it feels awful weird to be signing that ISO a year after we learned of that problem.

Mrs. BROOKS. And I noticed in the document that Dr. Burgess had there was some of that, that the ISO was a year after the arrest even.

Mr. PATTERSON. Correct.

Mrs. BROOKS. Although at the time of the arrest, typically that individual would be under their medical licensing procedures as well. Is that correct?

Mr. PATTERSON. Correct.

Mrs. BROOKS. But wouldn't it make more sense to in many ways implement an ISO in the middle of the criminal investigation because those can take months if not years, and in the meantime we've got all of these people dying.

Mr. PATTERSON. I couldn't agree with you more and, quite frankly, even in the absence of the ISO, my concern is is that why aren't we trying to get a voluntary surrender as quickly as we have. And we have a lot of offices that do that in a very expeditious manner.

Mrs. BROOKS. And will your proposed guidelines impose a cap on the length of time it can be delayed? Is that the kind of discussion you're having. You're looking at, like, 30 days? Forty-five days?

Mr. PATTERSON. I think, striking that balance, we have to figure out where the days are. There will probably always be that exception that comes up and I think as long as people are willing to—

whether it's a U.S. attorney or a states' attorney that is willing to put in writing why we need to delay and we can evaluate that, I think that's something.

The process itself I think we have to work through. Like I said, we have new head of diversion control. This is an issue that has been bothering me greatly. Since October I've seen these and I've signed them and I have generally the same question every time, which is why are they taking so long.

Mrs. BROOKS. And for the record, I would just like to acknowledge when I became a U.S. attorney in 2001 one of the very first huge cases we did was against a doctor, Dr. Randolph Lievertz, for over-prescription of oxycodone, and DEA in 2001, 2002 and beyond said prescription drugs were going to be the next crisis in this country. Didn't start in 2010, didn't start in 2011. It was back in 2001, 2002, and we had a huge focus on it during that period of time and it's just really been very devastating, seeing that we fell off of that commitment it feels like in the last several years. I yield back.

Mr. HARPER. Gentlewoman yields back.

The chair will now recognize the chairman of the Full Committee for some follow-up questions. Mr. Walden.

Mr. WALDEN. Thank you. I appreciate the indulgence of the committee.

You raise an interesting issue about the U.S. attorneys weighing in here and saying to the DEA, stop—don't do your ISO—we want to proceed with the criminal investigation.

One question—do they have the authority to override your ISO authority? That would be one. And then I want to know the who, what, when, where, why.

Who are the U.S. attorneys that interceded on which cases in what areas and told the DEA suspend, and do they have that authority? Because, to Mrs. Brooks' point, people continue to die during this period, and I want to know this—this is part of our public policy debate here is does a U.S. attorney's office somewhere have the authority to tell you don't do the ISO, don't stop the death because we got to investigate and go criminal, which will have a bigger penalty, which I respect.

But is it one agent somewhere? One U.S. attorney in one state, is that why West Virginia went off the rails? And so I would like you to get back to the committee with answers to those questions.

Mr. PATTERSON. I would be happy to do so, sir. And look, what I can assure this committee is I think this is a topic that we have had some robust discussion on lately as we've gone through these and I will also assure you that the direction of this administration is to stop the harm as quickly as possible.

Mr. WALDEN. But I think you should be able to answer the one question. Do the U.S. attorneys have the authority to overrule your agency's decision making? I know you weren't there running it at the time.

Mr. PATTERSON. I would believe that we could issue the ISO even against the wishes of a U.S. attorney or a state's attorney. It probably doesn't help relationships to take those kinds of unilateral actions.

But, that said, I think part of this is the education of us holding up these things, why they look at either criminal or civil actions.

Mr. WALDEN. I would go back to Mr. Griffith's analogy. If you have got a drunk driver driving down the road, you don't wait until they have the fatal accident to pull them over and stop them.

Mr. PATTERSON. I couldn't agree with you more.

Mr. WALDEN. You can prosecute them along the way and I would think you could make the case, going backwards, because the prescriptions have been written. The pills have been sent out.

These two pharmacies we raised with you months ago are, my understanding, still operating in West Virginia. Are they not?

Mr. PATTERSON. I don't know. Those are the ones I have to go——

Mr. WALDEN. They're not operating. All right.

Well, if you can get back to us on the who, what, when, where, why on these U.S. attorneys that would be good.

Thank you.

Mr. HARPER. Gentleman yields back.

The chair will now recognize the gentleman from Georgia, Mr. Carter, for 5 minutes.

Mr. CARTER. Thank you, Mr. Patterson.

Mr. Patterson, I suspect you know that currently I am the only pharmacist serving in Congress, and Mrs. Brooks makes a good point. This is not something that started in 2010 or 2011. It was going on in 2001 and 2002. I was practicing back then. Now, granted, I haven't practiced in quite a while. It's probably been 4 or 5 years since I practiced. But I still know what's going on out there.

We've been kind of nibbling or you have been nibbling around the edges here. There have been great questions asked here but I want to follow up on the questions that Representative Collins asked about the beginning of where this problem starts and that's the doctors who are writing these prescriptions.

Now, I am not naive enough to believe that there aren't pharmacies out there that are in collusion with doctors or filling fraudulent prescriptions. But I want to talk about the doctors who are writing these prescriptions who are obviously out of control and why it's taken DEA so long to get them in control or under control.

I will just give you an example. I served in the Georgia State legislature for 10 years. I sponsored the legislation that created the prescription drug monitoring program back in 2009. I was jumping up and down then, saying this is a problem, we've got to get it under control, and it was falling on deaf ears. There are doctors right now in our community that our pharmacists won't fill prescriptions for. They just say no, that doctor's out of control, I don't fill for that doctor.

I was working one President's Day. We were out during our session. On President's Day we are always out. I had someone come into my pharmacy, a young lady who had the holy trinity of drug abuse—180, oxycodone, Xanax, and Soma, three prescriptions there. I looked at them. She gave me her driver's license from Florida. I said, I am not filling these prescriptions. She drove off in a car with Kentucky driver's license plates.

Now, I am not going to fill those prescriptions unless I have a legitimate prescription, OK, and I didn't want to fill that. But you're putting me in the position where I've got to judge whether that patient is legitimate or not. I am not trained in law enforcement, but as a pharmacist. But I want to know why, when there are doctors out there who are writing these prescriptions why can't you get them quicker?

Mr. Collins is right. You ought to be able to turn that around in 48 hours. The first time I get three prescriptions for 180 of the oxycodone, Xanax, and Soma I know that doctor is out of control.

Something's wrong there.

I had a doctor who we didn't fill for, Dr. B. I went home about a year ago and some of the pharmacists were telling me, oh, they finally busted Dr. B. I thought, wow, why did it take them 5 years to bust him? We never filled his prescriptions for 5 years but he kept on practicing. Well, they didn't exactly bust him. They got him for Medicare fraud. Didn't even get him for writing those prescriptions—never did.

Another example here, Dr. D.N. He got literally thousands of people addicted to these medications, and then he goes before the Composite Medical Board and gets slapped on the wrist, and they come back and they make him practice under the supervision of another doctor. That's his penalty. Now he lives on the waterfront, a beautiful home, beautiful cars, and yet thousands of people have been addicted because of these prescriptions that he has written.

We wouldn't fill his prescriptions. He's a rogue doctor. We are not filling those. Tell me why it takes you so long to get to the alpha, to the beginning, to the doctors who are writing these prescriptions who are out of control. Explain that to me, because I don't understand it.

All you have to do is go into a community and say, what doctors do you not fill for, and the pharmacists will tell you, we don't fill for this doctor and we don't fill for that doctor.

Mr. PATTERSON. Well, and that's, quite frankly, what we have to rely on. Look, the one thing I am not going to do in this space is shift blame anyplace. This is a collective——

Mr. CARTER. Well, it appears to me that that's what you're doing because Mr. Collins is right. You can turn this around in 48 hours. Just get those doctors out of there.

Mr. PATTERSON. But in the cases of these doctors, look, when we do our reviews we ask information, try and solicit people to essentially, in the registrant community to come in and talk about the registrants they have problems with.

If that doesn't happen, then our next course is someone that's been arrested that says, this is what's happening in a criminal case.

Mr. CARTER. But you can understand our frustration. When we don't fill prescriptions for that doctor but for years—literally, 4 or 5 years, they continue to practice.

Mr. PATTERSON. I understand, and this is where PMP data becomes absolutely critical and it's because that isn't——

Mr. CARTER. But what can we do to help you to be able to get these doctors under control? What can we do? Tell me what we can do in Congress.

Mr. PATTERSON. The PMP data is really what it boils down to.

Mr. CARTER. We've had the PDMP since 2009 in Georgia.

Mr. PATTERSON. But, sir, DEA doesn't have access to that data.

It depends on the state.

Mr. CARTER. Can you shut the doctor down? Can DEA shut the doctor down or is that up to the Composite Medical Boards of the states?

Mr. PATTERSON. No, if we had someone that was showing us that a doctor was over-prescribing then——

Mr. CARTER. But when you get this information of pill dumping you know that that pharmacy is getting those prescriptions from somewhere. Then that ought to be an indication to you. We need to go to that community and we need to find out what's going on here. They're coming from somewhere.

Mr. PATTERSON. Understood.

Mr. CARTER. Thank you, Mr. Chairman. Mr. HARPER. Gentleman yields back.

The chair will now recognize the gentleman from West Virginia, Mr. McKinley, for 5 minutes.

Mr. MCKINLEY. Thank you, Mr. Chairman. As not a member of this committee, I appreciate you giving me the opportunity to raise some issues with that.

Again, Mr. Patterson, thank you for being here. Are you familiar with this book written by John Temple called "American Pain?"

Mr. PATTERSON. No, sir.

Mr. MCKINLEY. This is about the clinic down in south Florida that was the epicenter of the opioids. I really would suggest that you and everyone else that's paying attention to this read that book.

But anyway, because with all due respect for the way some of your testimony has gone on this about ARCOS, he was able to assemble all of this book about drug abuse without access to ARCOS.

So for someone to say that we couldn't access it, we couldn't use it because it was manual, it was too much information, this man was able to put it together and be able to demonstrate this "American Pain" clinic down in south Florida prescribed two times the amount of medicine of all the doctors combined in the State of Ohio. He was able to put that together long hand, and he's not an agency with all the resources you have to be able to do that. He also was able to put together all of the pill mills in Florida combined. So nine times the amount of pain medicine that was issued by every state in the country. He did that long hand.

So with all due respect, I don't think you can hide behind the fact that you didn't have the resources to be able to do this because it was coming in manually.

If I could, I am curious about the production quotas with it because in the book he talks about how speed pills back in the 1970s were becoming a problem, and DEA stepped up and they cut the production by 90 percent and the problem went away.

And then in the 1980s we had a problem with Quaaludes—same thing. They cut the production and it went away. Now, fast forward to today or what we've been dealing with over the last 10 years or so, the opioids.

We continue to increase the production of opioids, continue to distribute those. Didn't we learn anything from the past experience, that we should be cutting back? And it wasn't until 2017 that we actually had our first reduction. But it's still nearly 50 percent more than we were 10 years ago in production of opioids.

How would you respond to that? Didn't we learn anything?

Mr. PATTERSON. No, I understand that, sir.

And look, the quota numbers are set, unfortunately, to ensure access to the patients and you can see the disturbing trend that happened with quotas. The industry said more and more people needed these prescriptions.

We worked aggressively in the last year and a half to try and work on the quota issue and pull this back. I give a lot of the credit to the states.

Mr. MCKINLEY. If I could recover my time, because I think that perhaps I know you're meaningful to do this, to correct it, but it failed, because I am coming from that state that has 52 drug overdoses per 100,000 people. We are leading the Nation with this. Someone has to get to this.

So I am just curious, I know you have the ability to transfer resources and funds within DEA. So my question goes back to you— have you made any transfer back into West Virginia? Are you going to put more resources there in West Virginia as a result of your ability to do transfer?

Mr. PATTERSON. We have, and we are continuing to do so.

Mr. MCKINLEY. We just put in a year or so ago down, a tactical diversion squad in Clarksburg. I think that's the second one we have in West Virginia. Is that correct?

Mr. PATTERSON. That's correct.

Mr. MCKINLEY. Leading the Nation—is that sufficient? Do you think that you have diverted enough attention into West Virginia that you don't need to divert any more funds and resources into West Virginia?

Mr. PATTERSON. Sir, the creation of the Louisville division, which polled three states all struggling with this same problem: Tennessee, West Virginia, and——

Mr. MCKINLEY. I am sorry. I am just dealing with West Virginia.

It's the epicenter. You know that and I know that——

Mr. PATTERSON. Sir, so we——

Mr. MCKINLEY [continuing]. It has been there for nearly 10 years. It's been the highest level and we've not seen the resources come in to West Virginia.

And now I appreciate very much that you put a tactical diversion squad, or your predecessor did, into Clarksburg. But I've got to think there is a lot more attention needs to go with it because if this man can do this by long hand, can put this information together, I think you all could do it. With your resources, you could do a far better job and save a lot of lives and turn some families around.

So I am asking you, please, to look at more diversion into West Virginia—some of the funds and resources that you can to help out in this situation.

Mr. PATTERSON. Again, sir, we've been working on that and we are continuing to put more resources into that particular division.

Mr. MCKINLEY. So what are the optics on this, in the 10 seconds I've got left? How am I going to be able to measure whether you're successful with what you're doing?

Because just last year in county we've already had a 50 percent increase in overdose drug—overdose deaths in West Virginia in my county. How are we going to measure this? Are we going to see a drop next year?

Mr. PATTERSON. Look, the concern we have had is that we've seen the shift into fentanyl and other illicit substances. The goal is to continue to drive down the prescription rates and the diversion of prescription pills, and we are going to have to work this licit market and, frankly, the place——

Mr. MCKINLEY. Again, what are the optics? Am I going to see a decline next year?

Mr. PATTERSON. I would hope we see declines across the board.

I think some states are going to take longer than others, sir.

Mr. MCKINLEY. Thank you. Yield back. Mr. HARPER. The gentleman yields back.

The chair will now recognize the vice chairman, Mr. Griffith, for follow-up questions.

Mr. GRIFFITH. Thank you very much, Mr. Chairman. Appreciate it, and this question was from Mrs. Brooks, who, unfortunately, had to step out for a minute.

Do the Medicaid fraud control units run by the state AG's offices still exist in many states?

Mr. PATTERSON. I would have to find out, sir.

Mr. GRIFFITH. All right, because what she was indicating was was that these particular MFCUs who are going after Medicaid fraud often can also pick up over prescribing data and that that's a collaborative unit that you all ought to be looking at in the various states to figure out who the rogue doctors are and that would help you in that regard as well.

Mr. Patterson, moving on, can you explain to me how can you all maintain that voluntary registration surrender can be as effective a tool in protecting the public safety as an ISO if it takes years to get the voluntary surrender as in the case of the owner of the Sav-Rite No. 1 in Kermit, West Virginia?

Mr. PATTERSON. I would assume in that case and, again, I need to get the particular facts on it—the voluntary surrender probably came as part of the criminal case.

Mr. GRIFFITH. And so what you would do is you would reverse that order and have the voluntary surrender or an ISO happening early on?

Mr. PATTERSON. Absolutely, sir.

Again, I can't go back and necessarily understand why certain people did certain things——

Mr. GRIFFITH. But you can make sure, going forward, that we shorten the time?

Mr. PATTERSON. Absolutely, sir.

Mr. GRIFFITH. All right. In your written testimony, you mentioned prescription drug monitoring programs as a tool that can be used to combat prescription drug diversion.

How does the DEA currently utilize the PDMP data in its investigations?

Mr. PATTERSON. So this varies state to state because the concern is, again, is our access to this data and how we can access this data and that is a state by state decision. And so every state varies.

This is one of the big conversations that we've had with the 48 states that are parts of these two coalitions.

Mr. GRIFFITH. All right. Let us know how we can help.

Your written testimony also mentioned that law enforcement access to PDMP data varies widely from state to state, as you have just told us. Can you tell me what the DEA is doing to address those concerns and to address any access barriers the agency currently faces with respect to the PDMPs?

Mr. PATTERSON. Again, working with all the states individually on these issues and to the extent that we can leverage the coalitions to help us in that.

Look, in a perfect world we have a federal PDMP process that we can take all this data and put together. I think in a less than perfect world at a minimum the states all need to be able to share this data with each other.

Mr. GRIFFITH. And in your experience, are there areas—and you just have gone over some of it—but is there some other areas that we might be able to improve the PDMP process?

Mr. PATTERSON. I think that's the key piece. Mr. GRIFFITH. All right.

I appreciate it, Mr. Chairman. I yield—— Mr. HARPER. The gentleman yields back.

Mr. Patterson, just to give you a little update, I am going to recognize Mr. Carter in just a minute for a follow-up question. Then Ms. DeGette and myself will have concluding questions and we'll be done shortly. So thank you for being here with us today.

The chair will now recognize Mr. Carter, the gentleman from Georgia.

Mr. CARTER. Thank you, Mr. Chairman. I will be very brief.

I just want to follow up, Mr. Patterson. You're correct, you can't do anything about what happened years ago. But you can do a lot about what's happening now. I want to give you a sincere caution here.

What's happening with the wholesalers when they are limiting the pharmacies from getting a certain amount of drugs whereas that has all the best of intentions—what it causes sometimes is for some of our patients not to be able to get the medications that they need and I just warn you to please be careful with that. There are patients out there, i.e., hospice patients, who truly need these medications.

We found ourselves running out and we couldn't order it from the wholesalers because we'd already used up our limit for that month. So that put these people in a very precarious position and it's not a good position.

It's a very bad feeling for a pharmacist to have to profile and have to go out and say, oh, this patient doesn't need pain medication. Who am I to say that the long-haired tattooed body-pierced person is not in pain? That's not fair.

We've got to make sure that we get this under control and I still maintain that starting with the physicians and tell me what I can do to help you, to give you the tools that you need so that you can react quicker and get them under control when they get out of control.

That's all I am asking you to do is tell me what you need because I promise you I will do my best to get you those resources so that you can get these rogue physicians—and they're not all of them but some of them—a good amount of them are out of control and they get out of control quickly and it gets out of control very, very quickly.

Thank you, Mr. Patterson.

Mr. PATTERSON. Understood.

Mr. HARPER. The gentleman yields back.

The chair will now recognize the ranking member, Ms. DeGette, for concluding questions.

Ms. DEGETTE. Thanks, Mr. Chairman, and I want to echo, this is a rough topic, Mr. Patterson, and we know you haven't been there that long. But we also know that it's urgent that we get this right. It's just urgent for the safety of our constituents.

There's just a couple of areas I wanted to clarify. Mr. Collins was asking you some questions about these—the settlement that the DOJ has had with some of the distributors because of issues—reporting suspicious orders and it's really important that they report these suspicious orders to you because you can't do your job unless you get this reporting. Isn't that right?

Mr. PATTERSON. Absolutely.

Ms. DEGETTE. Now, for example, the DOJ has reached two settlements with Cardinal Health. In 2008, Cardinal agreed to pay $34 million to resolve allegations that it shipped large quantities of opiates to pharmacies without reporting those orders to the DEA.

And then in 2012 again, Cardinal agreed to pay $44 million to resolve similar claims. Now, do you know, broadly speaking, why the Department of Justice decided to pursue these cases against Cardinal?

Mr. PATTERSON. I don't, ma'am. I know that, from the documents I have seen on the 2012 case, the frustration was is that the MOUs or MOAs in that scenario essentially they had gone back and violated again.

Ms. DEGETTE. Right.

Mr. PATTERSON. So that is probably the basis for——

Ms. DEGETTE. That's your understanding?

Mr. PATTERSON. Yes, ma'am.

Ms. DEGETTE. Now, McKesson similarly reached two agreements with DOJ agreeing to pay $13.25 million in 2008 and again $150 million in 2017 to resolve allegations that it failed to report suspicious orders. Would you suspect it's the same kind of a situation that you talked about a minute ago?

Mr. PATTERSON. Yes, ma'am.

Ms. DEGETTE. Now, do you agree that suspicious order reports are a key part of preventing diversion?

Mr. PATTERSON. Absolutely, because, again, I go back to the fact that the manufacturers and distributors are the key registrants that we need to hear from.

Ms. DEGETTE. Right. Right.

Now, if distributors fail to report suspicious orders, they really do undermine your ability to oversee the supply chain. Is that right?

Mr. PATTERSON. Yes.

Ms. DEGETTE. One more topic, and this is following up on something Ms. Walters was asking you about, and I don't think maybe you understood her question.

On this website that you have been talking about that you have for distributors to look at, it lets other distributors see if other distributors are providing to these pharmacies. But it does not tell volume. Isn't that correct?

Mr. PATTERSON. I would have to check it. I believe it does. It goes back a 6-month window. But I would get back to you on that particular issue.

Ms. DEGETTE. I think so, because it's my understanding that the distributors object to disclosing volume. Here, your associate's handing you something.

Mr. PATTERSON. No volume.

Ms. DEGETTE. No volume. OK. And, from my perspective I can understand what they're saying about that impacting trade secrets and so on.

But the problem, from my perspective, is if you're just saying, OK, we are going to have a website where you can see if other distributors are providing in that area, if you don't know the volume then it's really hard for somebody to see whether there's an abuse going on or not. Wouldn't you agree with that?

Mr. PATTERSON. Yes, ma'am.

Ms. DEGETTE. I think this website is something we should probably talk about more and maybe you can supplement your answers to see how we can use that effectively, because just knowing if other people are going in there I don't think that's going to solve our problem.

Thanks, Mr. Chairman. I yield back.

Mr. HARPER. The gentlewoman yields back.

Just for clarification, it appears in 2008 that Cardinal Health paid $34 million in civil penalties and then again in 2016 an additional $10 million was paid out through one of its subsidiaries, Kinray—if that clarifies that.

Through our investigation, Mr. Patterson, the committee has learned certainly that as early as 2008 the DEA received almost daily suspicious order reports, which received millions of opioids that had been tied to known pill mill physicians like Mr. Collins' neighbor that he referenced. Yet, most continue to remain in operation and it's unclear to what extent, if any, DEA followed up on the suspicious order reports it received.

So tell us what is the process that the DEA takes when evaluating suspicious order reports it receives and the actions that the agency takes in response?

Mr. PATTERSON. So, sir, when those come in they're currently reviewed by and looked at for investigation by the divisions. This is one of the changes that we are making by bringing this into headquarters process.

Some of these companies, obviously, have districts all throughout the country. One of the reasons why we want to look at them is because we want to look at them as a corporation, not just as individual entities or other problem areas.

So that is a change that we are doing. I would be happy to go back and look at specific issues on——

Mr. HARPER. Sure.

Mr. PATTERSON [continuing]. Any of SORS database and what was or wasn't done. I think the decentralization—we have had structural problems, I would say, in terms of how we used not just some of this information but how we looked at it.

Those structural changes we are rapidly trying to get a handle on to make these—especially in the suspicious orders reports more beneficial because, one, we need them for the registrants, but two, we have to do something with them when we get them. And you have discussed implementing the process to improve and to process those suspicious orders at DEA headquarters.

Has DEA identified breakdowns in the way its field division processes suspicious order reports in the past and what corrections or adjustments have been made or do you anticipate being made?

Mr. PATTERSON. So, again, I think the uniformness of how we look at these things and the accountability that we hold the people to when we get these reports is critical.

So that's one of the big changes for us to make sure that as we are looking at these—I have had conversations with all of the staff in this space, whether, it goes back to the ALJ or the folks in chief counsel that do it with our expectations, to go back to what Mr. Collins was talking about.

It has not been comfortable conversations. But we have to essentially do the things that we are supposed to be doing each and every day and personalities can't play a role in this.

Mr. HARPER. And when you were making decisions at DEA headquarters, the personnel at the headquarters probably have field experience in some level in DEA. Would that be a fair assessment?

Mr. PATTERSON. That's correct.

Mr. HARPER. And as you're looking at these, are you also taking into consideration those that are in the field now maybe that have never been to headquarters to try to get their input on the actual boots on the ground?

Mr. PATTERSON. I think it's important and, look, I haven't spent years in this diversion world. In fact, I've really only done it for about the last 18 months as the deputy and now as acting.

What I will tell you is that fresh sets of eyes on problem sets are always critically important.

Mr. HARPER. OK.

You talked about well, what do we do—prevention, education, treatment. Your role is really in enforcement and prosecution, at least laying the groundwork for that.

The problem that we see as we look at this in great detail is local law enforcement does not have the capability to take care of this issue. That's why you see many of these cases coming out of rural areas. So we would certainly want to make sure that you're doing things to pivot, to take care of the rural areas in this country as you're looking at that.

Now, there were a number of times that you referenced, I will get back to you or we'll get you that information. So just know that we'll have follow-up on that.

Mr. PATTERSON. Absolutely.

Mr. HARPER. And we'll look for that.

We should be able to work together on this, and just know that we are not happy that the chairman of the full committee, Chairman Walden, had to even call for a press conference.

So we want to make sure, going forward, there are things that we need to know or things that we need to inquire on or things that you have for us. We would prefer more openness between the committee and the DEA, going forward.

And with that we thank you for your time today, for what turned into a fairly long time for you. It's been helpful to us and we look forward to the follow-up questions that we have.

I want to thank the members who have attended today and participated in today's hearing and I will remind members that they have 10 business days to submit questions for the record and I would ask, Mr. Patterson, if you would see that those are responded to promptly as you receive those.

With that, the subcommittee is adjourned.

[Whereupon, at 12:23 p.m., the committee was adjourned.]

[Material submitted for inclusion in the record follows:]

U.S. House of Representatives,
Committee on Energy and Commerce

March 16, 2018

TO: Members, Subcommittee on Oversight and Investigations

FROM: Committee Majority Staff

RE: Hearing entitled "The Drug Enforcement Administration's Role in Combating the Opioid Epidemic."

The Subcommittee on Oversight and Investigations will hold a hearing on March 20, 2018, at 10:00 a.m. in 2322 Rayburn House Office Building, entitled "The Drug Enforcement Administration's Role in Combating the Opioid Epidemic." The purpose of this hearing is to discuss the response of the Drug Enforcement Administration (DEA) to the opioid crisis, including the detection and investigation of suspicious orders of opioids, and DEA's enforcement approach to the opioid epidemic.

Witness

Robert W. Patterson, Acting Administrator, U.S. Drug Enforcement Administration.

Background

The U.S. continues to experience an opioid epidemic, with opioid-involved overdose deaths currently being the leading cause of injury death in the U.S., taking the lives of 115 Americans per day.[28] According to a recent report issued by the Centers for Disease Control and Prevention (CDC), prescription or illicit opioids were involved in nearly two-thirds of all drug overdose deaths in the U.S. during 2016, a 27.7 percent increase from 2015.[29] In total, more than 351,000 lives have been lost since 1999 due to an opioid-involved overdose.[30]

Beginning in April 2014, through numerous hearings, the Subcommittee has undertaken a comprehensive examination into the root causes of the opioid epidemic and explored possible solutions to enable greater access to effective, evidence-based treatment for substance use disorders. On May 8, 2017, the Committee launched an investigation into the distribution of prescription opioids, initially sending letters to the three largest wholesale drug distributors in the U.S. as well as the DEA.[31] The Committee expanded this investigation to include two additional wholesale drug distributors, and sent a second letter to the DEA on October 13, 2017.

Role of the DEA in Combatting the Opioid Epidemic

The DEA was established within the Department of Justice by Executive Order on July 1, 1973, when the Office of National Narcotics Intelligence and the Office for Drug Abuse Law Enforcement were merged, and the Attorney General was granted additional authority to coordinate federal efforts to combat illicit drug abuse.[32] Today, the DEA is

---

[28] Centers for Disease Control and Prevention, *Understanding the Epidemic, Opioid Overdose*, Aug. 30, 2017, https://www.cdc.gov/drugoverdose/epidemic/index.html.

[29] Centers for Disease Control and Prevention, *Vital Signs: Trends in Emergency Department Visits for Suspected Overdoses* – United States, July 2016-September 2017, Mar. 9, 2018, https://www.cdc.gov/mmwr/volumes/67/wr/mm6709e1.htm.

[30] Centers for Disease Control and Prevention, Data Brief 294. *Drug Overdose Deaths in the United States*, 1999-2016, https://www.cdc.gov/nchs/data/databriefs/db294_table.pdf#page=4.

[31] *See* H. Comm. Energy & Commerce, *Letters to Distributors and the DEA Regarding Alleged Pill Dumping in West Virginia*, May 9, 2017, https://energycommerce.house.gov/news/letter/letters-distributors-and-dea-regarding- alleged-pill-dumping-west-virginia/.

[32] Reorganization Plan No. 2 of 1973, 3 C.F.R. 785 (1971 – 1975 Comp.) *reprinted at* 21 U.S.C. § 801.

the federal agency principally responsible for enforcement of the Controlled Substances Act (CSA), enacted under Title II of the Comprehensive Drug Abuse Prevention and Control Act of 1970.[33] The CSA established the schedules for controlled substances[34] and provided authority for the DEA to register entities engaged in the manufacture, distribution, or dispensation of these substances as well.[35] The CSA also established registration requirements[36] and provided the authority for the DEA to deny, revoke, or suspend such registration(s) if it determined the registrant to be out of compliance with the mandates of the CSA.[37] The CSA was designed to combat diversion by providing for a closed system of drug distribution, in which all legitimate handlers of controlled substances must obtain a DEA registration and, as a condition of maintaining such registration, must take reasonable steps to ensure their registration is not being used as a source of diversion. The DEA regulations require all distributors to report suspicious orders of controlled substances.[38] In addition to reporting all suspicious orders, a distributor has a statutory responsibility to exercise due diligence to avoid filling suspicious orders that might be diverted to non-medical, scientific, or industrial channels. Failure to exercise such due diligence could provide a statutory basis for revocation or suspension of a DEA registration.[39]

The CSA also authorized the DEA to establish annual production quotas for controlled substances.[40] According to the CDC, the number of prescription opioids sold to pharmacies, doctors' offices, and hospitals in the U.S. nearly quadrupled from 1999 to 2010, yet there was no increase in the number of patients treated for pain during this time period.[41] In August 2017, the DEA announced its intention to reduce the amount of controlled substances, including opioids, manufactured in the U.S. by 20 percent in 2018.[42] The reduced 2018 production figures were finalized by DEA in November 2017.[43] Recently, the Attorney General issued a memorandum to DEA, directing the agency to examine its regulations governing aggregate production quotas and noting "[s]tudies have indicated that the United States is an outlier in the number of opioid prescriptions issued each year."[44]

---

[33] Comprehensive Drug Abuse Prevention and Control Act of 1970, Pub. L. 91 – 513, 84 Stat. 1236, 1296 (1970).
[34] 21 U.S.C. § 812.
[35] 21 U.S.C. § 822.
[36] 21 U.S.C. § 823.
[37] 21 U.S.C. § 824.
[38] 21 C.F.R. 1301.74(b).
[39] 21 U.S.C. § 823(e) and 21 U.S.C. § 824(a).
[40] 21 U.S.C. § 826.
[41] Centers for Disease Control and Prevention, *supra* note 1.
[42] Press Release, U.S. Drug Enforcement Admin, DEA proposes reduction to amount of controlled substances to be manufactured in 2018 (Aug. 4, 2017) *available at* https://www.dea.gov/divisions/hq/2017/hq080417.shtml.
[43] Established Aggregate Production Quotas for Schedule I and II Controlled Substances and Assessment of Annual Needs for the List I Chemicals Ephedrine, Pseudoephedrine, and Phenylpropanolamine for 2018, 82 Fed. Reg. 51873 (Nov. 8, 2017).
[44] *Memorandum from Hon. Jefferson Sessions, Attorney Gen., United States of America, to Robert Patterson, Acting Adm'r, U.S. Drug Enforcement Admin.*, Mar. 1, 2018, https://www.justice.gov/file/1040226/download.

According to its Fiscal Year (FY) 2019 budget request, the DEA regulates more than 1.73 million registrants that are licensed to manufacture, distribute, and prescribe controlled substances.[45] Among the tools available to DEA to ensure compliance with the CSA, and to protect the public health and welfare, are Immediate Suspension Orders (ISOs) and Orders to Show Cause (OTSCs), the latter of which require a registrant to prove to the DEA Administrator why the registrant's DEA registration should not be revoked or suspended.[46] If, however, the DEA Administrator determines that a DEA registrant's activities constitute an imminent danger to the public health or safety, the Administrator may issue an ISO, which requires the immediate surrender of the registrant's DEA registration, pending the final resolution of an accompanying OTSC.[47]

Decline in Enforcement Actions Initiated by DEA

Throughout the last two decades, the opioid epidemic has worsened. In 2016, opioids were involved in 42,249 overdose deaths – an amount five times higher than the number of opioid-involved deaths reported in 1999.[48] The impact of the opioid epidemic has become so pronounced that it has caused the overall life expectancy in the U.S. to decline during the past two consecutive years.[49] The opioid epidemic has also received widespread media coverage and elicited responses at every level of government. Yet, since 2011, the number of ISOs issued by the DEA has significantly declined.

According to data provided by the DEA, the number of ISOs issued by the agency declined from 65 in 2011, to six in 2017.[50] The DEA has publicly stated that the high number of ISOs issued during the 2011 and 2012 time frame were due to actions the DEA took to shut down numerous rogue "pill mill" pharmacies in Florida.[51] However, statements and allegations made by current and former DEA officials suggest the number

---

[45] U.S. Dep't of Justice, FY 2019 Budget and Performance Summary – Drug Enforcement Administration (DEA), https://www.justice.gov/jmd/page/file/1033151/download (last visited Mar. 11, 2018).

[46] *See* 21 U.S.C. § 824(c) and 21 C.F.R. § 1301.37(b).

[47] *See* 21 U.S.C. § 824(d) and 21 C.F.R. § 1301.36.

[48] Centers for Disease Control and Prevention, *Drug Overdose Death Data*, Dec. 19, 2017, https://www.cdc.gov/drugoverdose/data/statedeaths.html.

[49] Lenny Bernstein and Christopher Ingraham, Fueled by drug crisis, U.S. life expectancy declines for a second straight year, *Wash. Post*, Dec. 21, 2017, https://www.washingtonpost.com/national/health-science/fueled-by-drug-crisis-us-life-expectancy-declines-for-a-second-straight-year/2017/12/20/2e3f8dea-e596-11e7-ab50-621fe0588340_story.html?utm_term=.9b960a164076.

[50] See Office of Sen. Orrin Hatch, DEA Immediate Suspension Orders 2008-2017, https://www.hatch.senate.gov/public/ _cache/ files/ 80f96e98-6c08-4bd8-bdec-ee8c99cf7596/ISO%20&%20Show%20Cause%20Order%20Charts%20for%20the%20Record.pdf.

[51] See *Oversight of the Ensuring Patient Access and Effective Drug Enforcement Act Before S. Comm. on the Judiciary*, 115th Cong. (2017) (statement of Demetra Ashley, Acting Assistant Adm'r, U.S. Drug Enforcement Admin). In her written testimony, Acting Assistant Administrator Ashley stated, "DEA issued 104 ISOs between FY2011 and FY 2012, with all but four being issued against practitioners . . . and pharmacies. Those actions were largely attributed to significant efforts to combat pill mills in Florida . . . The number of ISOs issued in FY 2011 and FY2012 were seen as atypical by historical DEA data."

of ISOs issued by the agency also declined because of internal policy changes.[52] To date, the DEA has not addressed these allegations directly.

Prescription Opioid Distribution Investigation

In May 2017, the Committee opened an investigation into the distribution of prescription opioids by wholesale drug distributors, with a specific focus on unusually large opioid shipments to small pharmacies in West Virginia. Between 2007 and 2012, distributors sent more than 780 million hydrocodone and oxycodone pills to the state.[53] In that timeframe, 1,728 West Virginians fatally overdosed on those two drugs.[54]

While the investigation is ongoing, the Committee uncovered additional statistics that raise questions about the adequacy of due diligence performed by wholesale drug distributors, and the companies' adherence to the CSA's requirement that they implement a suspicious order monitoring program and report any suspicious orders to DEA.[55] The statistics also raise questions about the DEA's oversight of its registrants in West Virginia as the opioid crisis continued to worsen.

Among the Committee's findings: a single pharmacy in Mount Gay-Shamrock, West Virginia—population 1,779—received more than 16.5 million hydrocodone and oxycodone pills between 2006 and 2016; distributors sent 20.8 million opioid pills to Williamson, West Virginia—population 2,900—during the same period; a pharmacy in Kermit, West Virginia— population 406—ranked 22nd in the entire country in 2006 in the overall number of hydrocodone pills it received, with a single distributor supplying 76 percent of its hydrocodone pills that year.

Issues

The following issues may be examined at the hearing:

- What is DEA's role in responding to the opioid epidemic?

---

[52] See e.g., Lenny Bernstein and Scott Higham, Investigation: The DEA slowed enforcement while the opioid epidemic grew out of control, *Wash. Post*, Oct. 22, 2016, https://www.washingtonpost.com/investigations/the-dea-slowed-enforcement-while-the-opioid-epidemic-grew-out-of-control/2016/10/22/aea2bf8e-7f71-11e6-8d13- d7c704ef9fd9_story.html?utm_term=.f19aef7fe849; Bernstein and Higham, 'We feel like our system was hijacked': DEA agents say a huge opioid case ended in a whimper, *Wash. Post*, Dec. 17, 2017, https://www.washingtonpost.com/investigations/mckesson-dea-opioids-fine/2017/12/14/ab50ad0e-db5b-11e7-b1a8-62589434a581_story.html? hpid=hp_rhp-banner-low_mckesson-603am-hed% 3Ahomepage%2Fstory&utm_term=.f620afa9efdc; and Bill Whitaker, *Whistleblowers: DEA Attorneys Went Easy on McKesson, the Country's Largest Drug Distributor*, CBS News 60 Minutes, Dec. 17, 2017, https://www.cbsnews.com/news/whistleblowers-dea-attorneys-went-easy-on-mckesson-the-countrys-largest-drug- distributor/.

[53] Eric Eyre, *Drug firms poured 780M painkillers into WV amid rise of overdoses*, Charleston Gazette-Mail, Dec. 17, 2016, https://www.wvgazettemail.com/news/cops_and_courts/drug-firms-poured-m-painkillers-into-wv-amid- rise-of/article_99026dad-8ed5-5075-90fa-adb906a36214.html.

[54] Ibid.

[55] See 21 C.F.R. § 1301.74.

- Why did the number of enforcement actions initiated by DEA decline while the opioid epidemic continued to worsen?
- What changes, if any, did DEA make to the evidentiary standards or policies related to Immediate Suspension Orders or Orders to Show Cause?
- How has DEA learned from past practices in order to improve its response to the opioid epidemic?

From:
To: Rannazzisi, Joseph T.
Sent: 5/6/2011 4:59:39 PM
Subject: RE: Bates

Joe,

Well said! That's been my contention from the start. The activities by Bates are egregious and the company took no efforts to protect the public or to change their operating methodologies (especially after they had some official notice from the DEA). Our first and most prominent social responsibility government officials in the DEA is to "protect the public." I think that trumps all other activities.

I think that's what Congress/citizens would expect us to do. As such, your position is right on target!

From: Rannazzisi, Joseph T.
Sent: Friday: May 06, 2011 1:33 PM
Cc: Masumoto, Scott S; Harrigan, Thomas M.
Subject: FW: Bates

FYI

From: Rannazzisi, Joseph T.
Sent: Friday, May 06, 2011 4:31PM
To: Gleason, Robert (Chris)
Cc: Goggin, Wendy H.;
Subject: RE: Bates

Chris,

I've discussed the case with division management and I've been informed that the criminal section agrees with pushing forward toward the PI hearing.

The A made a finding of that threat based on her knowledge and experience and the facts before her, and there is no evidence that her finding was unfounded.

I would much rather have a record showing the agency attempted to defend its authority but lost.

Joe

From: Gleason, Robert (Chris)
Sent: Friday May 06, 2011 2:32 PM
To: Rannazzisi, Joseph T.
Cc: Goggin, Wendy, H.;
Subject: Bates

Joe,
Thanks,
Lee

C. Lee Reeves
Associate Chief Counsel
U.S. Department of Justice
Drug Enforcement Administration
Diversion & Regulatory Litigation Section

From:
Sent: Monday, August 19, 2013 5:24 PM
To: Reeves, Less
CC:
Subject: CCD Interpretation of Policy

Good Afternoon!

I was in DEA HQ last week and met with a number of OD Section Chiefs. Several of them advised me that on a number of recent occasions., CCD *has* required them *to* submit an "expert witness" report and review of documents (e.g., prescription monitoring programs data, patient files, etc.), prior to submitting either (or both} requests for Immediate Suspension Orders and Orders to Show Cause.

I informed my colleagues that we (in the Houston Division) had not encountered this issue in the past, but given that we have a ease we plan on sending up to you shortly, where we will be seeking one or both of those, I thought I should write to ask you whether that is a requirement and/or CCD policy?

As you might guess. if the "expert witness" review process is now a mandatory requirement and practice, given the current fiscal climate we all face, as the Diversion Program Manager, it will be difficult if not impossible for me to justify and authorize expenditures for expert witness review on a case(s) which has not been at least tentatively accepted by your office, so…I thought it prudent to touch base with you on this ahead of time (prior to our sending up the case I referred to above) and seek any guidance or or other suggestions you might have.

If it would be more productive/efficient, perhaps we can discuss this by telephone, at your convenience.

Thank you.

Diversion Program Manager

From: Reeves, Lee
To: [redacted]
Sent: 8/22/2013 4:07:00 PM
Subject: FW: CCD Interpretation of Policy

As an FYI, I've sent this to OD/Russ Holske.

From: Reeves, Lee
Sent: Tuesday, August 20, 2013 11:48 AM
To: [redacted]
Cc:
Subject: RE: CCD Interpretation of Policy

[redacted]

Thank you for your email regarding the use of and need for medical experts. I appreciate the opportunity to clear up what I believe may be some misconceptions on the nature and origin of the need for medical experts in diversion cases involving allegations of improper prescribing.

Here's some background:

A prescription for a controlled substance is not "effective" unless it is "issued for a legitimate medical purpose by an individual practitioner acting in the usual course of his professional practice." 21 C.F.R. § 1306.04(a). Under the Controlled Substances Act, it is fundamental that a practitioner must establish a bona fide doctor-patient relationship in order to act "in the usual course of . . . professional practice" and to issue a prescription for a "legitimate medical purpose." *See United States v. Moore*, 423 U.S. 122, 142-43 (1975); *United States v. Lovern*, 590 F.3d 1095, 1100-01 (10th Cir. 2009); *United States v. Smith*, 573 F.3d 639, 657 (8th Cir. 2009); *see also* 21 C.F.R. § 1306.04(a) ("an order purporting to be a prescription issued not in the usual course of professional treatment . . . is not a prescription within the meaning and intent of [21 U.S.C. 829] and . . . the person issuing it, shall be subject to the penalties provided for violations of the provisions of law related to controlled substances").

As the Supreme Court has explained, "the prescription requirement . . . ensures patients use controlled substances under the supervision of a doctor so as to prevent addiction and recreational abuse. As a corollary, [it] also bars doctors from peddling to patients who crave the drugs for those prohibited uses." *Gonzales v. Oregon*, 546 U.S. 243, 274 (2006) (citing Moore, 423 U.S. 122, 135, 143 (1975)). Both DEA and federal courts have held that "establishing a violation of the prescription requirement 'requires proof that the practitioner's conduct went "beyond the bounds of any legitimate medical practice, including that which would constitute civil negligence."' *Laurence T. McKinney*, 73 Fed. Reg. 43,260, 43,266 (2008) (quoting *United States v. McIver*, 470 F.3d 550, 559 (4th Cir. 2006)). Establishing that a practitioner's conduct exceeded "the bounds of any legitimate medical practice" necessarily requires an understanding of what conduct would, or arguably would, constitute legitimate medical practice. Because such determinations require specialized knowledge, training, and/or judgment, expert testimony is generally necessary to sustain allegations of improper prescribing.

** ** **

To be clear, this is not a Chief Counsel's Office requirement/policy. This is the requirement of the Administrator and the courts, as evidenced by decisions they have issued on this subject, including the Administrator's very recent decision in *Ruben* (in which the Administrator rejected evidence related to undercover buys which were not supported by expert testimony). I cannot tell you in advance, without knowing the facts of a case, whether expert testimony will be needed to support a particular allegation (whether in an ISO or an OTSC). However, we are and remain willing to assist you in determining whether an expert is required in a given case, and urge you to please contact us so that we can discuss the merits of proceeding without or with an expert. To reiterate, there is no Chief Counsel/CCD requirement or policy that there needs to be a medical expert in every case. It depends on the nature of the allegations as well as the facts underlying that case.

It is important to note that Chief Counsel has brought cases and prevailed without expert testimony where the evidence that the practitioner knew that he was engaged in a blatant drug deal. *See, e.g., Robert F. Hunt*, 75 Fed. Reg. 49,995, 50,003 (2010) (holding, without expert testimony, that physician lacked a legitimate medical purpose in issuing prescriptions to undercover officers in view of physician's admission that he falsified medical records "just to cover [his] ass" and that practitioner's notation in patient's medical file of a history of osteoporosis that "has nothing to do with [the undercover], it just has to do if the State ever comes in to monitor my charts that I have a reason for prescribing [controlled substances]"). As a general matter, however, these cases are the exception rather than the rule.

I understand and appreciate the cost concern that you have raised, and I have raised this issue with OD here. Given that diversion-related activities (including the retention of experts) are fee-funded, the fact of sequestration is not relevant. It is my understanding from OD that obtaining funds for an expert should be not be a significant hardship. I encourage your office to submit a request to OD for expert witness funding when appropriate.

Please don't hesitate to let me know if I can answer any other questions.

Thanks,

Lee

Greg Walden, Oregon
Chairman

Frank Pallone, Jr., New Jersey
Ranking Member

One Hundred Fifteenth Congress
Congress of the United States
House of Representatives
Committee on Energy and Commerce
2125 Rayburn House Office Building
Washington, DC 20515-6115

May 10, 2018
Mr. Robert W. Patterson
Acting Administrator
Drug Enforcement Administration
870l Morrissette Drive
Springfield, VA 22152

Dear Mr. Patterson:

Thank you for appearing before the Subcommittee on Oversight and Investigations on March 20, 2018, to testify at the hearing entitled "The Drug Enforcement Administration's Role in Combating the Opioid Epidemic."

Pursuant to the Rules of the Committee on Energy and Commerce, the hearing record remains open for ten business days to permit Members to submit additional questions for the record, which are attached.

To facilitate the printing of the hearing record, please respond to these questions with a transmittal letter by the close of business on Thursday, May 24, 2018.

Thank you again for your time and effort preparing and delivering testimony before the Subcommittee.

Sincerely, Greg Harper
Chairman
Subcommittee on Oversight and Investigations

cc: The Honorable Diana DeGette, Ranking Member, Subcommittee on Oversight and Investigations

Attachment
U.S. Department of Justice
Office of Legislative Affairs

Office of the Assistant Attorney General
Washington. D.C. 20530
OCT 23 2018

The Honorable Gregg Harper
Chairman
Subcommittee on Oversight and Investigations
Committee on Energy and Commerce
U.S. House of Representatives
Washington, D.C. 20515

Dear Mr. Chairman:

Enclosed please find responses to questions for the record arising from the appearance of Robert W. Patterson, former Acting Administrator of the Drug Enforcement Administration, before the Subcommittee on Oversight and Investigations on March 20, 2018, at a hearing entitled "The Drug Enforcement Administration's Role in Combating the Opioid Epidemic." We apologize for our delay and hope that this information is of assistance to the Committee.

The Office of Management and Budget has advised us that there is no objection to submission of this letter from the perspective of the Administration's program. Please do not hesitate to contact this office if we may be of additional assistance regarding this or any other matter.

Sincerely,
Prim F. Escalona
Principal Deputy Assistant Attorney General

cc: The Honorable Diana DeGette Ranking Member

QUESTIONS FOR THE RECORD, DRUG ENFORCEMENT ADMINISTRATION, FOR A HEARING ENTITLED "THE DRUG ENFORCEMENT ADMINISTRATION'S ROLE IN COMBATING THE OPIOID EPIDEMIC," SUBCOMMITTEE ON OVERSIGHT AND INVESTIGATIONS, COMMITTEE ON ENERGY AND COMMERCE, U.S. HOUSE OF REPRESENTATIVES, MARCH 20, 2018

Questions from Chairman Gregg Hamer

1. How do you define "success" in improving DEA's efforts to combat the opioid epidemic? What performance metrics is DEA using to track such progress?

Response. Due to the complexity of the Drug Enforcement Administration's (DEA) regulatory program, the Diversion Control Division has worked aggressively to improve its communication and cooperation with its nearly 1.8 million registrants, who represent medical professionals, pharmaceutical drug manufacturers, and those in the drug supply chain. DEA works with its registrant population by: (1) hosting Pharmacy Diversion Awareness Conferences and Practitioner Diversion Awareness Conferences (PDACs) throughout the country; (2) administering the Distributor Initiative Program with a goal of educating distributors on how to detect and guard against diversion activities; and (3) maintaining an open dialogue with various national associations such as the National Association of Boards of Pharmacy (NABP),

American Medical Association (AMA), Federation of State Medical Boards, and other groups to address diversion problems and educate the medical community on improving prescribing practices. By the end of 2017, DEA had hosted 100 PDACs in 50 states (as well as the District of Columbia and Puerto Rico) training more than 13,1 00 pharmacists, pharmacy technicians, and others on the important role they play in ensuring that valid prescriptions for controlled substances are filled. In early May 2018, DEA initiated a nationwide program to offer similar training to individual practitioners.

In addition to the training opportunities offered to registrants, DEA has also begun a program to proactively send targeted email messages to various segments of its registrant population on matters of mutual interest. For example, in February 2018, DEA sent correspondence to 1.3 million prescribers nationwide alerting them of the Centers for Disease Control and Prevention's (CDC) recommendation (part of CDC's Prescribing Guideline for Chronic Pain) for opioid prescribing for acute pain and alerted practitioners to a free training webinar available from CDC. DEA will be sending similar correspondence alerting these same practitioners about resources available from the Substance Abuse and Mental Health Services Administration (SAMHSA) on locating a substance abuse treatment provider in their state. We have also sent targeted messages to DEA's Schedule I research population on enhancements made to streamline the registration process, as well as to the manufacturer and distributor populations on new enhancements to assist them in fulfilling their regulatory responsibilities to identify and report suspicious orders. In the coming months, DEA will send targeted messages to certain practitioners on how they may utilize telemedicine to treat opioid use disorders.

Over the last several years, DEA has also noticed a downward trend in the amount of prescriptions for controlled substances being written by prescribers. At the same time, DEA has increased the number of administrative actions (e.g., Immediate Suspension Orders (ISOs), Memorandums of Agreement (MOAs), Letters of Admonition). DEA has also seen an increase in reports through Rx Abuse Hotline, and higher participation and amounts collected at National Prescription Drug Take Back Initiatives (NTBis)). Specifically, combined ISO and Order to Show Cause (OTSC) actions in Fiscal Year (FY) 2017 and FY 2018 have more than doubled since 2014.

Year	Orders to Show Cause Filed	Immediate Suspension Orders Filed
2014	32	8
2015	62	5
2016	57	9
2017	79	6
2018	71	20

2. What is the process that the DEA takes when evaluating the suspicious order reports it receives and the actions the agency takes in response? How long has this evaluative process been in place and how does it differ from DEA's previous suspicious order evaluation process?

Response. Since the enactment of the Controlled Substances Act (CSA) in 1970, all DEA registrants who distribute controlled substances have a statutory duty to "maintain effective controls against diversion" of controlled substances into other than legitimate medical, scientific, and industrial channels. The first regulations implementing the CSA in 1971 contained a provision regarding "suspicious orders of controlled substances." This provision, which has remained essentially unchanged since 1971, currently appears in 21 CFR § 1301.74(b) and reads as follows: "The registrant shall design and operate a system to disclose to the registrant suspicious orders of controlled substances. The registrant shall inform the Field Division Office of the Administration in his area of suspicious orders when discovered by the registrant. Suspicious orders include orders of unusual size, orders deviating substantially from a normal pattern, and orders of unusual frequency."

These Suspicious Order Reports (SORs) are currently fielded and verified by DEA personnel and can be used as a tool to identify and pinpoint vulnerabilities throughout the closed system of drug distribution. Since 2010, DEA has found that certain distributors were not adequately following their internal controls or not reporting suspicious orders. Through negotiated settlements involving civil penalties, compliance agreements, and other remedies, DEA has worked with DEA-registered manufacturers and distributors to strengthen suspicious order monitoring and reporting. DEA is also exploring ways to require that suspicious orders are submitted to a central database. Centralized reporting would provide for a more efficient review, dissemination, and investigation of suspicious activity.

In addition, we have launched a new tool within the Automation of Reports and Consolidated Orders System (ARCOS) to assist drug manufacturers and distributors with their regulatory obligations under the CSA. The tool will allow a distributor or manufacturer to enter the DEA registration number of a prospective purchaser (e.g., pharmacy, hospital, or doctor), as well as a drug code for the controlled substance it wishes to purchase. The ARCOS application will return a count of the number of registrants who have sold that particular controlled substance to that prospective purchaser in the last six months. This new query application will help distributors identify red flags indicative of suspicious orders.

Finally, DEA's Diversion Control Division urges DEA registrants and the public at large to "submit a tip" regarding possible CSA violations, including illicit drug distribution or trafficking; suspicious online pharmacies selling controlled substances over the internet; and the illegal sale and distribution of a prescription drug by individuals, including doctors and pharmacists. These tips are submitted through the

Diversion Control Division website at https://www.deadiversion.usdoj.gov/tips_online.htrn. DEA also maintains a telephone hotline (877-RxABUSE) for the community to submit tips that may establish leads relating to the potential diversion of controlled substances. These tips are submitted to a DEA Field Division for prompt action by either a DEA Special Agent or a professional staff member.

3. What is the current guidance on the amount of time it should take the DEA Chief Counsel's Office to review and respond to an Immediate Suspension Order request?

Response. The Office of Chief Counsel does act and always has acted with expediency when reviewing and processing requests for ISOs. The Office of Chief Counsel, Diversion and Regulatory Litigation Section routinely collaborates with investigative personnel to guide and assist them before the ISO request is submitted to the Diversion Control Division, Pharmaceutical Investigations Section. As part of the case intake process, the Diversion and Regulatory Litigation Section, Pharmaceutical Investigations Section, and investigative personnel from the field work collaboratively to ensure that the requisite evidence has been collected and to confirm the strategy moving forward. Whether and how quickly an ISO can be charged varies from case to case, and necessarily depends on several factors, including whether the requisite evidence has been gathered, the restrictions (if any) on the administrative case placed by the prosecutor's offices handling parallel criminal or civil matters, as well as other investigative needs (e.g., timing the service of the ISO with search and arrest warrants).

4. Does DEA compare the number of opioids a pharmacy receives during a given period of time to the regional average that are received by nearby pharmacies?

If so, how long has that been part of DEA's monitoring practice and how does the agency determine the applicable region? If not, why not?

Response. When DEA initiates a case against a registrant, the investigators use all of the tools available and gather as much information as possible in order to build a strong case. The comparison of opioids received between a targeted pharmacy and regional average received by nearby pharmacies is taken into account; however, there may be legitimate mitigating circumstances that can explain a sudden surge (e.g., the establishment of a long-term care facility nearby). As such, this calculation is only one method used by law enforcement officers and diversion investigators in determining if a registrant is in violation of the CSA.

5. What does the DEA believe it means for a drug distributor to "know your customer?" What kind of due diligence are the distributors expected to exercise over their customers and how often should they be conducting this due diligence?

Response. It is fundamental for sound operations that distributors and manufacturers take reasonable measures to identify their customers, understand the normal and expected transactions typically conducted by those customers, and, consequently, identify those transactions conducted by their customers that are suspicious in nature.

Some states have restrictions on distribution practices that are more stringent than the federal rules. The extent of compliance with state law is taken into consideration when civil, administrative, or criminal actions against a distributor are under consideration. It is required that any regulated person or entity verify that a customer for controlled substances possesses a valid DEA registration or is exempt from that requirement.

The granting of a DEA registration signals only a proper application, the establishment of the required records system, and the required security system at the time of the on-site inspection by DEA. The registration is not a confirmation of proper ongoing business practices and does not relieve the registrant of the responsibility to evaluate such transaction.

Certain regulations also speak to the duty of a registrant. For example 21 C.F.R. § 1301.74(a) states, "[b]efore distributing a controlled substance to any person who the registrant does not know to be registered to possess the controlled substance, the registrant shall make a good faith inquiry either with the Administration or with the appropriate State controlled substances registration agency, if any, to determine that the person is registered to possess the controlled substance."

Further, 21 C.F.R. § 1301.74(b) states, "[t]he registrant shall design and operate a system to disclose to the registrant suspicious orders of controlled substances. The registrant shall inform the Field Division Office of the Administration in his area of suspicious orders when discovered by the registrant. Suspicious orders include orders of unusual size, orders deviating substantially from a normal pattern, and orders or unusual frequency."

6. If a distributor is supposed to know their customer, how is it possible that pharmacies, located in rural West Virginia communities, had orders for egregious volumes of opioids filled by these distributors for years?

Response. DEA defers to the distributors to provide the response to this question. The distributors are best suited to address this matter as it involves their business practices.

7. How many DEA diversion investigators were assigned to West Virginia in 2006, and how did DEA make this staffing determination? How many DEA diversion investigators are assigned to West Virginia currently?

Response. In 2006, there were two diversion investigators assigned to West Virginia, and currently, there are six diversion investigators assigned to West Virginia. DEA considers many factors when compiling its submission for the President's Budget. Our analysis included the development of proposals that identify priorities focused on anticipated program needs and that will allow DEA to continue to target the most significant drug trafficking threats including Consolidated Priority Organization Targets (CPOTs), Priority Target Organizations (PTOs), and other significant drug trafficking organizations (DTOs).

As you may know, between 2006 to 2010, a handful of DEA-registered practitioners in West Virginia turned their practices into pill mill operations by writing prescriptions indiscriminately to individuals for an opioid (in this case hydrocodone combination products), often in combination with a benzodiazepine. These illegitimate prescriptions were submitted to and filled by a pharmacy.

DEA, along with its federal, state, and local partners, identified the individuals involved in violations of the CSA and worked with the U.S. Attorney's Office for the Southern District of West Virginia to arrest the following individuals, all of whom were sent to jail for their crimes.

Date of Arrest	Individual	Registration Number
December 19,2011	William F. Ryckman, MD Owner, Mountain Medical Center	BR5346033 (surrendered 5/13110)
February 2, 2012	James Wooley, Pharmacist Owner, Strosnider, DBA: Sav-Rite Pharmacy	FS1092787 (surrendered 4/7/2009 BS7437064 (surrendered 2/2/2012)
May 24, 2012	Diane E. Shafer, MD	BS6435780 (surrendered 12/16/09)
March 19,2013	Myra Sue Miller, employee of William Ryckman	Not applicable

In addition to the above mentioned arrests and license revocations, the following individuals' registrations were revoked:

Individual	Registration Number
Augusto Abad, MD	FA1136806 (surrendered 2/26/10)
John Tiano, MD	BT7431884 (surrendered 12/15/09)
Katherine Hoover, MD	BH0267890 (retired 7/10/10)

The six DEA registrations noted above were revoked following a voluntary surrender (in some instances pursuant to the terms of a plea agreement). That means that DEA did not need to use its OTSC or ISO authority in these cases, and therefore they do not contribute to the OTSC and ISO statistics that we have previously shared with the Committee. In this way, voluntary surrenders can be just as effective at stemming the diversion of controlled substances as OTSCs and ISOs.

Following these investigations, in December 2013, a total of$1.5 million in assets were seized from these pill mill operators. Myra Miller forfeited her interest in the Mountain Medical Center's two commercial buildings valued at approximately $610,000 along with over $475,000 in cash seized from her residence. Another $413,000 from a bank account in William Ryckman's name was also forfeited. Diane Shafer forfeited $134,000, and Katherine Hoover forfeited $88,000. Funds seized by the Federal Government were then awarded to the West Virginia State Police as part of the Department's Asset Forfeiture Equitable Sharing Program which disperses seized funds to various state and local law enforcement agencies involved in federal investigations.

In addition to the above, the Diversion Control Division has also taken numerous steps to examine sales and monitoring processes. For example, the Diversion Control Division utilizes various reports and records to monitor trends or determine anomalous transactions which can then be developed into investigative leads.' A unit within the Diversion Control Division's Pharmaceutical Investigations Section uses aggregated ARCOS data to identify patterns and trends in the flow of narcotic controlled substances through the closed system of drug distribution. This unit is now proactively preparing quarterly threat assessment reports for each of DEA's 23 Field Divisions to prioritize DEA's limited resources in furtherance of criminal, civil, and regulatory investigations against DEA registrants.

DEA has devoted additional resources to West Virginia by increasing its presence in the state. In 2016, DEA established an Assistant Special Agent in Charge in Charleston, WV. This senior level manager now oversees the entire state from the State Capitol, rather than from Washington, D.C. Also in 2016, DEA added a second Tactical Diversion Squad (TDS) in Clarksburg. In 2017, DEA headquarters deployed one of its two "mobile" TDS groups to West Virginia, which pursues criminal investigations against those who traffic controlled prescription drugs. On January 1, 2018, DEA established the new Louisville Field Division, its 22nd Division Office in the United States. This office covers Kentucky, Tennessee, and West Virginia and will enhance DEA enforcement efforts within the Appalachian mountain region and unify drug trafficking investigations under a single Special Agent in Charge. DEA anticipates that this change will produce more effective investigations on heroin, fentanyl, and prescription opioid trafficking, all of which have a significant impact on the region. The division will also better align DEA with the U.S. Attorney's Offices in those areas, similar to current Bureau of Alcohol, Tobacco, Firearms and Explosives (ATF) and Federal Bureau of Investigation (FBI) offices, and also to the Appalachia High Intensity Drug Trafficking Areas (HIDTA) Program.

Finally, after the explosion and subsequent demise of illegal pill mills in Florida, DEA analyzed and reallocated several hundred positions from its Miami Field Division to other offices across the country, including West Virginia, to better utilize its limited resources.

8. The press reports and the Committee's investigation show internal conflicts between DEA lawyers and DEA investigators that apparently went on for years. Where was the DEA Administrator, and later the Acting Administrator who followed her, during this conflict? Why didn't the former head of the Agency resolve this dispute and unite the agency?

Response. Then DEA Chief Counsel, Wendy Goggin, addressed this issue with the subcommittee staff during her interview on March 23, 2018. We believe the information shared in meeting addressed this concern.

9. What actions are you taking to improve morale at the DEA?

Response. Many of the issues highlighted regarding morale are not reflective of the current state of DEA. Within the last two years, DEA has undergone senior leadership changes within the office of the Administrator, Chief Counsel, and Diversion Control Division. DEA does not believe that there are any overarching morale concerns within the organization.

10. How does the DEA currently utilize PDMP data in its investigations?

Response. As you are aware, prescription drug monitoring programs (PDMPs) are state-run electronic database systems used by practitioners, pharmacists, medical and pharmacy boards, and law enforcement, but access varies according to state Jaw. These programs are established through state legislation and are tailored to the specific needs of each state. DEA strongly champions robust PDMPs and encourages medical professionals to use this important tool to detect and prevent doctor shopping and other forms of diversion. Law enforcement access to request, view, and utilize PDMP data in support of ongoing investigations in a manner that protects personally identifiable information is vital. However, access to information in support of active state and federal investigations varies widely from state to state, with some states requiring a court order in order for law enforcement to obtain data.

DEA utilizes PDMP data in support of its ongoing investigations, particularly to bolster its cases against prescribers or other entities that are acting outside of the law. This data is only one piece of the totality of circumstances that are considered when DEA is pursuing a case against a DEA registrant.

11. What is the DEA doing to address any access barriers the agency currently faces with respect to PDMPs?

Response. DEA and law enforcement face many challenges when trying to access and utilize PDMP data. As mentioned in the response to Question 10 above, law enforcement access to request, view, and utilize PDMP data in support of ongoing investigations in a manner that protects personally identifiable information is vital. However, access to information in support of active state and federal investigations varies widely from state to state, with some states requiring a court order in order for law enforcement to obtain data.

While PDMPs are valuable tools for prescribers, pharmacists, and law enforcement agencies to identify, detect, and prevent nonmedical prescription drug use and diversion, PDMPs do have some limits in their use for detecting diversion at the retail level. For example, drug traffickers and drug seekers willingly travel hundreds of miles to gain easy access to pain clinics and physicians that are operating unscrupulously and outside of the law, making interconnectivity between PDMPs vital. As a result, the Office of National Drug Control Policy (ONDCP) and the Department's Bureau of Justice Assistance (BJA) currently offer assistance for interstate and state-tribal PDMP linkages. CDC's Prevention for States program supports states' advancements to identify and prevent prescription drug overdoses, which includes activities focused on improving interoperability between PDMPs and Electronic Health Record (EHR) technology and providing real-time provider access. Forty-four states are currently able to exchange prescription data between certain states. In some instances, data sharing may be limited to a single neighboring state. In other instances, data sharing may span states within a specific region.

There are currently two interstate data sharing hubs in operation: RxCheck, BJA's open standards solution developed and operated in partnership by the IJIS Institute (IJIS) with funding from BJA; and PMP Interconnect (PMPi), a proprietary solution operated by the National Association of Boards of Pharmacy (NABP). As of August 2017, nine states are live or are implementing interstate data sharing using both hubs, 36 states are live or are implementing interstate data sharing using the PMPi hub only, and 4 states are live or are implementing interstate data sharing using the RxCheck hub only.

Federal partners are working to address interoperability. Brandeis University's PDMP Training and Technical Center, funded by BJA, has assisted the IHS to improve interoperability between IHS, its pharmacies, and PDMPs. BJA currently provides funding to 30 states through the Harold Rogers PDMP Program for implementation, enhancements, or enhanced data sharing, including interstate data sharing. CDC supports work in states to enhance and maximize PDMPs as a public health and clinical tool.

In addition, DEA has entered into information sharing agreements with multiple coalitions of state Attorneys General and an individual state Attorney General. Pursuant to those agreements, each of which have confidentiality provisions, state Attorneys General have committed to assisting the DEA obtain PDMP information from their states. Law enforcement access to this data is crucial to help build the strongest cases possible against those actors who are acting outside of the law.

Question from the Honorable Michael C. Burgess

12. I recently reviewed a document published by the Drug Enforcement Administration's Diversion Control Division listing all of the DEA investigations of physician registrants that resulted in the arrest and prosecution of the registrant. I was surprised to see that this list, despite going back to the early 2000s, is only 103 pages long. This list also shows that recent activity has been diminishing, despite that the number of opioid deaths has substantially increased in recent years. What is the reason for the decline in data regarding arrests and prosecution of physician registrants since 2010?

Response. DEA has seen an increase of doctors in voluntarily surrendering registrations, which results in the diminishing numbers of prosecutorial actions being taken against prescribers.

Questions from the Honorable Tim Walberg

13. How long from start to finish should it take to issue an Immediate Suspension Order (ISO)?

Response. How quickly an ISO can be charged varies from case to case, and necessarily depends on several factors, including whether the requisite evidence has been gathered, the restrictions (if any) on the administrative case placed by the prosecutor's offices handling parallel criminal or civil matters, as well as other investigative needs (e.g., timing the service of the ISO with search and arrest warrants).

14. Do you expect the field division to act with expediency when they identify a situation that could warrant the use of an ISO?

Response. Yes, the Office of Chief Counsel, Diversion and Regulatory Litigation Section routinely collaborates with investigative personnel before the ISO request is submitted to the Diversion Control Division, Pharmaceutical Investigations Section. As part of the case intake process, the Diversion and Regulatory Litigation Section, Pharmaceutical Investigations Section, and investigative personnel from the field work collaboratively to ensure that the requisite evidence has been gathered and to confirm the strategy for moving forward.

15. If too much time passes between a field division's request for an ISO and a DEA lawyer's approval of the ISO, could that undermine the original evidence and justification the field relied upon in their request for an ISO?

Response. DEA personnel routinely collaborate to make sure that all administrative actions (including OTSCs and ISOs) are supported by the requisite evidence and are processed as quickly as possible. Specifically, the Office of Chief Counsel, Diversion and Regulatory Litigation Section routinely collaborates with investigative personnel before the ISO request is submitted to the Diversion Control Division, Pharmaceutical Investigations Section. As noted above, whether and how quickly an ISO can be charged can and does vary from case to case, and necessarily depends on several factors.

16. Would you expect the Chief Counsel's office to act with expediency when they receive an ISO request from the field?

Response. The Office of Chief Counsel does act and always has acted appropriately when reviewing and processing requests for ISOs.

17. I'd like to draw your attention to a case that originated in my home state of Michigan. This case shows the practical consequences of some of the questions my colleague from Virginia, Mr. Griffith, asked you.

In December 2013, Dentist Mark Kamp agreed to pay $125,000 to settle claims that he wrote hundreds of illegitimate prescriptions for hydrocodone and other drugs this includes drugs given to at least two Birmingham Public School bus drivers. According to emails obtained by the Committee, DEA agents wanted to issue an ISO against Mr. Kamp at least eight months earlier, presumably because of the immediate danger to the community. But an email sent Apri123, 2013 from a senior attorney evaluating the case appears to indicate that the Office of Chief Counsel believed a medical expert would be needed to review prescriptions and patient charts and render an expert opinion before the issuance of an ISO.

On the same day the attorney made that assessment, someone involved with the case we don't know who because the name is redacted wrote back to ask whether DEA attorneys would require the field to obtain a medical expert before submission of any ISO. The person flagged both the associated cost and delay and stated this was not required in past cases brought against physicians and pharmacies. That email seemingly went unanswered for more than a month, until DEA attorneys finally provided the requested guidance. According to Dr. Kamp's settlement, he continued issuing illegitimate prescriptions for controlled substances through September 2013, though he eventually surrendered his DEA registration.

a. But in a case in which an ISO is being sought, do you expect the Chief Counsel's Office to respond to questions about the case in a timely manner? Does this seem like an undue delay to you both on the part of the Chief Counsel's office for not responding to the question, but also on the part of the field for waiting a month to follow up?

Response. As previously mentioned, the Office of Chief Counsel does act and always has acted appropriately when reviewing and processing requests for ISOs. The Office of Chief Counsel, Diversion and Regulatory Litigation Section routinely collaborates with investigative personnel before the ISO request is submitted to the Diversion Control Division, Pharmaceutical Investigations Section. Whether and how quickly an ISO can be charged can and does vary from case to case, and necessarily depends on several factors noted above.

18. Another email obtained from DEA seems to indicate that the Chief Counsel's Office provided some internal guidance on deadlines for responding to an ISO request from the field. One email from May 2013 references a 3-day window in which DEA attorneys should review and act on ISO requests if the evidence submitted was stale. The unknown author of the email also poses a question to Lee Reeves about whether DEA attorneys are required to act on all ISO requests within 7 days. What is the current guidance on the amount of time it should take the DEA Chief Counsel's Office to review and respond to an ISO request?

Response. As previously mentioned, whether and how quickly an ISO can be charged can and does vary from case to case, and necessarily depends on several factors, including whether the requisite evidence has been gathered, the restrictions (if any) on the administrative case placed by the prosecutor's offices handling parallel criminal or civil matters, as well as other investigative needs (e.g., timing the service of the ISO with search and arrest warrants). However, the Office of Chief Counsel does act and always has acted appropriately when reviewing and processing requests for ISOs.

Questions from the Honorable Frank Pallone, Jr.

19. How many instances has DEA identified using proactive analysis of ARCOS data- of distributors shipping potentially excessive amounts of opioids in the last two years? How many instances has DEA identified using proactive analysis of ARCOS data- of pharmacies receiving potentially excessive amounts of opioids in the last two years?

Response. DEA identified 160 distributors that shipped potentially excessive amounts of opioids from January 2016 to June 2018 using proactive analyses of ARCOS data.

DEA identified 7,680 pharmacies that purchased potentially excessive amounts of opioids in the last two years: 2,073 in 2016, 4,228 in 2017, and 1,379 from Jan June, 2018 using proactive analyses of ARCOS data. These pharmacies were identified in top purchaser or above average listings, in the United States, a state, county, or zip code. DEA also utilized a Department of Health and Human Services (HHS) dataset (Medicare Part D) to identify 181 pharmacy outliers.

20. What types of proactive ARCOS analytics does DEA now perform that would identify a pharmacy that received amounts of controlled substances from each of its distributors that would not raise red flags, but when aggregated among all of its suppliers would total a sufficiently large amount that could be considered suspicious? In how many instances has DEA performed such analyses and identified such pharmacies in the last two years? What actions, if any, did DEA take after identifying such information in those instances?

Response. In the ARCOS online system, pharmacy totals are automatically aggregated among all of its suppliers unless distributor totals are needed separately. The ARCOS system aggregates continuously, and supplier totals are automatically generated. Additionally, all Diversion Investigators (Dis) have access to the ARCOS system and can run their own reports and analysis. All ARCOS leads and analytical results are sent to DEA Field Offices and/or our federal, state, and/or local law enforcement partners for further investigation.

21. What types of proactive ARCOS analytics does DEA now perform that would identify a geographic region (e.g., by three-digit ZIP code preflx) that received suspiciously high amounts of opioids? In how many instances has DEA performed such analyses and identified such geographic areas in the last two years? What actions, if any, did DEA take after identifying such information in those instances?

Response. DEA currently sends out proactive Targeting Analysis packages to the various field offices when a red flag has been raised through a review of ARCOS data and has not been resolved by the registrant. Those leads are continuously generated and used by the field, in addition to and with other sources of information, to determine if the registrant is acting outside of the closed system of distribution. DEA also sends out an annual threat assessment to the various field offices that can be used to help identify areas where potential diversion may be occurring within those geographic locations. ARCOS data is not the sole determining factor in deciphering if diversion is occurring but can be a useful tool when combined with other investigative tools to determine if a registrant is a bad actor. The actions taken by DEA as a result of these investigations has varied depending upon the discovery of diversion and if the registrant was continuing to be non-compliant.

22. How many full time equivalent (FTE) employees does DEA have dedicated to proactively analyzing ARCOS data for the purposes of identifying troubling trends (such as potential diversion, fraud, or abuse) and potential investigations into distributors and pharmacies?

Response. DEA currently has two units that are dedicated to analyzing ARCOS data the Targeting and Analysis Unit and the ARCOS Unit. The Targeting and Analysis Unit is responsible for reviewing ARCOS reports, running various analytics, and sending targeting packages out to the field offices for further investigation or to support any current on-going investigations that were initiated in another manner (e.g., a tip from a Confidential Source or a report into our RX Abuse Hotline). The ARCOS Unit is responsible for verifying the information that is input by the manufacturers and distributors who are required to report to ARCOS on a quarterly basis.

23. To what extent does DEA share ARCOS data with state law enforcement agencies, attorneys general, public health agencies, and other state agencies? How often does DEA share this data, and what amount of granularity does DEA provide (e.g., does the data identify distributors and pharmacies)?

Response. It has long been DEA policy to share ARCOS data (and other DEA information) with state law enforcement agencies, state Attorneys General, state public health agencies, and other state agencies involved in active civil or criminal cases involving controlled substances. The frequency and nature of the information shared varies and is dependent upon the number of active investigations.

In April 2018, the Department filed a motion to participate as a "friend of the court" in the ongoing Multi-District Litigation (MDL) against opioid manufacturers and distributors.

That litigation, which has been consolidated in the Northern District of Ohio, involves more than 900 lawsuits brought predominately by state and local governments against opioid manufacturers and distributors. DEA has provided the MDL parties ARCOS data concerning the most commonly abused prescription opioids. The shared ARCOS data encompasses transactions between January 1, 2006 and December 31, 2014 and is not redacted. Therefore, it identifies distributors, manufacturers, and pharmacies The DEA also provided the parties with select SORs. All of the information the DEA provided in the MDL is covered by a protective order.

DEA also recently entered into information sharing agreements with two separate coalitions of state Attorneys General and an individual state Attorney General. Each agreement has a confidentiality provisions. DEA intends to provide the state Attorneys General who enter into those agreements the same information it provides the parties in the MDL.

24. During your testimony, you stated that DEA intends to change the way it uses suspicious order reports that it receives from distributors. What does DEA now do with the suspicious order reports it receives from distributors? What changes does DEA intend to make with the suspicious order reports?

Response. Since the enactment of the CSA in 1970, all DEA registrants who distribute controlled substances have a statutory duty to "maintain effective controls against diversion" of controlled substances into other than legitimate medical, scientific, and industrial channels. The first regulations implementing the CSA in 1971 contained a provision regarding "suspicious orders of controlled substances." This provision, which has remained essentially unchanged since 1971, currently appears in 21 C.F.R. § 1301.74(b) and reads as follows:

The registrant shall design and operate a system to disclose to the registrant suspicious orders of controlled substances. The registrant shall inform the Field Division Office of the Administration in his area of suspicious orders when discovered by the registrant. Suspicious orders include orders of unusual size, orders deviating substantially from a normal pattern, and orders of unusual frequency.

This information is currently fielded and verified by DEA personnel across its 22 Field Divisions and can be used as a tool to identify and pinpoint vulnerabilities throughout the closed system of drug distribution. Since 2010, DEA has found that certain distributors were not adequately following their internal controls or not submitting suspicious orders. Through fines and other remedies, DEA has developed agreements with DEA-registered manufacturers and distributors to strengthen suspicious order monitoring and reporting.

25. How many suspicious order reports does DEA now receive from distributors annually?

Response. DEA currently has one active MOA with a distributor pursuant to settlement agreement that requires them to submit SORs electronically to DEA headquarters. Over the years there have been a number of registrant distributors and manufacturers who have also been under MOA's as a result of administrative actions taken against them. DEA headquarters has received 1,204,400 electronic SORs from 135 distinct registrants from 2007 to 2018.

DEA is also in the process of creating a centralized reporting system in which all manufacturers and distributors would be required to report suspicious orders, therefore creating a quicker turnaround time for investigation into verified suspicious orders.

26. How many cases has DEA initiated against registrants as a result of suspicious order reports it received in the last two years?

Response. SORs are regularly used as one element to build a case against a registrant that appears to be acting outside of the regulations set forth in the CSA. These reports are used in conjunction with various other elements to support taking criminal, civil, or administrative action against a registrant and are not enough in and of themselves to make a case against registrant.

27. What is the status of DEA' s draft regulations that would require suspicious orders to be reported electronically and to DEA's central office?

Response. DEA regulations requiring a suspicious order to be reported electronically to DEA headquarters are in the process of being drafted and will undergo the required inter and intra-agency review.

28. Has DEA provided any additional guidance or outreach to registrants regarding what constitutes a suspicious order? If so, please provide details of such guidance or outreach, including copies and the date such guidance was provided or outreach was conducted.

Response. DEA continues to provide guidance on what constitutes a suspicious order through formal training and informal interactions with registrants. Since the enactment of the CSA, all DEA registrants who distribute controlled substances have a statutory duty to "maintain effective controls against diversion" of controlled substances into other than legitimate medical, scientific, and industrial channels. The first regulations implementing the CSA in 1971 contained a provision regarding “suspicious orders of controlled substances.” This provision, which has remained essentially unchanged since 1971, currently appears in 21 C.F.R. § 1301.74(b) and reads as follows: “The registrant shall design and operate a system to disclose to the registrant suspicious orders of controlled substances. The registrant shall inform the Field Division Office of the Administration in his area of suspicious orders when discovered by the registrant. Suspicious orders include orders of unusual size, orders deviating substantially from a normal pattern, and orders of unusual frequency.”

29. Which DEA division is responsible for determining what recommendation to provide the Administrator to take a particular administrative action against a registrant (e.g., Order to Show Cause or Immediate Suspension Order)?

Response. Each DEA Field Division is responsible for determining which recommendation to provide to the Administrator with regards to a particular administrative action (e.g., OTSC or ISO) that will be taken against a registrant within their own division. That recommendation is then reviewed by the Office of Chief Counsel prior to obtaining concurrence or nonconcurrence from the Assistant Administrator of the Diversion Control Division. Under regulation, OTSCs may only require concurrence at the Diversion Control Division level. ISOs require concurrence or nonconcurrence from the Administrator.

30. During your testimony, you stated that DEA has begun to use ARCOS data in a more proactive manner to identify potential diversion cases. In an April2, 2018 press

release, DEA announced that in February and March, "DEA surged the efforts of special agents, Diversion investigators, and intelligence research specialists to analyze 80 million transaction reports from DEA-registered manufacturers and distributors" that resulted in 366leads and 188 active investigations, culminating in 28 arrests, 54 other enforcement actions, and 283 administrative actions. However, during your testimony, you referred to "approximately 400 targeted leads" that DEA developed based on ARCOS and other data, and that "of those 400 packages that went out, a good majority of what we saw in that data and the outliers and what they identified were ongoing cases that we already bad."

a. To clarify, how many of those 188 investigations were initiated as a result of DEA identifying leads through proactive analysis of its ARCOS data (as opposed to analyzing ARCOS data to support already ongoing investigations)? What actions were taken in those cases?

Response. The cited investigative data is derived from DEA's case management system, which does not track the initiating factor (e.g., a tip from the public, information that is discovered in a different investigation, ARCOS information provided to an office, etc.), so we are unable to provide that information. The reference to ARCOS data helped to underscore the fact that investigations are supplemented by ARCOS data and that ARCOS data is not used as the sole determining factor in the initiation of investigations.

Questions from the Honorable Yvette Clarke

31. How can the DEA take a more nuanced approach to managing the supply of legal schedule II opioid medications? As we are seeing, simply cutting legal production is going to cause irreparable harm to hospice and palliative care patients and families in the New York 91h and nationwide?

Response. The quota system is a nimble regulatory tool in which DEA establishes individual quotas for manufacturers based on a variety of information. The quota is then used to produce all drug products that contain that controlled substance. The manufacturer determines the allocation of that quota to the various products (and strengths) it produces. It is outside DEA's regulatory authority to compel a manufacturer to use its quota to manufacture a specific drug product that may be in shortage. In situations where DEA is made aware of the need for an increased quota and an increase can be adequately justified, DEA works quickly to make the necessary adjustments. However, since the Food and Drug Administration Safety and Innovation Act of 2012 (FDASIA) was enacted in July 2012, no special requests for expedited quota review have been forwarded to DEA.

32. How does the DEA plan to deal with the shortage of both injectable opioids and benzodiazepines?

Response. Since January 31, 2018, the Diversion Control Division has received comments from hospital groups and stakeholders. These groups have expressed serious concerns regarding the shortages of injectable products that contain Schedule II controlled substances, namely fentanyl, meperidine, hydromorphone, and oxymorphone. In response to the concerns raised by these groups, the Diversion Control Division established a "working group" to assess the alleged shortages, began holding conference calls with various vested entities from industry to cancer centers, and continues to keep stakeholders apprised of its efforts.

Early in 2018, the working group discovered that two companies, who had requested additional procurement quota, alleged that the drug shortages were being created by DEA. We take such claims seriously and have researched this issue. Based upon that research, DEA has determined that these two manufacturers had significant discrepancies in reports they submitted to DEA. DEA relies upon the information in those reports when establishing each manufacturer's quota, specifically their Year-End Report (YERS) and quarterly reports submitted to ARCOS. In order to address the deficiencies in those reports, DEA is currently performing administrative inspections at both companies to resolve these inaccuracies.

Since mid-February, three DEA-registered manufacturers of injectable products have received increases to their respective procurement quotas in accordance with DEA regulations (21 C.F.R. § 1303.12). DEA is communicating directly with these manufacturers and will continue to adjust individual procurement quotas as necessary. DEA is working tirelessly, in coordination with the Food and Drug Administration (FDA)'s Drug Shortage team, and will continue to review all potential solutions to help address the issue.

Questions from the Honorable David B. McKinley

33. On March 1, 2018, Attorney General Sessions issued a directive for you to reform DEA's drug quota regulations, including a potential interim final rule with immediate effectiveness that would govern quotas for next year. When can we expect this and can you provide my office with an update?

Response. DEA final rule titled "Controlled Substances Quotas" was published on July 16, 2018 and became effective on August 15, 2018. *See* 83 F.R. 32784.

34. Does federal law require that drug quotas must be based on legitimate patient needs, not what drug makers want in terms of production?

Response. Data and considerations utilized by DEA to establish quotas includes: total net disposals (i.e., sales) for the current and preceding two years; estimates of medical need (provided by the FDA); actual and estimated inventory; U.S. export requirements; product development requirements; manufacturing losses and other factors that affect "yield"; and documented theft and loss data (i.e., diversion). 21 U.S.C. § 826(a) requires the Attorney General to determine the total quantity and establish production quotas to be manufactured each calendar year for each basic class of controlled substance in Schedules I and II, and ephedrine, pseudoephedrine, and phenylpropanolamine. These aggregate production quotas (APQs) provide for the estimated medical, scientific, research, and industrial needs of the United States, for lawful export requirements, and for the establishment and maintenance of reserve stocks. DEA is charged with the management of controlled substances and chemicals for scientific, medical, research, and industrial applications, while also preventing diversion of these same substances and chemicals. To manage this complex system, DEA requires that manufacturers of Schedule I and II controlled substances and the importers and manufacturers of ephedrine, pseudoephedrine, and phenylpropanolamine (Combat Methamphetamine Epidemic Act (CMEA) List I chemicals) apply for quotas to control the quantity of material produced or procured per calendar year.

35. Does the Controlled Substances Act require quotas to be set at the amount America "needs" or quotas be set at the amount that drug makers "want"? [*see* 21U.S.C.§ 826(a) ("total quantity ... to provide for the estimated medical ...needs of the United States")]

Response. As set out in the response to Question 34 above, DEA considers a variety of factors when proposing the APQs for the following year. Please note that the APQs are established through notice and comment rulemaking procedures after an assessment of the factors described in 21 C.F.R. § 1303.1l(b), including:

(1) Total net disposal of the class by all manufacturers during the current and two preceding years;
(2) Trends in the national rate of net disposal of the class;
(3) Total actual (or estimated) inventories of the class and of all substances manufactured from the class, and trends in inventory accumulation;
(4) Projected demand for such class as indicated by procurement quotas requested pursuant to 21 C.F.R. *§* 1303.12; and
(5) Other factors affecting medical, scientific, research, and industrial needs in the United States and lawful export requirements, as the Administrator finds relevant, including changes in the currently accepted medical use in treatment with the class or the substances which are manufactured from it, the economic and physical availability of raw materials for use in manufacturing and for inventory purposes, yield and stability problems, potential disruptions to production (including possible labor strikes), and recent unforeseen emergencies such as floods and fires.

In this way, the APQs represent more than retail sales resulting from prescriptions issued by practitioners nationwide. The APQs include quantities required for product development, manufacturing losses, research, exports, various categories of non-saleable materials, and inventory levels of 50 percent for bulk manufacturers. The APQ values can vary based on the number and status of new products being researched (material set aside and not saleable), international contracts (for exports), manufacturers establishing contracts with backup active pharmaceutical ingredients (API) suppliers, and new manufacturers entering the market.

36. Is the current quota system flawed because it relies too heavily on drug maker's estimate of how many pills they can sell?

Response. No, as highlighted in the responses to Questions 34 and 35 above, DEA takes into account multiple data points and considerations when establishing quotas.

37. As I referenced in my testimony, the DEA cut the supply to methamphetamines and other drugs that were being abused in the 1970's and 1980's and had success in reducing abuse problems. Yet the quota for prescription opioids was consistently raised by the DEA from the 1990's to present day. Would it not be accurate to say that these unchecked increases in opioid quotas were one of the root causes of this crisis?

Response. The APQ for each year is established on the best actual and forecasted data provided to the DEA in the Spring of the previous year, from various sources as required by 21 C.F.R. § 1303.11. Throughout the course of the following calendar year, each individual manufacturer's quota request is analyzed using actual year-to-date data at the time of submission and annualized for the remainder of the calendar year. This quota review process allows DEA to administer quota allotments based on current trends and recent changes in an individual manufacturer's national rates of disposal, FDA notifications, changes in production cycles, current inventory position, as well as yield, stability, and recall issues *(see* 21 C.F.R. §§ 1303.23-1303.26 and 1303.12). This individualized analysis typically results in lower individual quota allotments than originally predicted by the DEA, which were based on actual and forecasted data received from the various sources during the initial APQ analysis completed prior to the start of the calendar year.

Since 2014, DEA has observed a decline in prescriptions written for certain Schedule II opioids. These declines have led to overall reductions in licit demand that in turn, have directly impacted the factors DEA considers when establishing the APQs for Schedule II opioids. In October 2016, DBA announced a 25 percent reduction (or more) in the 2017 APQs for many prescription opioids, including oxycodone, hydrocodone, fentanyl, hydromorphone, and morphine. Hydrocodone was reduced to 66 percent of the previous year's (2016) level. In late 2017, DBA announced a nearly 20 percent reduction in the 2018 APQs (from the 2017levels) for controlled substances, and these reductions included the aforementioned opioids as well as oxymorphone, codeine, and meperidine. These decreases can be attributed to combined local, state, and federal activities and interventions, including creating new partnerships, enforcing current regulations, and dissemination of provider education and guidance documents, including the CDC Guideline for Prescribing Opioids for Chronic Pain released in March 2016. In addition, we are encouraged that more states have enacted and enforced laws mandating the use of PDMPs by medical providers and pharmacists which provides prescribers with valuable information to guide their medical decisions.

38. When the quotas were being set, wasn't in DEA's responsibility to ensure that they were being used for legitimate patient needs? Did patients in Williamson, West Virginia, population 2,900 need 21 million opioids over a 10 year period (2006-2016)? Was there not negligence on the part of the DEA in increasing these quotas and if so, who is being held responsible?

Response. DBA is responsible for determining the total quantity and establish production quotas for each basic class of controlled substance in Schedules I and II to be manufactured each calendar year to provide for the estimated medical, scientific, research, and industrial needs of the United States. However, the quota provisions of the CSA were not designed to work in isolation in combatting the diversion problem. Under the full scheme of the CSA, the nearly 1.8 million registrants must work in concert with DEA for an effective diversion control program. A prescription for a controlled substance must be issued for a legitimate medical purpose by an individual practitioner acting in the usual course of his professional practice. Therefore, when noncompliant registrants willfully write fraudulent prescriptions for controlled substances, reductions in quota would simply reduce the total amounts of controlled substances being supplied to both the licit and illicit markets.

39. If the quotas are based on legitimate patient need, then why can't we be more transparent in terms of the manufacturer's justification for how many pills they want to make?

Response. DEA supports transparency and continues to make strides to increase transparency in many different facets across the agency. In instances pertaining to quota justification, DEA is required to protect the commercial information of innocent parties. It is the policy of the United States Government--enforced by the threat of criminal sanction-to protect as confidential the business records commercial enterprises are compelled to give the government *See* 18 U.S.C. § 1905 ("Whoever, being an officer or employee of the United States or of any department or agency thereof ... publishes, divulges, discloses, or makes known in any manner ... any information coming to him in the course of his employment or official duties or by reason of any examination or investigation made by, or return, report or record made to or filed with, such department or agency or officer or employee thereof, which information concerns or relates to the trade secrets, processes, operations, style of work, or apparatus, or to the identity, confidential statistical data, amount or source of any income, profits, losses, or expenditures of any person, firm, partnership, corporation, or association; or permits any income return or copy thereof or any book containing any abstract or particulars thereof to be seen or examined by any person except as provided by law; shall be fined under this title, or imprisoned not more than one year, or both; and shall be removed from office or employment.") For this reason, generally DEA does not disclose information to the public that it believes is either confidential or proprietary. An important exception to this rule is when DEA cooperates with and shares information with local, state, tribal and federal Agencies. *See* 21 U.S.C. § 873.

In: Battling the Opioid Epidemic
Editor: Vincent Hardy

ISBN: 978-1-53615-548-8

Chapter 3

CARTELS AND THE U.S. HEROIN EPIDEMIC: COMBATING DRUG VIOLENCE AND PUBLIC HEALTH CRISIS*

The Subcommittee on Western Hemisphere, Transnational Crime, Democracy, Civilian Security, Human Rights, and Global Women's Issues

Thursday, May 26, 2016
U.S. Senate,
Subcommittee on Western Hemisphere, Transnational Crime, Civilian Security, Democracy, Human Rights, And Global Women's Issues,
Committee on Foreign Relations

The subcommittee met, pursuant to notice, at 9:03 a.m. in Room SD–419, Dirksen Senate Office Building, Hon. Marco Rubio, chairman of the subcommittee, presiding.

Present: Senators Rubio, Gardner, Boxer, Kaine, Menendez, and Markey.

* This is an edited, reformatted and augmented version of Hearing before the Subcommittee on Western Hemisphere, Transnational Crime, Democracy, Civilian Security, Human Rights, and Global Women's Issues, Committee on Foreign Relations, United States Senate, One Hundred Fourteenth Congress, Second Session, dated May 26, 2016.

OPENING STATEMENT OF HON. MARCO RUBIO, U.S. SENATOR FROM FLORIDA

Senator RUBIO. Good morning. This hearing on the Subcommittee of the Western Hemisphere, Transnational Crime, Civilian Security, Democracy, Human Rights, and Global Women's Issues will come to order. I thank you for being here today.

The title of this hearing is "Cartels and the U.S. Heroin Epidemic: Combating Drug Violence and Public Health Crisis."

Before we begin the meeting, on a matter of personal privilege, I wanted to acknowledge the contributions of a loyal and a dedicated staffer because behind every one of us here in the Senate, there are loyal and really hardworking people. Literally they sit behind us at these meetings, and they do all the hard work behind the scenes to make sure that we are briefed and prepared to cast votes and advance public policy that makes a difference.

Since 2011, Maggie Dougherty has been an instrumental part of our policy team, and she has logged in countless hours working on all sorts of complex and important issues for our office. She has also logged in countless hours sitting behind us here in these committee meetings, but no longer. Today is Maggie's last Senate Foreign Relations Committee meeting. In a week's time, she will depart our office to even a bigger and better opportunity. So I just briefly wanted to thank her for everything she has done for us. We are very proud of her work. [Applause.]

Senator RUBIO. So the title of this hearing, "Cartels and the U.S. Heroin Epidemic"—we have two panels testifying. The first is an official panel that will feature Mr. Daniel Foote, the Deputy Assistant Secretary of State for the Bureau of International Narcotics and Law Enforcement at the U.S. Department of State, and Mr. Kemp Chester, the Associate Director for the National Heroin Coordination Group for the Office of National Drug Control Policy.

The second panel will present the Honorable Teresa Jacobs, the Mayor of Orange County, Florida, and Mr. Steven Dudley, the Co- Director of InSight Crime.

Thank you all for being here today. We appreciate your time. We appreciate your dedication. I would also like to thank all of those who worked alongside my staff and making this hearing possible.

Drug cartels operate out of countries in the western hemisphere, and they do so by using sophisticated distribution systems that move narcotics into and across the United States. Heroin supplied by these cartels has created a public health epidemic and fueled drug violence across this country.

The heroin epidemic, drug war, and fight against drug violence are, unfortunately, becoming part of everyday events in our society. It is our duty to find the best possible avenues and allocate resources to provide the best tools to equip those on the front lines to fight this public health crisis. We need to examine what the United States, Mexico, and other regional partners are doing to cooperatively address the rise in heroin and in drug trafficking. Promoting the efficacy and proper execution of U.S. initiatives to stop the spread of heroin and combat the drug cartels should be one of our top priorities.

Here are some facts. One of the primary culprits in this fight is called fentanyl. It is a synthetic opiate that is 25 to 40 times more potent than heroin and it may be used to treat pain associated with advanced cancer. While fentanyl is legally prescribed in the United States, the CDC states that most cases of fentanyl-related overdoses are associated with non-pharmaceutical fentanyl. It is a type used as a substitute for heroin or mixed with heroin or other drugs, sometimes without the user's knowledge.

In 2015, the DEA's National Drug Threat Assessment Summary reported that Mexico and China have been cited as the primary source country, though some analogs of fentanyl are manufactured in China. These supplies are often trafficked into the United States across the southwest border or delivered through mail couriers. Transnational criminal organizations also use Florida as the point of arrival for South American cocaine and heroin. Much of the illegally diverted and produced fentanyl is found in the same U.S. markets where white powder heroin is found.

According to the Substance Abuse and Mental Health Services Administration, the estimated number of individuals who used heroin was 914,000 people in 2014.

In addition, there are about 586,000 individuals, or basically .2 percent of the 12 and older population, who had a heroin disorder in 2014.

While there has been an increase in heroin overdoses and heroin- related deaths across the United States, the Midwest and the Northeast regions have been areas of particular concern. To this day despite the administration's efforts, heroin-related overdose deaths increased by 244 percent between 2007 and the year 2013.

The U.S. has responded to such findings by launching the Heroin Response Strategy, leveraging upon the 15 high intensity drug trafficking areas across the country.

Mexico, our regional partner, has displayed willingness to cooperate with U.S. authorities, but despite these operations, the International Narcotics Control Strategy Report estimates that less than 2 percent of cocaine that comes through Mexico is seized by this country's authorities. Under the Merida Initiative, Congress has provided billions in funds to the Mexican Government to improve security and the rule of law, and I applaud the continued efforts of the Mexican Government to continue its drug crop eradication efforts and to arrest drug kingpins. However, we are still far from the finish line.

I think the Congress can continue to work in constructive ways to promote legislation addressing opiate abuse. I am proud to be the cosponsor of the Comprehensive Addiction and Recovery Act, a bipartisan bill that overwhelmingly passed the Senate. I also applaud the House for working to address this issue, and I hope soon we will be able to send this legislation to the President's desk.

It is my hope that today's hearing will shed light on the consequences that this epidemic will have in our society and future generations if left unaddressed and not given proper attention. I am optimistic this hearing will serve as the opportunity to learn about the administration's priorities in combating the heroin epidemic and drug violence. And I hope you will address these issues in your testimony as well.

With that, I will now turn it over to our ranking member, Senator Boxer, for her opening statement.

STATEMENT OF HON. BARBARA BOXER, U.S. SENATOR FROM CALIFORNIA

Senator BOXER. Mr. Chairman, thank you so much for holding this important hearing.

The abuse of illegal and legal drugs in America is an absolute crisis, and to fight it, we need to act on many fronts.

Take the case of opioids. These are legal prescription drugs that are killing approximately 125 people every single day here at home. The CDC says that in 2014, 47,000 people died from opioid abuse. Just imagine that.

We need to do much more than we have done so far to put real dollars behind the effort to stop this madness.

Then there is the issue we will focus on today of illegal drugs being transported into this country.

Recently I visited Costa Rica, and I learned that this peaceful country is very alarmed about drug cartels infiltrating their population. We must help them stop this real threat. And I hope to ask a question about that.

And while we are working cooperatively with the Mexican Government, specifically an initiative called the Merida Initiative, and while we have to date seized more than $4 billion in narcotics and illicit currency, let us face it. That is a drop in the bucket. We simply have to address the demand in the United States for these lethal products. And I know that is not your job, and I am not going to even ask you about that. But I am making a statement as a United States Senator. We have to address the demand in the United States for these lethal products.

Supply and demand go hand in hand. A long time ago, I was an economics major. It is like economics 101. When people demand a product, we know what happens. The supply will come. And when even more people demand a product, the price will go up and it goes around in a circle.

Years ago, too many to even mention—so I do not even know where my chairman was at that time it was so long ago, very long—when I first came to Congress, I wrote a bill called Treatment on Demand because what I found out, Mr. Chairman and members, is that when there is a person in America with a terrible addiction, at that time—and it is so true today—they wake up one day and they say I have done it, I have had it, I need a new life. They cannot get in anywhere. So people say, very good, come back in 2 weeks. This is an emergency circumstance in many ways, but it is not considered that. So they will go in. Maybe they will get a pat on the back. Come back in 2 weeks. And by then, maybe they have even overdosed.

Now, I know we are working with Colombia and Guatemala helping farmers develop alternatives to opium production. But again, we need to be even more aggressive in our policies regarding drug production, trafficking, and consumption here at home.

In California, we have four of those areas that my chairman spoke about that are designated as high intensity drug trafficking areas by the Obama administration. I am extremely grateful to the administration. We had that help under George Bush as well. When you identify an area, it means you are going to get some attention, some Federal dollars, some Federal help because a lot of these local people, our police forces and so on, really do need that help. So I am very grateful for that.

We have also discovered tunnels from Mexico to San Diego, which act as conduits for thousands of pounds of cocaine. And this points to the continuous challenges we face in dealing with these dangerous cartels. They are really good at what they do, and they intimidate everyone. And that is why this fight is so critical. We need even stronger partnerships with Mexico and other countries in the region.

And I want to say this. Alienating our Latin American neighbors and our Latinos here at home is the worst possible thing we can do, first of all, on a human level because in my view it is prejudice and bigotry. But it does not make sense if we are really trying to crack down on these cartels. We need our friends to work with us. We do not need to escalate some kind of ridiculous debate about walls and all the rest.

I do want to thank our witnesses for being here today. There is a lot of burden on you, and this is very difficult. The war on drugs has not been a success. And I think the reason is we have not done enough on the demand side or on any side. We need to do much better.

And I want to thank my chairman because I think this is really well-timed given what we are facing with the opioid crisis. Thank you.

Senator RUBIO. Thank you, Senator Boxer.

Before we begin with the testimony, I did want to recognize the senior Senator from New Jersey, who has done an extreme amount of work on western hemisphere issues but also issues regarding transnational crime, if he wanted to give any opening comment.

Senator MENENDEZ. No, thank you.

Senator RUBIO. With that, please join me in welcoming our first witness, Mr. Foote. Thank you for your testimony before us here today.

STATEMENT OF DANIEL L. FOOTE, DEPUTY ASSISTANT SECRETARY OF STATE, BUREAU OF INTERNATIONAL NARCOTICS AND LAW ENFORCEMENT U.S. DEPARTMENT OF STATE, WASHINGTON, D.C.

Mr. FOOTE. Chairman Rubio, Senator Boxer, Senator Menendez, Senator Gardner, thank you for this opportunity to appear before you to discuss the work of the State Department's Bureau of International Narcotics and Law Enforcement Affairs to combat the production and trafficking of heroin particularly by Mexican-based drug trafficking organizations that are responsible for the vast majority of the heroin on America's streets today.

In the United States, we face an epidemic of opioid abuse. Well over half of the more than 47,000 American deaths from last year were due to either domestically produced controlled prescription pain relievers or heroin, which is often combined with other deadly drugs such as fentanyl.

In Mexico, drug trafficking organizations have killed tens of thousands of citizens, and these organizations continue to foment violence, instability, corruption, and addiction.

This scourge is broader than just the United States, and we will not solve it alone.

The overwhelming majority of the heroin in the U.S. is produced or distributed by Mexican drug trafficking organizations. For many years, they have been trafficking not only heroin but also much of the cocaine, methamphetamine, and other illicit drugs that enter our country. Most of these drugs enter through our border with Mexico.

The United States and Mexico developed the Merida Initiative in 2007 with major focus on combating the production and trafficking of illicit drugs across our borders. Today the Pena Nieto and Obama administrations remain committed to Merida's strategic goals. Our Merida partnership, which brings together significant investments and capabilities of both countries, continues to help build Mexico's capacity to fight narcotics trafficking, organized crime, and violence. Together, we are aggressively responding to this threat by putting the leaders of drug trafficking organizations in jail, by seizing their drugs and money, and by dismantling their organizations. Today, through Merida, INL is professionalizing and building the capacity of Mexican law enforcement agencies, supporting the Mexican Government's efforts to strengthen border management and security, and helping advance reform across Mexico's justice sector.

Bilaterally we have agreed that targeting the production and trafficking of heroin, as well as fentanyl and other dangerous synthetic substances, is a top shared priority. To that end, INL and DEA are providing training to law enforcement officers, investigators, and analysts increasing Mexico's ability to identify, investigate, and dismantle clandestine heroin and fentanyl labs.

With our interagency partners, we are also improving information sharing between our governments on heroin and fentanyl working together to get better assessments on opium poppy cultivation and heroin and fentanyl production in Mexico and continuing to explore other avenues to enhance our bilateral cooperation and effectiveness.

Building strong, effective Mexican justice sector institutions, capable of confronting organized criminal enterprises, is a difficult, long-term challenge. This work must be sustained, for it is only through a committed, coordinated effort that sustainable capacity to deter the cultivation, production, and trafficking of illicit drugs will be strengthened. The significant investments of both of our governments are producing results, and with your continued support, this successful collaboration with Mexico will continue.

Thank you.

[Mr. Foote's prepared statement is located in the Additional Material Submitted for the Record section at the end of this transcript.]

Senator GARDNER [presiding]. Thank you, Mr. Foote.

Mr. Kemp Chester, Associate Director for the National Heroin Coordination Group, please begin your testimony. Thank you.

STATEMENT OF KEMP CHESTER, ASSOCIATE DIRECTOR FOR THE NATIONAL HEROIN COORDINATION GROUP, OFFICE OF NATIONAL DRUG POLICY, WASHINGTON, D.C.

Mr. CHESTER. Chairman Rubio, Ranking Member Boxer, and members of the subcommittee, thank you for inviting me here this morning to discuss the public health and public safety issues resulting from heroin use, the Government of Mexico's efforts to reduce the availability of heroin in the United States, and U.S.-Mexico cooperation to address heroin issues in both countries.

In 2014, the most current year for which we have data, more than 47,000 Americans, or approximately 129 people each day, died from a drug overdose. Of the overdose deaths in 2014, 22 percent involved heroin.

The threat posed by heroin has continued to grow dramatically over the past several years, and since 2007, deaths involving heroin have risen 340 percent from 2,402 in 2007 to 10,574 in 2014.

Heroin use has spread into suburban and rural communities and is growing among most socioeconomic classes, age groups, and races.

Mexico is currently the primary supplier of heroin to the United States with Mexican drug traffickers cultivating opium poppy, producing heroin, and smuggling the finished product into the United States. Poppy cultivation in Mexico has increased substantially in recent years, rising from 17,000 hectares in 2014 to 28,000 hectares in 2015, which could yield potential production of 70 metric tons of pure heroin.

The heroin crisis is being compounded by the reemergence of illicit fentanyl, a powerful synthetic opioid more potent than heroin.

Illicit fentanyl is sometimes mixed with powder heroin to increase its effects or mixed with dilutants and sold as synthetic heroin. Increasingly fentanyl is being pressed into pill form and sold as counterfeit prescription opioid pills. The majority of the illicit fentanyl in the U.S. is clandestinely produced in Mexico or in China.

Fentanyl is extremely dangerous and deadly. In 2014, there were more than 5,544 drug overdose deaths involving synthetic narcotics other than methadone, a category that includes fentanyl. This number has more than doubled from 2 years earlier.

U.S.-Mexico engagement regarding heroin has been robust. In October 2015, ONDCP Director Michael Botticelli participated in a bilateral security dialogue where the importance of increased poppy eradication efforts by the Government of Mexico, as well as drug interdiction, clandestine laboratory destruction, and the disruption of precursor chemical trafficking were all highlighted.

In early March, Director Botticelli, Ambassador William Brownfield, the Assistant Secretary of State for International Narcotics and Law Enforcement Affairs, and I met with the Mexican Attorney General Gomez, and she announced her role as the synchronizer of Mexico's efforts to disrupt the production of heroin and illicit fentanyl. Importantly, we agreed then to jointly develop a focused national plan to concentrate Mexico's efforts against heroin and fentanyl.

The urgent need to sustain progress toward addressing the Nation's heroin and fentanyl crisis requires increased collaboration between Federal agencies and with our partners working at the State, local, and tribal level where the crisis is felt most deeply.

In November 2015, the team that I lead, the National Heroin Coordination Group, was created within the Office of National Drug Control Policy to form the hub of a network of interagency partners who will leverage their home agency authorities and resources and to harmonize interagency activities against the heroin and fentanyl supply chains to the United States.

The ONDCP-funded high intensity drug trafficking areas, or HIDTA program, the locally based program that responds to drug trafficking issues facing specific areas of the country, has also been instrumental. In August 2015, ONDCP committed $2.5 million in HIDTA funds to develop a heroin response strategy. This innovative project combines prevention, education, intelligence, and enforcement resources to address the heroin threat through seven regional HIDTAs covering 17 States and the District of Columbia.

So while we have laid a firm foundation to address the heroin crisis, much remains to be accomplished. For example, we do have gaps in our capability to detect illicit fentanyl at our borders, and our Mexican partners could certainly do more in the areas of opium poppy eradication and clandestine laboratory identification and neutralization.

And while my remarks have focused on addressing the supply side of the opioid crisis, we must address opioid use disorders with a balanced approach that also regards addiction as a public health matter, using substance abuse prevention and treatment strategies and recovery support services. In his fiscal year 2017 budget, President Obama proposed $1 billion in new mandatory funding to expand the availability of evidence-based strategies such as medication-assisted treatment and to extend the availability of substance abuse treatment providers.

ONDCP will continue to work with our international partners, Federal Government Departments and agencies, and our partners at the State, local, and tribal levels to reduce heroin and fentanyl production and trafficking and the profound effect these dangerous drugs are having in our communities.

Thank you for the opportunity to testify today, and I would be happy to answer any of your questions.

[Mr. Chester's prepared statement is located in the Additional Material Submitted for the Record section at the end of this transcript.]

Senator RUBIO [presiding]. Thank you.

And I am going to defer my questions because I know members need to be in other places, and I will basically be here throughout the duration. And so I will turn over to the ranking member for her questions.

Senator BOXER. Thanks. I just have two questions for Mr. Foote. So, Mr. Chester, breathe. You are off the hook here.

Mr. Foote, in 2008, Mexico's Congress passed a series of significant reforms to its criminal procedures, new laws to promote greater access to justice, and strengthened measures to combat organized crime, measures that would make the Mexican justice system look a little bit more like our own. These reforms were intended to be implemented by 2016. Where does the implementation of these judicial reforms stand, and how has the United States assisted in this process? And how do you feel about whether they are really doing what they committed to do?

Mr. FOOTE. Thank you, Senator.

As you know, Mexico committed and passed legislation to implement a new criminal justice system which is an accusatorial justice system, much like ourselves. At this point, of the 32 Mexican states, 24 have implemented this with federal level crimes and I believe 9 have implemented it at state level crimes. Obviously, this is a long-term process, and some of the states in Mexico will not meet next month's deadline.

We remain committed and continue to work closely with them on a number of issues. Thanks to the gracious appropriations of Congress, we have dedicated approximately $250 million to these efforts between the Department of State and USAID through issues such as training judges, prosecutors, courtroom personnel, law students. Over 4,000 have been trained to date through Department of Justice's OPTAT prosecutorial training program. We also have a number of law school and institutional exchange programs through the American Bar Association and a number of universities here in the United States.

We are preparing law enforcement for their new roles in the accusatorial justice sector. For instance, our Department of Justice partners in ICITAP have trained thousands of law enforcement in crime scene investigations, provided equipment for units and forensics, fingerprinting, and other collection there so that Mexico can comply with international standards.

Senator BOXER. Okay. Thank you. What I am getting from you is that there is progress being made, although not everyone will meet the deadline. It is an optimistic report.

And so that leads me to my final question, which I alluded to in my statement. As we continue to work with the Mexican Government—and that is just critical. We have to. We have to work here at home to reduce the demand. We have to work across the border to reduce the supply. And that is where the rubber meets the road in both of these areas where we need to work with Mexico.

I am concerned about the rhetoric in the presidential campaign describing our relationship with Mexico. I know it is a tough question for you. I just want you to say what you feel in your heart because we need to know. Mexican officials have said on the record that some of the proposals mentioned on the campaign trail—we know who we are talking about here, a candidate who is talking about building a wall, having Mexico do it, insulting Mexican Americans here at home—that some of the proposals would have a cataclysmic effect on our bilateral relations.

Has this divisive rhetoric affected diplomatic relations with Mexico at this point? Has it impacted the United States' ability to work with the Mexican Government to combat drug trafficking? And are you concerned that that type of rhetoric could just completely undermine what we are trying to do here?

Senator RUBIO. Just for the record, she is not talking about me. [Laughter.]

Senator BOXER. I am so not talking about you.

Mr. FOOTE. Excellent. Well, I will try to strike a balance between answering your question and not entering too deeply into our own domestic politics here.

Senator BOXER. I know it is a tough one, but you know what? When people talk, it has real-life impacts, especially presumptive nominee.

Mr. FOOTE. You have all seen some of the reactions from south of the border from our Mexican brothers and sisters. You have seen President Vicente Fox's reactions and others.

From the embassy bilateral level to date, we continue to work very closely together. In my personal opinion, I do not believe it has gravely affected our ability to do business together. Mexico in the last several months has reiterated its commitment to continuing with the Merida Initiative. Where the populace of Mexico stands on this may be another matter. But we continue to be able to work closely together bilaterally on all——

Senator BOXER. So the words have not had an impact on what is going on at the very top levels in your opinion on the work that you were doing at this point.

Mr. FOOTE. Not in their dealings with us.

Senator BOXER. That is excellent.

Now we have to make sure that those policies never come into effect.

Thank you very much.

Senator RUBIO. Thank you, Senator Boxer.

Senator Menendez?

Senator MENENDEZ. Thank you, Mr. Chairman, for calling the hearing. It is an important one.

And thank you both for your service to our country.

Mr. Foote, how many agencies are involved in interdiction and eradication efforts with respect to Mexico's border with us in our efforts to stop interdiction, stop flows, use intelligence? How many agencies are involved?

Mr. FOOTE. U.S. agencies I hope is what you are asking?

Senator MENENDEZ. U.S. agencies.

Mr. FOOTE. Thank you. INL, Department of State. You have Department of Justice, DEA, FBI to a certain extent. Department of Homeland Security is heavily involved through Customs and Border Protection, Immigration and Customs Enforcement, Homeland Security investigations. Our military supports some of the border efforts of Mexico's military. And then we have some ancillary agencies who are based in Mexico City, but while their chief focus is not the border, they do peripherally work on it such as ATF and the U.S. Marshals.

Senator MENENDEZ. And if you had to guess how much money has been spent on interdiction and eradication efforts in Mexico since the start of the epidemic that we are experiencing here, would you put it at?

Mr. FOOTE. My understanding is $2.5 billion has been appropriated, of which approximately $1.5 billion has been obligated or committed to specific projects, of which we still have at this point new initiatives for about $700 million.

Senator MENENDEZ. Now, are you speaking just Merida specifically?

Mr. FOOTE. Pardon me?

Senator MENENDEZ. Are you speaking just of Merida specifically? Mr. FOOTE. Largely.

Senator MENENDEZ. There is money spent far beyond Merida.

Mr. FOOTE. There certainly is, Senator. I am not in a position to comment on Department of Justice's appropriation. I just do not have the figures. That is something we could get for you.

Senator MENENDEZ. I was not looking just at appropriation. I look at all the agencies you mentioned, your own, INL, Department of Justice, DEA, FBI, Homeland Security, Immigration, military, Alcohol, Tobacco and Firearms. And I think to myself it has to be billions collectively. And I was one of the architects of the Merida Initiative, which I support.

But $1.5 billion later, billions between all of our respective agencies, and what we have is an opioid epidemic. And as a policy-maker, one has to take a step back and say to themselves, what is not working because something is not working. If billions of dollars later what you see is a spike versus a trend in the other direction, then something is not working. So if I were to say to you, what is not working, what do we need to change, your answer would be?

Mr. FOOTE. First of all, Senator, I think we have in the past few years come to the realization that this is a shared responsibility between the United States and source countries and trafficking countries. I am heartened by the Senate's recent passing of the opioid legislation. It is something that is going to help us. Certainly Mexico-specific, their capacities are far greater than they were when we started the Merida Initiative in 2007. Information sharing and collaboration has led our own U.S. law enforcement agencies to interdict significantly more on our southern border due to Mexico cooperation.

We still do have a way to go. I think we also need to get better here in the United States at demand reduction and treating the health issues of addicted people. It is a shared responsibility and it is no longer just a supply-side issue.

Senator MENENDEZ. So as I listened to your response, it is everything that we are doing except for a more significant effort on demand reduction, but it is not suggesting that there is anything that we are not doing. And all I can look at and say if you are spending billions and instead of the trend going the opposite direction, it is rising, you have to raise the question what is it that we are either doing wrong or what is it that we are not doing that we need to do in order to meet the challenge because otherwise we can appropriate billions and billions, but still find ourselves in a trend that is undesirable.

So the only thing I heard from you in your response to me was doing more demand reduction, which I certainly believe is true. But I did not hear about anything else. So you know, you have to question whether or not the continuation of this type of expenditure in this manner is the right policy.

Let me ask you this. Do you believe that there is sufficient coordination, a seamless coordination between at least on our side of the border as it relates to all the agencies that you suggested are engaged in this fight?

Mr. FOOTE. Senator, obviously, we can always get better at everything we do. Department of State kind of works from the southern border south. So I do not feel that it is our position to comment on interagency coordination north of the border. South of the border, we have robust interagency coordination through the country team at Embassy Mexico City. We can always get a little better there.

Senator MENENDEZ. Your Mexican partners—are they doing everything that they can in order to meet the challenge on their side of the border?

Mr. FOOTE. During the beginning part of President Pena Nieto's administration, there was a pause in Plan Merida as I think we did a mutual assessment of the security relationship, particularly on their side, and over the past year and a half, we have seen much closer collaboration, an unprecedented openness and frankness in our bilateral dialogue.

To answer your question, is Mexico doing everything that they can, they could improve. Some of their efforts are not yet at the optimal level, but we remain optimistic and positive that they are moving in the right direction.

Senator MENENDEZ. Well, I appreciate the optimism, but I am seeking to introduce a little dose of realism into it. And so part of the challenge is that you have lawless states in some of the northern part of Mexico where I have heard U.S. citizens from the region who have come to talk to me say that many who had businesses, longtime relationships on the immediate other side of the border, that basically cannot operate there because the federal government's presence—i.e., the federal government of Mexico's presence—is not there. So if you have lawlessness and if you have uncontrolled states, then you have the opportunity for drug traffickers to avail themselves of that. And it seems to me that while I am an incredibly strong and have been for 25 years supporter of the U.S.-Mexico relationship, we need to be honest in this relationship in order to make sure that we are making the progress that we need here and for Mexico to be able to regain its sovereignty over parts of northern Mexico that it presently does not have.

Thank you, Mr. Chairman.

Senator RUBIO. Thank you.

Let me use some of my time that I yielded just to interject, to follow up on that.

Secretary Foote, how would you assess the assertion made by a group of experts from the Inter-American Commission on Human Rights that there may have been another bus involved in the incident in which 43 students disappeared in Guerrero, Mexico that was packed with heroin bound for the U.S.?

Mr. FOOTE. Senator, thank you for that question. Given that we have not seen the results of the final investigation from Mexico, I am not in a great position to answer that question right now. We would be happy to answer that for the record in writing.

[The material referred to above was not available when this transcript went to press.]

Senator RUBIO. Okay.

Senator Kaine?

Senator KAINE. Thank you, Mr. Chair, and thanks to the witnesses.

First, to get an idea of the scope of this challenge on the Mexican side in terms of the black tar heroin, is the poppy production for this heroin still significantly confined to the state of Nayarit or is it more broadly distributed? Mexico is a big country. So when we talk about a problem in Mexico, I worry that we are not being specific enough.

Mr. CHESTER. Yes, Senator. Our latest crop estimate that was produced about 2 months ago shows two major growing areas in Mexico, one in the state of Guerrero and then another in what is called the tri-border region up in the northern part of the country. Those are the two major growing areas in Mexico, with very, very small kind of sporadic spots in other parts of the country, but they are basically concentrated in those two areas.

Senator KAINE. And then the fentanyl is made in labs, and I gather that most of the fentanyl that comes in is either coming in— it is made in China and may be transited in through Mexico or also made in labs in Mexico. Are those the two main sources for fentanyl?

Mr. CHESTER. That is correct.

And I will tell you that our understanding and our awareness of fentanyl traffic has evolved dramatically over the last 6 months as we have seen the crisis rise. So in order of magnitude, I cannot tell you, but what I can tell you is that China is a significant supplier of fentanyl to the United States or it is ordered by individuals on the dark web around the Internet and then, using parcel post or the Postal Service, shipped directly to them.

We also know that fentanyl is shipped into Mexico in some cases mixed with dilutants and smuggled across the Southwest border and that there are precursor chemicals that are shipped into Mexico that can be used for the production of clandestine fentanyl in laboratories in Mexico. So as you look at the vectors coming into the United States, those are the two main ones that we see for finished fentanyl coming into the United States or its manufacture in Mexico.

Senator KAINE. I want to talk, Mr. Chester, about your written testimony. I am sorry I did not get here for your entire oral testimony.

But on page 1, there are several principal factors contributing to the current nationwide heroin crisis: the increased availability of heroin in the U.S. market, the availability of pure forms of heroin that allow for non-intravenous use, its relatively low price, and a relatively small percentage of non-medical users of opioid prescription drugs transitioning to heroin.

I am trying to unpack that statement, and I am wondering if your statement puts enough of a finger on the prescription opioid problem. I have heard it stated through Michael Botticelli and others that 80 percent of those who OD on heroin in this country, not fatal ODs but total ODs, started their addiction to opioids by being addicted to prescription opioids and then transition to heroin because they could get it for a lower price. Is that an accurate statement?

Mr. CHESTER. No, Senator. And I am glad you asked that question. Of the numbers of individuals who non-medically use opioids and then transition into heroin, that number is actually relatively small. It is about 3.6 percent.

Senator KAINE. For non-medical use.

Mr. CHESTER. That is correct. So the non-medical use of a prescription opioid like OxyContin and kind of the traditional "got it from the medicine cabinet, got it from friends or family members"—the percentage of those individuals who transition to heroin use is relatively low. It is about 3.6 percent.

But conversely, of individuals who are non-treatment users of heroin, 80 percent of them actually abused a prescription opioid in the past. So while there is not a direct causation between the two, the non-medical use of opioids is a strong risk factor for eventual heroin use.

Senator KAINE. And even the medical use of opioids can be a risk factor for eventual heroin use. Correct?

Mr. CHESTER. Yes, Senator, that is right. So an opioid in and of itself and its effect on the body—obviously, it is a very addictive drug and affects the body in unique ways, as an opioid. So those individuals who take opioids, whether they get them from a doctor or whether they get them from a friend or a family member for non-medical reasons are at risk for eventual opioid addiction if not used properly. That is correct.

Senator KAINE. And you cite in the testimony the relatively low price of heroin—and that is relatively low compared to past trends but also compared to the cost of opioid-based prescription drugs. Correct?

Mr. CHESTER. That is correct. So the street price of a gram of heroin compared to the street price, if you will, of an opioid pill or an oxy pill or something of that nature, that is correct. That is what we consider to be one of the contributing factors. So it is the availability and the general low price and then the purity that have all been contributing factors to the current crisis that we are in with heroin. That is correct.

Senator KAINE. Mr. Foote talked about the work that we have done in this body and we are trying to harmonize with the House in this recent CARA, Comprehensive Addiction and Recovery Act. We really believe it here—and I think it is now bipartisan—we are seeing in all of our States that if we do not get a hold of the culture of over-prescription of opioid-based prescription drugs, we are just hollowing out communities, rural, urban, suburban, rich and poor. And this was a drug addiction that came out of the medicine cabinet. In many instances it was a trusted professional in a white coat that was handing somebody this prescription saying this is going to do you good and it is not going to do you harm, driven by inadequate science, driven by frankly marketing scams. And that is inextricably related to this heroin issue. And so I think it is kind of hard to deal with the heroin issue in the abstract without talking about this culture of over-prescription, that hopefully we are working together to reel in.

Last question I want to ask—and it is probably too early to know this. But in terms of the growth of the number of hectares of poppy production in Mexico, do we have any evidence to suggest whether that is at all connected with marijuana legalization in the United States? I actually kind of like this notion of the States as labs and they can experiment and we can see what happens. But I have heard it said—and I do not know whether there is any evidence to back it up—that the legalization of marijuana in some States that has allowed marijuana to be grown has taken hectares of land that were used for marijuana cultivation and, well, we do not have a market for our marijuana anymore because there is competition, so we will switch to something like poppies to produce black tar heroin. Is there any evidence of that?

Mr. CHESTER. We have actually looked closely kind of at the crop transference to see if there is anything there, and I can tell you at this time, whether it is too early or whether it does not exist, we cannot definitively say that farmers have decided to switch from one crop to another in Mexico. We cannot say that with any degree of authority at this point.

Senator KAINE. But that is something that you are going to continue to monitor.

Mr. CHESTER. It is something that we do watch, yes.

Senator KAINE. Great.

Thanks, Mr. Chair.

Senator RUBIO. To interject on that point, it is my sense—and you are both experts at this—that very few people wake up in the morning and say I am going to go shoot heroin just for the first time. There is a gateway to the heroin use. A lot of it is being driven by people that were prescribed prescription opiates. They now become physically dependent. The prescription opiate is cut off. They are going through severe withdrawal, and the only thing that addresses that withdrawal, if they are not in treatment, is access to heroin, and that brings all sorts of problems.

Absent that, what is the other gateway? How does someone get dependent on heroin minus the prescription drug gateway, which we have already discussed?

Mr. CHESTER. Senator, it is a difficult question just because you are dealing with a number of variables down at the individual level as to the reasons why people engage in the behavior. We do know a couple things. Heroin in general terms is kind of at the end of a trajectory of long-term drug use and that a high number of heroin users are actually poly-drug users. And so they are not an exclusive heroin user. They get the drugs that are available to them, and because of the high availability of heroin, a lot of times that is heroin.

The other thing that we look at—and we do a number of surveys to look at this. But what we realize is that youth behavior from the ages of about 13 to about 18 is a very strong factor in terms of risk- taking behavior, in terms of underage drinking, tobacco, marijuana, things of that nature in shaping youth attitudes eventually that they carry with them for the rest of their lives in terms of risk-taking behavior for using other drugs.

So what we cannot say is that we can put a finger on this or that particular reason why a person does something, but we do know that the availability of drugs in society obviously increases the chances that an individual who is inclined to use them is going to intersect them at some particular point. And I think that is one of the—with the discussion we had about the availability of heroin being the driving factor.

Senator RUBIO. So just to understand your testimony, we understand the pill problem that leads to that. But what you are basically saying is if someone, especially at some point earlier in their life, begins to use a substance, alcohol, whatever it may be, an intoxicant of some sort, there now starts a potential trend where the next thing is, well, what is out there that is better, what is out there that is stronger. Once you have crossed that barrier, it could unleash this cycle of basically a set of dominoes that ultimately lead you to the heroin point.

Mr. CHESTER. Yes, sir. And again, it is not direct causation, but it certainly is risk-taking behavior and patterns of behavior.

And that is why the prevention strategies, particularly through programs like the Drug Free Communities Program that ONDCP manages are incredibly important because they are locally based, and they allow trusted individuals to be able to speak to people at very, very young ages about things just like that and their attitudes about drugs and foreign substances in the body and things of that nature. So they, through evidence-based prevention strategies, are able to talk to people at those young ages when they are vulnerable in shaping their ideas about drug use that they carry with them for the rest of their lives.

Senator RUBIO. Senator Markey?

Senator MARKEY. Thank you, Mr. Chairman, and thank you for this hearing. I think this is the most important hearing we are going to have on our relations with Mexico and with China this year in the Congress, and I thank you for it.

This issue of fentanyl is to my way of thinking kind of the most important threat that we have to families in the United States at this time. I will just give you some numbers. In Massachusetts, in 2015, 57 percent of the opioid-related overdose deaths in Massachusetts had a positive screen for fentanyl. Specifically of the 1,319 individuals whose deaths were opioid-related in 2015 where a toxicology screen was available, 754 of them had a positive screen for fentanyl. So we can talk about prescription drugs. We can talk about heroin, but fentanyl is now the issue.

And we—that is, New England—are at the epicenter of it. It comes up from Mexico to Lawrence, Massachusetts, and then it goes out into New Hampshire, other States, but Massachusetts as well.

So the pathway is China into Mexico, then into Lawrence, Massachusetts, into Ohio, into Virginia, into Florida. And when it is over half of the deaths now in Massachusetts, it is clearly a looming threat that is a preview of coming attractions to every single city and town in our country.

So that is why this hearing is so important because it gets to the question of what is Mexico doing in partnership with China. We will start with that, Mr. Foote. What are specifically Mexico and China at the highest governmental levels doing in order to interdict this new synthetic formula that is lacing heroin with a drug 50 times more powerful than heroin, so powerful that the DEA does not even let its dogs any longer sniff for fentanyl for fear that the dog will just die with the first sniff of fentanyl. 3 grams, 3 equivalent of salt grams, could kill a human being if they gained access to it. What are Mexico and China doing in cooperation with you in order to interdict that drug?

Mr. FOOTE. Senator, first, I will touch on Mexico and China's bilateral relationship on this. With our support, Mexico and China are meeting and discussing fentanyl regularly every year. They are both involved in the multilateral side of things. Just last month at the U.N. General Assembly special session on drugs, they were both there. China—their minister of public security led the conclusion statement. They were fully on board. And they are a member, both countries, to the three international drug conventions.

We also sponsor in the United States two annual fentanyl and precursor chemical conferences with Mexico and China.

Senator MARKEY. So how successful is this effort so far?

Mr. FOOTE. That is a good question, Senator. Fentanyl is a new problem for the Department of State and INL, and it is one where we are applying lessons we have learned with other substances in other crime areas over the years, and at this point we are working as hard as we can to have success but I cannot quantify it.

Senator MARKEY. Has it been elevated to the highest level? In other words, with human rights and copyright infringement, is this issue now at the highest level of negotiations with the Chinese Government and with the Mexican Government?

Mr. FOOTE. It is. Mr. Chester went down in March with our folks and spoke to a large interagency group headed by the Attorney General in Mexico on this issue. We regularly engage with China. Our diplomats are going to China next week at a very high level diplomatic engagement where they will raise it. We raise it regularly in the joint liaison group on law enforcement, which has a counter-narcotics working group that meets throughout the year. We have actually seen some positive signs from China.

Senator MARKEY. What is the evidence? If you were going to convict them of doing something, what would the evidence be to convict them?

Mr. FOOTE. To convict?

Senator MARKEY. Convict China of actually doing something to block this from coming into Mexico and then into the United States. What would the evidence be to convict them of doing good?

Mr. FOOTE. Of doing good.

We have seen encouraging progress. There is still plenty to do. Last year, their ministry of public security officially controlled 116 new substances, including several analogs of fentanyl, and they have expressed high receptivity and continue to send information on new synthetic substances to help us to efficiently control them. So they are doing something. There is more that can be done, obviously.

Senator MARKEY. Clearly we have the evidence in 2015 in Massachusetts, and it is going to be worse this year in 2016. There is slim evidence that this thing is being slowed down. In fact, it is very clear that it is intensifying and it is going to kill. It is going to kill ultimately tens of thousands of Americans every year—every year. There is no other threat to our country that even matches that. Every single year, fentanyl is going to be able to do that. So if we do not stop it, it dwarfs every other issue. Every other issue will be a footnote compared to the magnitude of the impact on American families.

Mr. Chester, can we just go to Mexico? What is the level of cooperation that you are getting from the Mexican Government in interdicting fentanyl coming into the United States? We know it is el Chapo and his gang that is responsible for the traffic that comes up to Lawrence, Massachusetts, but pretty much for the whole country. What is your success level with the Mexican Government getting them to understand the magnitude of the threat to the American people?

Mr. CHESTER. Senator, I would tell you that I personally have been down there twice and then have dealt with the Mexican Embassy here in the United States. I will tell you that they understand how seriously we take this issue in the United States. They understand that this is our top illicit drug priority, and they also understand that it is not just heroin but it is heroin and it is fentanyl.

In a meeting down there in February, I put fentanyl on the table. And I will not say it was a "first heard" for them, but they were not really familiar with how serious the issue was in the United States. By the time we had gone down later with Director Botticelli and Ambassador Brownfield, that was part of the problem set that they agreed to work with us moving forward on.

So I will tell you that the Mexicans understand the importance that we place on this issue. They are very engaged on it, and they are willing to conduct a joint planning with us on the issues not only of poppy eradication, which addresses the heroin issue, but also lab identification and neutralization specifically on issues of either fentanyl creation or the milling of fentanyl with dilutants and other inert matter as it is transported across the border.

Senator MARKEY. Well, and it is a little bit disturbing to me if, from your testimony, it is a case of first impression for the principal law enforcement officials in Mexico, that they are just hearing about fentanyl, and it is just getting on their radar screen, and it is February of 2016, given the fact that more than half of all the people who died last year in Massachusetts, opioid-related, had fentanyl in their system. That is kind of a little bit disturbing to me. I am going to be very honest with you, and I do not like it to have just been introduced at that level.

I would like to have heard that President Obama has raised this issue with the president of Mexico, that President Obama has raised this issue with President Xi in China just because of the incredible level of fatalities all across our country. And we know specifically what the source of their death is.

So do you mind if I just continue a little bit? Thank you, Mr. Chairman.

So give me some hope here that there is an aggressive strategy in place on fentanyl and that it has been elevated to a level where there is a no-nonsense conversation going on in terms of what the expectations of our government is.

Mr. CHESTER. Right, Senator. In response to your concern, I know that the President did raise this with President Pena Nieto— the opioid issue with the Government of Mexico.

Senator MARKEY. He raised the fentanyl issue with——

Mr. CHESTER. I will check if it was specifically fentanyl, but I know the heroin issue was raised and the opioid issue——

Senator MARKEY. Well, I am asking about fentanyl here. Fentanyl is the epidemic. Fentanyl is the epidemic. It is not heroin. It is fentanyl. Fentanyl is 50 times more powerful. Fentanyl is what is showing up in a majority of the deaths. So you are not sure whether or not he has raised it.

Mr. CHESTER. And I need to make sure that fentanyl was part of that conversation between the two of them as well.

Senator MARKEY. How about you, Mr. Foote? Has the State Department specifically raised fentanyl at the highest levels with the Chinese Government and the Mexican Government?

Mr. FOOTE. We continue to raise it at the highest levels of dialogue that we have.

Senator MARKEY. What is the highest level?

Mr. FOOTE. Next week, our Deputy Secretary will be in China, and this is high on the agenda, if not top on the agenda. I cannot promise that President Obama raised it with President Xi, but certainly Secretary Kerry has raised it with the Chinese Government.

Senator MARKEY. Thank you, Mr. Chairman.

Senator RUBIO. Thank you.

Just a couple of points that I wanted to raise. First of all, why Lawrence, Massachusetts? Why New Hampshire? Why are these communities specifically targeted? In Florida, for example, central Florida, how does a community wind up targeted by these criminal gangs? What are the characteristics that are making them targets as opposed to some other part of the country?

Mr. CHESTER. Senator, there are a number of variables, one of which is the existing structure, the existing trafficker structure, that is in place in particular areas. In some cases, it is transportation networks. In some cases, the traffickers from Mexico have personal or business relationships with traffickers in a particular area or that geographically a place lends itself to further distribution. There are a lot of reasons why a particular——

Senator RUBIO. But the Northeast is far from the U.S.-Mexico border. I mean, my question is why did they not stop somewhere along I–95 and target there. Is it because of these existing structures that were there before?

Mr. CHESTER. We believe that there is very strong evidence that there are, that it is the existing structures that were there before.

When we specifically talk about fentanyl, one of the things that we have looked at as we have tracked the fentanyl crisis is why the Northeast, why the Eastern United States, why so much not the Western United States. And we believe that one of the strong contributing factors is the fact that fentanyl is more easily mixed into the white powder heroin which was preferred in the eastern part of the United States than it is in the black tar heroin which was preferred in the western part of the United States, and that has traditionally been the heroin market in the United States.

And so fentanyl is being mixed into powder heroin, and therefore it landed in the United States. And increasingly we are starting to see it be pressed into pill form and sold as counterfeit oxy or counterfeit opioids, but fentanyl has found a market in the Eastern United States probably because of those two reasons.

Senator RUBIO. I spent some time in New Hampshire over the last year and from that experience found myself in a lot of small townships, not large places, throughout New England that faced an overwhelming problem, almost as if they were specifically targeted perhaps because trafficking networks knew that they had smaller police departments. If you are a small township, you are not going to have a 1,000-officer department. Is there evidence that some of that is in play for these trafficking networks, that in essence, they look to set up in places where they can overwhelm local law enforcement with numbers and capabilities?

Mr. CHESTER. Senator, I do not know. I do not know whether the size of a population or the size of law enforcement was a particular reason why.

But to your point, it is a matter of deep concern that you find increasing numbers of heroin or fentanyl users in rural areas who are starting to use the product alone, and they are far from treatment and they tend to be further from first responders. Those are all things that make this particular crisis particularly pernicious. It is the fact that it has moved into a lot of rural areas, which is not something that we have seen in previous outbreaks of heroin or——

Senator RUBIO. And I know what I am asking—and perhaps it is more appropriate to the second panel—is more of a domestic issue as opposed to a transnational one. But some of the stuff we used to hear—because the supply is also driving the demand. They are interrelated. In essence, the supply meant these traffickers, who now had the supply on their hands, had to be more aggressive in finding market share. And one of the things I kept hearing a lot were that they were specifically targeting treatment centers, especially outpatient treatment centers where they knew people were getting treatment because of addiction, and they were waiting for them outside to tempt them to buy, that they specifically were targeting recovering individuals for the sale of this. And this is a pernicious, disgusting industry that we are dealing with here.

In that realm, I wanted to ask—you know, since the arrest of el Chapo, Secretary Foote, this is part of Mexico's, I believe, concerted policy to conduct high profile arrests of drug lords. And while it is positive that these organizations are being decapitated, have we seen any evidence that the arrest of a high profile individual impacts the ability of these organizations to continue to function specifically since el Chapo's arrest? Is there any evidence that the operation has been impacted by it, or is it just one of those things that is now functioning the way a corporate entity would, irrespective of who is at the top?

Mr. FOOTE. Senator, my personal experience is far more robust with Colombia where I led our programs several years ago. We have seen where the kingpin being arrested does certainly affect an organization. The question is how big is the structure, how organized is it, and how quickly can it recover. That is a question far better posed to our Drug Enforcement Administration guys than State.

Senator RUBIO. Let me ask you about Colombia. It is not directly related to the opiate issue, but nonetheless cocaine. They suspended their aerial eradication program ostensibly for fear of the impact that the defoliants would have on the population environmentally. There is a counter-argument out there that some have made, in which I find some credibility, that this is also part of the peace process, that in essence, this deforestation effort and the eradication effort was an irritant in the peace process with the FARC and other elements.

As a result, we now see numbers where for the first time in a long time there has been a massive increase in the amount of cocaine production in parts of Colombia that we had not seen in a while, and the assumption is that that cocaine is going to get sold. It is going to go somewhere and that we should expect at some point within the next couple years to see a spike in cocaine sales in the United States.

Do you have a view, irrespective of the reason why they are doing it, of what these new numbers mean for the U.S. in the years to come?

Mr. FOOTE. We are concerned about the suspension of aerial eradication. It is a sovereign decision of President Santos and the Colombian Government obviously. We believe while eradication and aerial eradication are not magic pills, they are valuable tools in any supply-side intervention on narcotics. It has long been a big part of our strategy in Colombia. We continue to work closely with the Colombians on the successor to Plan Colombia, which is Paz Colombia, Peace Colombia, and are in close contact to see which direction they decide to go if and when President Santos gets the peace process resolved.

Senator RUBIO. And here is my final question for the panel. And I thank you both for being here and for your testimony and for your work. The work you do is important and difficult.

We now have two separate but interrelated problems, as the Senators just pointed out a moment ago, the production of synthetic fentanyl, the growth of opiate poppies. My understanding is that the amount of poppy-based opiates grown in the western hemisphere is a small percentage of the overall production in the world. In your view—or do you know this—if a poppy-based opiate is produced or fentanyl is produced somewhere in the western hemisphere, Mexico or anywhere else, what percentage of that is destined for the United States in particular?

Mr. CHESTER. Senator, we believe that Mexico is the primary supplier of heroin to the United States and that the United States is the primary customer for Mexican heroin. That relationship in the western hemisphere is fairly solid. We do not see any widespread evidence of Southwest Asian heroin, Afghan heroin, Burmese heroin coming to the United States, although the Government of Canada does believe that Southwest Asia is its primary supplier of heroin.

So one of the things that we have discovered is a risk and we have identified as a risk is if we are successful against the Mexican drug trafficking organizations in bringing down the supply of Mexican heroin into the United States, do we open up the door for others.

Senator RUBIO. I think it is pretty clear that if you see a heroin overdose in the U.S., that heroin or that fentanyl came from Mexico or maybe in the case of fentanyl, China through the mail. I think that is pretty clear.

Here is my question. Are the opiates being grown or produced in the case of fentanyl in Mexico being sold anywhere else in the world or should we basically assume that virtually all of it that is being grown there—you can see it from the camera—pictures are being taken—all of that is headed to a city near you in the United States?

Mr. CHESTER. That is the assumption we make, Senator. Yes, that is correct.

Senator RUBIO. Well, I want to thank you both for being here. Did you have a final question, Senator Markey?

Senator MARKEY. Thank you so much. Again, for me this is the top topic. It does not get any bigger than this, and these are the gentlemen responsible for it in the United States. So to have them here and to know that they are the principal people working on the fentanyl issue I think is absolutely central.

So let me just ask you this, Mr. Chester. Your title is Associate Director for the National Heroin Coordination Group. Do you think it is time for us to just change the name to the National Heroin and Fentanyl Coordination Group? Do you think we should change the name just so it advertises correctly what is going on to the American people?

Mr. CHESTER. Senator, when we began our work this fall as the Heroin Coordination Group, and after Director Botticelli stood up this group within ONDCP in order to provide focused efforts against the heroin and the fentanyl problem. In our work what we determined was that we were going to handle heroin and fentanyl as part of the same problem set for a lot of different reasons. What has evolved over time in our work and in our planning and our work with the interagency is that we have discovered the incredible importance of fentanyl more so than what was identified 6 or 8 or 9 months ago.

The other important thing about fentanyl that I would like to bring up is the fact that the emergence and the visibility of fentanyl is driven almost entirely by the postmortem testing that is done on individuals in overdose deaths around the country. And in those areas where the testing is done and fentanyl is tested as part of the toxicology panel, you begin to see more. So it leads us to believe that in looking at both the heroin and fentanyl problem, we have a significant fentanyl problem, as you identified, that we believe was being masked by this increased availability in heroin. So we handled both of them as part of the same problem set simply because it allows us to be able to deal with the trafficking and the supply chain and the effects on communities in the exact same way.

Senator MARKEY. No, I appreciate that. So that is what I am asking. Should we add fentanyl to your title in your opinion? Does that make sense given what you now know and given how little Mexico, it turns out, knows when you had the conversation in February of 2016 about fentanyl? They did not have it on their radar. Did we raise it so that they understand? The same thing is true for the Chinese. What do you think?

Mr. CHESTER. The issue being raised to the Chinese——

Senator MARKEY. No, no. I am talking about Mexico. I am talking specifically here about Mexico right now. They did not know in February.

And by the way, even when I say 57 percent, a lot of experts think that is an understated number because of the poor reporting that goes on in terms of the total number of deaths.

And by the way, it is no secret why they do it. It is like a 300 percent markup—300 percent markup—in terms of their ability to make money off this as opposed to heroin or other drugs.

So again, from my perspective, this is the issue. This dwarfs any terrorist threat to the United States. This is what is going to kill people, tens of thousands, ultimately hundreds of thousands of Americans. It is going to be this fentanyl that comes into our country. You are the front line on this. Mexico just heard about it. I am not sure the Chinese understand the priority that we expect them to deal with this issue.

Mr. Chester, earlier today in your testimony, you said that there are gaps in the interdiction of fentanyl from Mexico coming into the United States. Could you explain in more detail what those gaps are?

Mr. CHESTER. We are speaking primarily about gaps in our ability to be able to detect fentanyl at borders, and what was brought up earlier is the ability of canines, canines being trained in order to be able to detect fentanyl because it is so deadly.

And we work very closely with CBP both in terms of intelligence and in terms of policy to address those gaps to better detect fentanyl not only at the Southwest border but in our air freight locations in the United States whether it is U.S. Postal Service or whether it is a commercial company. That has been an area of ongoing discussion for us so that we can better determine how much fentanyl is getting into the country and to be able to detect it when it does arrive, and whether that is detecting the chemical, the fentanyl itself, or the dilutant with which it is mixed.

Senator RUBIO. Gentlemen, I apologize. We have got to move to the next panel because in about 45 minutes, I have to preside over the floor and I turn into a pumpkin here. Not literally. [Laughter.]

Senator MARKEY. If I may just conclude. I would just strongly recommend to the administration that when the President meets with the president of Canada and Mexico, that he raises fentanyl to the highest level with them and lets them know that that is a threat to our country. And the same thing is true in any communications with the Chinese Government that it has to be at the highest level.

Thank you, Mr. Chairman.

Senator RUBIO. Thank you, Senator Markey. This is an important issue in the Northeast and for the country.

And I thank you both.

We are going to welcome our next panel.

As we will say at the end of the hearing, we keep the record open for a few days. If you receive any questions in writing, if you would respond as quickly as possible so we can close the record. We thank you both for being here.

So as they are getting seated and situated, I am going to, once again, reintroduce the members of our second panel. The Honorable Teresa Jacobs is the Mayor of Orange County, Florida, which we hope, if it has not yet been finalized, will be the site of the Pro Bowl in 2017. Right?

Ms. JACOBS. Yes, it is.

Senator RUBIO. Maybe you can give us an update on that too. We are excited about it.

And, of course, Mr. Steven Dudley, who is the Co-Director of In-Sight Crime.

Mayor, if you are ready—your testimony has been submitted in writing, and we look forward to hearing you as well. Thank you for being here.

STATEMENT OF HON. TERESA JACOBS, MAYOR OF ORANGE COUNTY, FLORIDA

Ms. JACOBS. Thank you, Chairman Rubio. And thank you for calling this very important hearing and allowing me to share a local perspective. The conversation this morning has certainly been informative for me, as I am sure it has been for everyone here.

First, a little background on Orange County, nothing that you do not know, but for the record. Orange County is home to the City of Orlando and 12 other municipalities. We have a strong economy and an exceptional quality of life. We have a population of 1.2 million people that call Orlando home, but we also have 66 million visitors on an annual basis and we continue to shatter national records for tourism. That is the good news.

The bad news and the very sad news is that we, like too many other communities across this country, have seen an alarming increase in the number of heroin overdoses and related deaths. I say heroin. When I say heroin, I mean opioids, opiates, I mean fentanyl, all of them combined. Last year, we lost 85 lives to heroin. We lost 62 lives to fentanyl.

We have heard this morning testimony about the increase in deaths related to opioids and opiates of anywhere from 200 to 400 percent since 2007. In Orange County, we have had a staggering 600 percent increase since 2011 alone, and already this year we have had 90 reported opioid overdoses, about 1 in 10 resulting in death.

Florida's fight against this current wave of opioid addiction began about 5 years ago. You may recall that in 2010, Florida was known as the "pill mill capital" of the country. Florida practitioners were prescribing oxycodone at levels that exceeded all the other States in our Nation combined. At a State and local level, we responded by outlawing unauthorized pain clinics. Yet, today the battlefront has moved. Today we fight heroin. Today we fight fentanyl.

Given the dramatic rise in the flow of heroin and fentanyl into our community, one can only surmise that drug cartels perceived us as a ripe marketplace. Unfortunately, it is nearly impossible to accurately assess the size of the heroin threat in Florida and across States in our Nation. But there are a few things that we do know.

In Orange County, we know that last year approximately 2,000 heroin users moved through our county jail alone, and on any given day, we treat roughly 200 heroin addicts in our jail. We know that in 2015 our county jail housed 100 expectant mothers who were addicted, whose babies will most certainly be born tragically addicted to heroin. We know that over 60 percent of overdose patients are uninsured, and yet we have only one inpatient facility with 26 detox beds available to the uninsured for all four counties in our region, with a combined population of 2.5 million people. Simply put, we know that our county jail has become the treatment center of last resort for far too many people who find themselves addicted to heroin, fentanyl, and other opiates and opioids.

For the good of our citizens, we are fighting back, and here is how. Last summer, we convened the Orange County Heroin Task Force, chaired by myself and our sheriff. Our joint work is having a positive impact, including the passage of the 2016 Florida legislature, which passed a measure allowing naloxone sales without an individual prescription. And while there is no single cure or solution, we know there are some universally effective approaches, many of which have been discussed here today. But I think at the heart of it is that we have to recognize that we must address the demand side while we attack the supply side, and an either/or policy simply will not work.

On the demand side, through our task force, we have joined forces with our K through 12 public education system, our universities, our faith-based communities, our medical communities. Together we are launching a social media campaign to educate the public on the risks of this highly addictive and deadly drug. We are trying to convince our citizens and warn them in advance that this is something that they want to avoid at all costs.

We are also not only treating heroin addicts in our jail, we are implementing a new medically assisted treatment program using Vivitrol. And this is an option for all of our addicts that are leaving our jail.

But we need the Federal Government's help to treat more addicts. As I mentioned a few minutes ago, we are woefully short on beds and other resources.

On the supply side, we are also doing our best to arrest traffickers on our streets. But our local efforts, no matter how highly leveraged and coordinated, are simply no match for the drug cartels and organized traffickers coming across our country's borders. And that is why we need your help to help stop the influx of drugs across our borders.

To end the crisis, to save lives, to save communities, we each have a role to play. Local governments have a crucial role to play. The State government does and the Federal Government does. But the efforts need to expand beyond government. We need every citizen that is a mother or a father or a friend of an addict—we need our entire communities engaged. We need doctors. We need the clergy. We need counselors. We need teachers. We need all of them to be informed. And that is why I think that we also need a nationwide awareness campaign.

And we have talked briefly about fentanyl. It needs to include the high risk of fentanyl and the low cost. Quite frankly, today it is less expensive for many of our addicts to get high on opioids than it is for them to go and get a Happy Meal. That is a sad state of reality that has to be addressed.

Thank you again so much for this opportunity, Mr. Chairman. Thank you for your and your committee's continued service and leadership on this issue.

[Ms. Jacobs's prepared statement is located in the Additional Material Submitted for the Record section at the end of this transcript.]

Senator RUBIO. Thank you, Mayor, and thank you for your work on this. You have been involved in this for a while now trying to deal with it back when the pill mill problem was going on, and we will talk about that in the questioning section.

Mr. Dudley, thank you for being here. We look forward to your testimony.

Statement of Steven Dudley, Co–Director, Insight Crime, Washington, D.C.

Mr. DUDLEY. Thank you very much, Chairman Rubio.

As we know, as U.S. consumption of heroin has increased significantly in the last few years, the U.S. portion of the world heroin market is quite small by comparison in terms of users but really outsized in terms of potential earnings. The RAND Corporation estimated in 2014 that U.S. consumers spent as much as $27 billion on heroin each year, an increase from $20 billion in the year 2000.

Mexican, Guatemalan, and Colombian criminal organizations have reacted to these changes by producing more heroin.

As noted already in the earlier panel, Mexico accounts for the bulk of the poppy production in the region.

Seizure data of heroin along the southwest border also indicate that Mexican criminal groups are moving increasing amounts of heroin into the U.S. market. Mexican criminal organizations are also the key transporters of Colombian heroin to the United States, and they manage and purchase the heroin produced in Guatemala or buy the opium gum wholesale to process it into heroin themselves in Mexico.

Inside the U.S., the trend appears to be the same. The DEA says that Mexican groups are seeking an increasing amount of the market share in the distribution business itself, displacing other wholesalers.

In sum, the picture we have is one of an increasingly lucrative, vertically integrated market with large Mexican criminal organizations managing the product from the point of production to the point of sale and seeking a greater market share of these sales.

The reality of the supply chain, however, is much more complex. While it helps us to use well-worn monikers when talking about these organizations, the truth is that they are not nearly as strong or monolithic as they once were. Names such as the Tijuana Cartel, the Juarez Cartel, the Zetas, or La Familia Michoacana may still evoke fear and sometimes awe, but they are not organizations as much as brand names. In many cases, the individual parts of the organization have as much contact with the bosses as a local Coca- Cola bottling plant manager might have with corporate headquarters.

Even the vaunted Sinaloa Cartel is more horizontally than vertically integrated. Take the recent case of the Flores brothers in Chicago. Before they were arrested, Pedro and Margarito Flores were said to be Sinaloa Cartel distributors in Chicago, one of the areas of greatest interest to this subcommittee. And they were. But as Federal intercepts of their conversations with cartel leaders show, the two brothers negotiated independently with each of the top two members of the Sinaloa criminal organization, obtaining different prices for the product that they were selling. Even after a war started between the Sinaloa Cartel and a rival group called the Beltran Leyva Organization, the Flores brothers continued to purchase drugs from portions of the Beltran Leyva organization and the Sinaloa Cartel.

The Flores case cuts at two different myths about the Sinaloa Cartel: number one, that this is one single organization; and number two, that it is tightly controlled by a single leader or a single group of leaders. The point is that as shipments get further and further from Mexico's wholesale points, the loyalties become more disperse and in some cases completely disappear. This is especially true in the U.S. market where violence is not a viable long-term option to ensure loyalty, win market share, or become a monopoly.

The effectiveness of U.S. law enforcement has made violence terrible for business and made the distribution chain a more democratic, capitalist affair. This is evident in other ways as well. While the amount of seizures indicates that there is more heroin available in the United States, it is still moved in very small quantities. The median seizure for the Los Angeles Field Division of the DEA in 2014, for example, was a single kilogram. In Denver, a 10- to 12-pound shipment is considered large.

The case of the Laredo brothers, recently indicted in the Eastern District of Pennsylvania, is indicative of these trends. The Laredo brothers are charged with moving 1 ton of heroin over a 6-year period. This is about 14 kilos per month. The organization was so subtle and, as one Mexican analyst put it, "mom-and-pop," the Mexican authorities were not even aware of the group.

This brings us to Mexico. The horizontal nature of the distribution chain makes it a difficult law enforcement problem in Mexico as well. As noted, the once monolithic criminal organizations are shells of what they once were. This is in part due to infighting of the type mentioned earlier but also Mexican law enforcement efforts. Many of the fragmented pieces have formed their own criminal organizations and brand names.

The upshot is that the chain of production in Mexico is broken into numerous pieces, including small and large producers of opium poppy plants, the opium gum producers, and processors, the wholesale purchasers, and the transporters. Production, transport, and distribution may all be different organizations. The Laredo brothers, for example, were purchasing opium gum from an independent broker, then processing it themselves, and distributing it in those small quantities in the U.S. for years without running into trouble with the large, supposedly all-controlling Sinaloa Cartel.

To be sure, violence is still a viable option in Mexico, so the pendulum may swing back towards more monolithic criminal organizations. But for the moment, the reality is that there are literally dozens of small criminal organizations involved in this trade from the point of production to the point of sale.

In sum, while the level of control that the Mexican production and transport groups exert over the supply chain is clear, we are not talking about one or two criminal groups, but dozens of interlocking organizations whose alliances are constantly shifting. The heroin supply chain appears to be a largely horizontal, diversified operation with multiple actors, and one that is obedient to market forces rather than one or two single vertically integrated distributors.

The result is that law enforcement efforts are largely muted. Whether you debilitate the Sinaloa Cartel or the Laredo brothers, you are hindering a small part of the overall production and distribution chain. Even if you did slow the heroin from Mexico, you would face an insurmountable task: stopping the flow from other countries, which would undoubtedly fill the void and account for the bulk of worldwide production anyway. Canada already gets up to 90 percent of its heroin from Afghanistan. And the United States once got all of its heroin from the Asian markets that supply the rest of the world.

Thank you for your time and attention. I look forward to your questions.

[Mr. Dudley's prepared statement is located in the Additional Material Submitted for the Record section at the end of this transcript.]

Senator RUBIO. Thank you both for being here.

I want to begin with one of the questions I alluded during the testimony, and that is—I cannot prove it. I guess it is anecdotal. We do not have a number behind this. But the notion that these criminal groups are specifically targeting people recovering. In essence, they basically station themselves outside of a rehabilitation outpatient center, even an inpatient center, knowing that these people are vulnerable and enticing them to fall back into addiction.

Mayor, have you seen evidence of this? Mr. Dudley, have you heard about this as a recurring issue, a specific practice at the local level of targeting people in recovery for sales?

Ms. JACOBS. Senator, I have not seen evidence of targeting our treatment facilities.

I will say that it certainly appears on the surface that there has been a targeting effort towards which communities to infiltrate with heroin, and certainly I look to the increase in heroin coming into our communities, the increase of fentanyl at the same time that we were restricting access to prescription drugs as suspecting that there is a strong correlation between those two and a causation between those as well. But I do not have direct evidence of it. It just seems hard to imagine that there would not be a direct relationship between them.

Mr. DUDLEY. Thank you, Senator.

I also do not have direct evidence of this activity on a local level. I will say in Mexico that criminal groups have targeted recovery facilities, but more as recruitment centers, not necessarily—— Senator RUBIO. Recruitment centers for?

Mr. DUDLEY. Recruitment centers for them, to basically build out their own criminal operations.

Senator RUBIO. You mean for like dealers?

Mr. DUDLEY. Not for dealers. Just for membership. So people who would participate in the criminal organization. So that has certainly happened especially with regard to La Familia Michoacana, a very famous group there.

The upshot of this is to say whether or not they are targeting to pushing drugs in certain areas I am not sure is as relevant as this sort of whole picture, which is what the Mayor alluded to, which is this idea that this is largely driven from people who use pharmaceutical drugs, and those people you can find all over. And that accounts also for the sort of dispersed nature of this epidemic as opposed to sort of the 1970s where you had it very concentrated in urban areas. Now we have it spread out throughout many different parts of the United States.

Senator RUBIO. So I want to share with you an anecdote. This weekend, I have a personal friend who is a police officer in Miami Dade County, and he recounted a story that he pulled up to a car that was kind of pulled over on the side of the road. And there was a woman in the driver's seat. She was kind of slumped over, and it caught his curiosity. So he pulled over and knocked on the window. This was a nice car, by the way. Obviously, this is a person of financial means. Knocks on the window and the person immediately pops to attention. And he can see that in her arm there was a needle. She was basically shooting up on the side of the road in a luxury vehicle. Knocks on the window. She rolls down the window. They begin to interact. Obviously, he had a decision to make about how to treat her. This is someone who said 10 years ago he would have arrested her and taken her in as a criminal using drugs in the street.

Today his perception has changed because he has had several interactions, including this interaction with a person who, by the way, is a member of the Florida Bar, is a successful, functional attorney whose husband apparently also has a problem. The fundamental challenge he faces: he does not want to take her to jail. He does not view her as a criminal. He views her as someone who has a disease and is in need of treatment to overcome it.

And by the way, her gateway into heroin was the use of a pharmaceutical pain killer for a surgical procedure 6 or 7 years ago, which she lost access to the medicine, and this is what has happened.

And so the concern that I have is twofold, and perhaps you can both opine on this.

Number one, if today you are dependent upon an opiate substance, irrespective of how you got there, but let us say in the case of this person because of the use of a pharmaceutical that led to this point, there is still an extraordinary stigma associated with it as if you are a bad person who is doing a really bad thing and needs to be punished for it.

And second, even if that stigma were to change so that we can get more people into treatment and accepting the fact that I am physically dependent on this substance, in many communities there is nowhere to take them. The only place you can take them potentially is to a jail where you hope their withdrawals are managed but may not be. And in essence, there is nowhere for them to go. We have many places. We just do not have the capacity to meet that reality.

Which leads to the third problem, and that is the number of people who end up in a jail cell for 15 days, go through withdrawal, do not realize they have lost their tolerance, even in that short period of time, and when they fall off the proverbial wagon, they go back to using the levels they were using before they went through withdrawal and it kills them because they lost their tolerance for an opiate.

So given that perspective, I am sure there are hundreds, if not thousand of cases like that. What are the impediments to getting someone who faces this now who—I do not think so, but could be watching C–SPAN at this very moment. Not many people watch C– SPAN—but are watching this or are hearing us talk about this. What is out there today or what is missing for someone who needs this treatment and just does not know what to do about it next? Because especially for the uninsured, there are not very many options from my understanding.

Ms. JACOBS. Thank you, Mr. Chairman. I think that is a key part of addressing the demand side. Part of it is to educate people and help them make the right choices to avoid overuse of prescription drugs, but the other part is how do we provide the resources to treat people that are addicted. And the treatment options are very limited. For the uninsured, as I pointed out, 26 beds for 2.4 million people. Our jail alone, one out of four jails in the region, we have on average 200 people that we are treating for withdrawal symptoms and offering them a treatment program when they leave. We need more treatment facilities.

When you ask me the question are traffickers, are dealers preying on people coming out of treatment centers, the reality is we do not have enough treatment centers to prey on.

Senator RUBIO. You said in your testimony—and I do not want to interrupt, but you said in your testimony you believe that Florida was specifically targeted because they knew we had the pill mill problem, and once that was cut off, these folks were going to need——

Ms. JACOBS. Exactly. That is what I believe. I do not have empirical evidence. What I have is the evidence of the increase in the flow of heroin and the increases in deaths related to heroin in correlation to our cutting off the pill mills.

Let me also say that while we were dispensing more oxycodone than the rest of the country combined out of Florida, most of that was leaving our State. And most of these pill mills—you could drive up and you could look in the parking lots. The parking lot would be full and only a small percentage of those were local license plates. So the cartels may have misjudged the appetite, but they, no question, have flooded us with very, very cheap drugs.

And the number of youth that I have seen that are struggling with addiction and have turned the corner and have had the good fortune and the money to find treatment, the insured portion of that population, to see that there actually is life after heroin addiction is very encouraging. But what is very discouraging is that most people that are addicts have no idea there is life, and most people that are addicts have no opportunity to get to those treatment centers.

Senator RUBIO. Just to fill in the gaps for those who may not be fully aware of the Florida pill mill problem, we had these facilities. You just basically pulled up and said my neck hurts or my back hurts, and by routine, they would give you a package of prescriptions. It was not just, by the way, oxy. They also put some other stuff in there. And people knew this, and you would have busloads of people actually come in sometimes. It was a huge problem. The Florida legislature closed that loophole that was allowing this to happen. So just to be fair, we are not talking about the oxy prescriptions being driven by a doctor at his or her office. It was these specific facilities that drove it.

Did you want to add something on the treatment part of it? Because I had one more question. I know that Senator Kaine——

Mr. DUDLEY. Just very quickly. I mean, this is obviously framed as a law enforcement debate. And certainly I was asked to talk about the criminal organizations.

But as you rightly pointed out, this is a public health issue. At the heart of it, this is a pharmaceutically driven epidemic, and it is a public health issue. And that is really the difficulty in facing up to this is that it is not necessarily strictly law enforcement. We are not talking about throwing people into jails. We need to be talking about how to get them better treatment.

Senator RUBIO. And my sense on the human side of it is I do not believe anyone wakes up in the morning and says today is the day I become a heroin addict or an opiate addict. It is not something somebody wants to happen. You just see growing evidence. People do not realize the power of this. There is no responsible way to use this, and its impact on everybody is a little different. We know some people are more sensitive or susceptible to addiction than others, but it basically restructures the brain's chemistry in a way a disease would and it has to be treated as that.

I look at these statistics, for example, in Florida as just an example. Orlando had 83 heroin deaths in 2014. Other communities have large numbers with West Palm Beach at 51, Miami at 60, Sarasota at 55. But that number pops out at you as a place that has been specifically targeted.

And then you see the rise in deaths and kind of the spike we have seen across the country in heroin and opiate deaths where the takeoff point is the introduction of fentanyl which, as we have already seen from testimony today, is an incredibly powerful and lethal substance, which in fact from my understanding is not prescribed outside of a hospital setting to begin with on the pharmaceutical side and is now being laced into——

I want to go to Senator Kaine. So I wanted to leave with this thought. I read the other day a report where someone who was a former—he is now a recovering addict—was asked about this and said, you know, when you hear that someone has died from an overdose that was sold by a particular dealer, it makes you want to buy from that particular dealer because you know what they are selling is the strong stuff. Now, maybe that is just one interview, one line somebody said. But it just kind of tells you the point we have reached here where it is a very difficult and debilitating condition that we have to try to understand here. And I think one of the keys is to remove the stigma associated with it.

And I think many of us would be very surprised at the number of people we interact with on a daily basis that at some level have a dependence problem, maybe not through street heroin, but of some sort as a result of what we have seen happen in this country. And hopefully we can make advances in pharmaceuticals so that we can draw the line and we will be able to treat pain effectively in this country without putting people at risk.

Senator Kaine?

Senator KAINE. Thank you, Mr. Chair.

And thanks to each of you. I am sorry I missed your opening testimony, although I read your written testimony.

And, Mayor, I will start with you. I was a mayor too in Richmond. And it was only when I was mayor that I really fully grasped the depths of the demand side of this challenge. You know, you can arrest a dealer and arrest another dealer and arrest another dealer, but if the demand for drugs is so potent, if it has its hooks in people so deeply, the next dealer will appear tomorrow.

We had a really tough problem in Richmond, and a lot of drug- related homicides were taking place in this little neighborhood near where the church that I go to is. And the number of stories that would appear on the front page of the paper about somebody from the suburbs coming in to buy drugs and getting shot at the corner of 2nd and Maryland or wherever, and you would think about five of those stories, people would quit driving in to buy drugs there. But, no, they would keep driving in to buy drugs.

And that just was evidence of how powerful addiction is, that you would have all this objective evidence that, wow, this is really going to be dangerous for me to go, but much less that the drugs could be dangerous, I could get shot, but the need is so intense that I am still going to go. And it sounds like you have seen that in your community. I was a mayor 20 years ago. The drugs were different. But it is the same thing of this addiction. And that is why the treatment issues are so important.

And the other thing we used to hear anecdotally—I am not an expert in this field, but when somebody who is under the grip of an addiction says I want treatment, that is a window that opens where the treatment, if it is not there, the window can close. And in a month from now when the bed opens up, the individual may be past the point of wanting treatment, may have ODed or may have lapsed back into behaviors not desiring treatment. So I do appreciate what the chair was saying and you were saying too about the need for treatment.

I am curious if you can talk about as a mayor the way to solve some of these challenges is definitely through how the partnership, State, Federal—talk a little bit about what you have done in your county on the partnership side. Do you have the right stakeholders around the table? Are there things we can do from a Federal level to ensure that if we are issuing funds, that we do it in a way that requires regional cooperation or multi-level stakeholder cooperation?

Ms. JACOBS. Thank you, Senator. In Orlando, one of the things that I think we have done very effectively is regional cooperation and collaboration. I think that that is crucial on tackling any large issue such as this. And so one of the reasons that we pulled together the task force that we did is we brought in so many different disciplines to make sure that we could attack this problem from all angles.

It is so important. We have limited resources at all government levels, and it always seems like the demand for resources outpaces supply. So it is important that programs are structured in a way that the funding is put to its best use.

And I do think that collaborative effort is important. We have a Metropolitan Bureau of Investigation that pulls together our FDLE, FDA, our local law enforcement, our police officers, our sheriff, our State attorney's office. That has been very effective for us on the enforcement side of this.

In terms of your comments about that window of opportunity for addicts, I cannot understand it either because I have never experienced a feeling of needing something so badly that I am willing to risk my life to have it. But I do understand that is the reality. I know enough people. Once we formed the task force, enough people came forward, literally walked up to me on the street. You know what it is like being a local mayor. People recognize you. They come up and they pour their heart and soul out to you. And it is a blessing to be at that level where you can really heard firsthand. And I have seen young people that you would never in your wildest imagination have thought were heroin addicts tell me their stories.

And what I also saw—I think I mentioned before you walked in here—was I also saw the other side. I saw that they came out the other side of heroin addiction, and they are living full lives and they are getting college degrees and they are going to be productive members of society.

And I think that most heroin addicts do not believe that is a possibility, and if they have that moment, if it is 15 minutes, if it is 2 hours, if it is 2 days, where they say, gosh, I want to kick this, reality is they are not going to be waiting for 2 weeks or a month. They are going to be waiting a lot longer in most of our communities to get into a treatment facility unless they have got a substantial amount of money. And that is a huge problem.

And as I said in my testimony, the best option is our county jail right now, and that is a lousy option. Not to say we have a bad jail. We do our best. But having a record does not help the situation.

So we really need to have options available. We need to have education. We need to have hope. We need to have whole communities that are engaged. And as you point out, it is destroying more than lives. It is destroying entire communities.

Thank you, sir.

Senator KAINE. We had, Mr. Chair, a chart recently placed before us at another hearing about opioid-based ODs per capita, the 50 States arrayed. It was unlike any chart I have ever seen ever. If you look at a chart that is usually about some kind of problem or crime or social breakdown, high income States will be at one part of the chart and low income States will be at the other part of the chart. If you looked at the top 10 most affected States, they included some of the poorest States in the country and some of the richest States in the country. And if you looked at the bottom 10 affected States, they included some of the poorest States in the country and some of the richest States in the country. This is really unlike any sort of similar epidemic or law enforcement problem I have ever seen in the traditional demographic data, not at all a predictor. It is rural over the suburban. It is all regions.

I went to a drug court graduation. Kind of the founding drug court in Virginia is in the Roanoke area, and the judge who founded it, who was this super, farsighted thinker about the need for drug courts, had a child who many years later was killed in a drug-related incident. And after I spoke at the graduation, one of the probation officers who helps the court run and has done so as a spectacular advocate for many years came up to me and said this is my second drug court graduation this week. I said, did you have another class? He said no. I went to my son's graduation in a community about 2 hours from here.

This affects every level, and that is why we are now spending the time that we are. But we have not spent time in this committee on it, and it is really important that we do so because this is not— just like it does not have demographic borders, this is not a problem that even has national borders. And we have got to grab a hold of some of the dimensions, Mexico, China, the other nations that are experiencing this, and build those partnerships not even in a metropolitan region, but we have got to build law enforcement and other partnerships internationally.

Thank you for being here, for your testimony.

Thank you, Mr. Chair.

Senator RUBIO. Thank you, Senator.

And I just wanted to ask you, Mr. Dudley, about these transnational groups that are targeting us. I think in your testimony you talked about this. So I just want to reiterate it. Whether it is fentanyl being produced synthetically or poppy-based opiates being grown in the Western Hemisphere, in particular in Mexico, they are coming here. This is the almost exclusive market for these trafficking networks. Is that correct?

Mr. DUDLEY. That is correct, absolutely. There is a small market, local market that they can satisfy, but it is minimal.

Senator RUBIO. Because you would think—so logically they are crossing the border, you would think the easiest from a logistical point of view is for them to flood it into Texas or flood it into California or into a border State. But you are hearing where the outbreaks are. And this is a national problem. There is no community in the country that does face it to some level, but you see these outbreaks in the Northeast in New Hampshire and Massachusetts and in places like central Florida. So it is not even I–10 alone where you would think they would come across.

What is your view of how is it winding up in these pockets? What are the distinguishing characteristics? You heard the previous testimony of the government witnesses. What in your view are the distinguishing characteristics that turn a community into a high- propensity, high-risk area?

Mr. DUDLEY. You know, it is such a new phenomenon because it is so disperse. But the fact that it is so disperse is really what leads to the criminal organizations being so disperse. And the notion that we have one single, all-encompassing enemy that is called the Sinaloa Cartel and once we incarcerate Chapo Guzman, then everything will be resolved is just simply not correct just because of the disperse nature of the market and the way in which these criminal organizations will satisfy that market.

It is an odd thing because in a way there are certain elements of this epidemic that we are victims of our own success. The fact that you would create ways so you cannot tamper with OxyContin, for example, you cannot store it anymore, the way in which it is distributed, well, then that makes it less available to people so then they start to search out other things.

The way in which the Mexican Government, in conjunction with the United States Government, has captured or killed several of the larger leaders of the larger criminal organizations has led to a fragmentation of these groups. So you have groups like you referred to Guerrero earlier. There is a Guerrero Unidos group, which was the group responsible for the massacre or supposed massacre of those 43 students that disappeared, 43 students currently still. You know, this is a group that was an offshoot of a larger group, the Beltran Leyva organization, and there are several like them.

So in order to wrap your hands around this as a law enforcement issue, it is incredibly difficult because the terrain is so much more horizontal than vertical. And even when you take out the larger leaders, what you are left with is a fragmented criminal landscape, and a landscape that does not necessarily—as in the cocaine market, they might depend on getting product from another country. In fact, they do from the Andes region. They need to get their product from other criminal organizations. But they do not have that dependency when it comes to the poppy production which is local and the heroin production which is local. So they can produce all of this themselves, which makes it much more difficult to wrap your hands around as well.

Senator RUBIO. Well, do you have anything further Senator?

I want to thank both of you for being here, for sitting through the previous testimony. I hope that was insightful as you go back and continue your work. And I want to thank you for coming here today and being a part of this hearing as well. This is an important issue. There has been a lot of debate about what is being done domestically on this issue. I am glad we touched on it.

I think this has to be dealt with. There is not like one law we can pass that deals with this. It has to be dealt with comprehensively whether it is on the treatment side for people to recover, on the prevention side, but also by targeting these organizations who are in the business of murder basically, which is what this ultimately is, and not just murdering each other for territory, but the direct murder of Americans by targeting us with the distribution of these products in our country.

So I want to thank all of you for being here.

I also want to ask consent to enter a statement for the record of Jack Riley, who is the Acting Deputy Administrator of the Drug Enforcement Administration. And without objection, I show that ordered.

[Mr. Riley's statement is located in the Additional Material Submitted for the Record section at the end of this transcript.]

Senator RUBIO. The record for this hearing is going to remain open until the close of business on Tuesday, May 31st. You might receive some questions in writing. If possible, I would ask you to respond just so we can close the record on this.

And with that I thank you both for being here, and this meeting is adjourned.

[Whereupon, at 10:55 a.m., the hearing was adjourned.]

Additional Material Submitted for the Record

Additional Questions Submitted for the Record by Members of the Committee, Responses to Questions Submitted to Assistant Secretary Daniel Foote by Senator Marco Rubio

Question 1. Mexico has been a very good partner but systemic corruption and other issues, including issues of trust, persist. What is the U.S. government's assessment of Mexico's commitment to truly stopping the Sinaloa cartel, in particular, and the flow of illicit narcotics to the U.S.?

Answer. Our partnership with the Government of Mexico on counternarcotics has led to enhanced collaboration on this important issue. The State Department's Bureau of International Narcotics and Law Enforcement Affairs (INL), under the Merida Initiative, is working with the Government of Mexico to help build the capacity of Mexico's law enforcement and rule of law institutions to disrupt drug trafficking organizations (DTOs) and to stop the flow of drugs from Mexico to the United States, including augmenting their ability to coordinate with U.S. law enforcement agencies. Through Merida, we have provided the Mexican government with the communications equipment and technical assistance to enable the Department of Homeland Security's Customs and Border Protection (CBP) and the Mexican Federal Police to conduct coordinated patrols of our shared border. Merida-supported implementation of the Cross Border Secure Communications Network and Cross Border Coordination Initiative provides direct communication between CBP Sector Offices and Mexico's Federal Police and State Command and Control Centers at ten locations along our shared border. INL also is working in partnership with CBP to provide training to Mexican Federal Police officers assigned to the northern border region.

The United States and Mexico are working to increase communication and information sharing on combating the production and trafficking of heroin and methamphetamine. In addition to discussions at the high level Security Cooperation Group meetings, in the last year INL supported U.S. Drug Enforcement Administration-led bimonthly counternarcotics meetings, which bring together experts from both countries to share information and strategies. These efforts to increase cooperation are paying off. Federal and state police in one of Mexico's northern border states recently arrested two suspects and seized 630 kilograms of methamphetamine, 80 kilograms of heroin, 48 kilograms of cocaine, one semi-automatic weapon, and two AK-47 assault rifles after acting on real-time intelligence provided by U.S. law enforcement. The federal police unit involved in the operation participates in the bimonthly counternarcotics meetings.

In recent years, the Government of Mexico has taken active steps to reduce corruption and other illegal activities in police forces and government institutions by vetting public officials through its Control de Confianza system. INL seeks to strengthen and accredit Mexican vetting institutions by establishing and deploying uniform standards for polygraph administration, background (socio-economic) investigations, and psychological assessments.

Question 2. Mexico has adopted a policy of high profile arrest of drug lords. While it is positive that these organizations are being decapitated, has the drug trade run by the cartels been impacted by these arrests in the way envisioned?

Answer. Capturing and successfully prosecuting high profile traffickers who have committed serious crimes and have operated with relative impunity is essential to maintaining the rule of law. High profile drug lords are responsible for the deaths of tens of thousands, and their sophisticated organizations create violence, generate illegal earnings and influence, and ultimately harm U.S. citizens and interests through cross-border flows of illicit drugs, goods, and people. We refer you to the U.S. Drug Enforcement Administration for additional details on the potential impact on the drug trade resulting from Mexico's high profile arrests.

Recognizing, however, that targeting high profile traffickers alone will not solve Mexico's security dilemma, the State Department's Bureau of International Narcotics and Law Enforcement Affairs (INL) supports Mexico's security and law enforcement efforts more broadly. Combating transnational criminal organizations requires a comprehensive approach that disrupts illicit financial and trafficking networks, combats government corruption, strengthens the rule of law, bolsters judicial systems, and enhances transparency. Under the Merida Initiative, INL focuses not only on disrupting organized criminal groups, but on institutionalizing rule of law, strengthening border security, and building strong and resilient communities in Mexico. INL's efforts to enhance state-level law enforcement professionalization, support Mexico's efforts along its northern and southern borders, and assist Mexico's transition to an accusatory justice system all augment the capacity of Mexico to effectively provide security, disrupt organized crime, and manage its borders.

Question 3. Since the arrest of Joaquin "El Chapo" Guzman, has there been a noticeable drop in narcotics trafficked by his organization? Specifically heroin?

Answer. At this time, the effect of El Chapo's arrest on the amount of narcotics trafficked by the Sinaloa Cartel is unclear. We refer you to the U.S. Drug Enforcement Administration for additional information on shifts in the trafficking of narcotics, including heroin.

The United States is fully committed to working with Mexico to combat the production and trafficking of illicit drugs. Over the past year, our bilateral dialogue, specifically on heroin, has reached an unprecedented level of openness and coordination and we are continuing to work closely with Mexico to increase these efforts.

Question 4. What successes can the U.S. government point to in cooperation with the Mexican government that have yielded concrete results?

Answer. For the past eight years under the Merida Initiative, the U.S. government has worked closely with the Government of Mexico to advance our shared security objectives and these efforts are demonstrating results, including:

Criminal Intelligence and Analysis Program

To support the Government of Mexico in improving criminal investigations to hold drug traffickers and other criminals accountable and boost public confidence in the rule of law, INL is supporting the professionalization of criminal intelligence analysts throughout Mexico. Initial programming has focused on equipping and training analytic units along the Mexico- U.S. border to serve as the primary state-level liaison with U.S. law enforcement entities to develop intelligence related to drug cultivation and trafficking, extortions, kidnappings, and homicides.

INL has trained and equipped five analytic units that have contributed to 1,900 investigations/citizen complaints resulting in more than 200 arrests as of the end of 2015. The units in the cities of Chihuahua and Ciudad Juarez provided intelligence that led to the arrest of a principal leader of the Sinaloa cartel. The Chihuahua unit also assisted in the identification and apprehension of two suspects responsible for an attack on a Ciudad Juarez television station, in addition to six kidnappings and five homicides. This unit also aided the apprehension of suspects responsible for the murder of the sons of two prominent Mexican journalists. The Sonora unit developed tactical intelligence, which led to the arrest of four suspects, identified as former Mexican military and enforcers for the Sinaloa Cartel. It also worked with ICE/HSI on an investigation that resulted in the seizure of five weapons, one grenade, three vehicles, and 450 kilograms of marijuana in Nogales, Sonora in 2015.

Anti-Money Laundering

To assist Mexico in disrupting transnational criminal organizations (TCOs), INL provided over $16 million in hardware, software, servers, and technical assistance to Mexico's Financial Intelligence Unit (UIF), a division of Mexico's Secretariat of Public Finance and Credit responsible for receiving, analyzing, and disseminating information on suspicious financial transactions. This assistance enhanced the Government of Mexico's ability to combat financial crimes and money laundering activity, resulting in the following successes:

In 2014 alone, the UIF froze 761 suspicious accounts.

Between March 2014 and May 2015, the UIF froze approximately $41 million in suspicious assets.

The UIF reports it collected as much data in 2015 as in the previous six years combined due to new IT platforms and additional data storage capacity principally provided by INL.

Corrections

Since 2008, the Department of State's Bureau of International Narcotics and Law Enforcement Affairs (INL) and the Government of Mexico have partnered to create a more effective, transparent, and humane prison system, including through accreditation by the American Correctional Association (ACA), which has helped to reduce escapism and mitigate the ability of imprisoned cartel members to fuel organized crime from behind bars. As of May 2016, a total of 30 Mexican correctional facilities have achieved ACA accreditation: six federal prisons, 22 state prisons, one state central office, and the federal training academy. INL plans to work toward having all federal prisons and one quarter of state prisons ACA-accredited by 2021. In a recent National Human Rights Commission (CNDH) evaluation of more than 150 federal and state prisons, ACA-accredited prisons received significantly higher average scores than non-ACA-accredited facilities. Of the top ten facilities, eight are either accredited or seeking accreditation, and none of the ten lowest scoring facilities in the CNDH evaluation are ACA-affiliated.

The state prison system in Chihuahua is an example of the program's success. In 2010, 216 prisoners in Chihuahua died as a result of prison violence, and the state reported more than 17 escapes. After achieving INL-sponsored ACA accreditation in 2013, there have been only three violent prison deaths, and no escapes from any accredited facility.

Question 5. I believe we should continue to expand military to military cooperation with the Mexican government as long as the Mexicans welcome our contributions. Maritime cooperation between our navies and coast guards seems like an underdeveloped area. Perhaps U.S. Northern Command should look at a role for Mexico to play in NORAD. The U.S. should also work to bring Canadian law enforcement into closer cooperation with Mexican law enforcement to stem illicit trafficking. What other opportunities exist where cooperation between the U.S. and Mexican governments can be improved?

Answer. We have an excellent relationship with the Mexican government and together we are continuously assessing our security relationship and working on ways to improve and enhance our cooperation.

The biannual "Security Cooperation Group" meeting, co-chaired by the National Security Council and Mexico's Center for Investigation and National Security (CISEN), serves as the primary forum for our senior policy makers to work with their Mexican counterparts to devise strategies to combat our shared security threats and identify and reassess strategic priorities, such as continuing the fight against organized crime, enhancing counternarcotics efforts, and jointly managing our 2,000 mile shared border. There are also multiple venues and working groups that facilitate operational and tactical security cooperation, including through the 21st Century Border Management Initiative, bilateral border violence prevention protocols, and other coordination mechanisms.

Specific to our military relationship, U.S. Northern Command works with Mexico on initiatives that not only assist in mitigating the current Transnational Criminal Organization (TCO) threat, but also focus on capacity building. They work with the Mexican Navy (SEMAR) and Army (SEDENA) to build specific capabilities, enhance our bilateral and regional engagement, and prioritize joint activities through programs in aviation, communications, and civil-military operations. SEMAR's participation in exercises, combined and multilateral, is increasing and planning is underway for joint U.S.-Mexican exercises next year that will increase interoperability with U.S. Naval Forces and bolster regional security.

The North American Leaders' Summit, to be attended by President Obama, Mexican President Peña Nieto, and Canadian Prime Minister Trudeau, will take place in Ottawa on June 29. The discussion of the effective exchange of information and coordination among law enforcement authorities will remain essential. We will also discuss continued coordination to pursue areas of cooperation to counter drug trafficking, trafficking in persons, and other illicit trade.

Question 6. Please summarize any progress that has been made as a result of the bilateral talks that have been occurring over the past year on how the U.S. and Mexican government can address heroin cultivation and production in Mexico.

Answer. Over the past year, our bilateral dialogue with the Government of Mexico on heroin has reached an unprecedented level of openness. This has led to enhanced U.S.-Mexico collaboration on this critically important issue, including increased communication and information sharing on heroin. In March 2016, Office of National Drug Control Policy Director Michael Botticelli and the State Department's Bureau of International Narcotics and Law Enforcement Affairs (INL) Assistant Secretary William R. Brownfield participated in meetings hosted by the Mexican Attorney General's Office with high-level officials from each of the Mexican federal government agencies involved in drug enforcement to discuss U.S.-Mexican collaboration on heroin and potential new areas of assistance. INL continues to increase the capacity of law enforcement and justice sector institutions to detect heroin distribution networks and prosecute those involved. INL has hosted seminars with several Mexican agencies to increase information sharing on heroin, and has facilitated a study trip with Mexican officials to Guatemala and Peru to examine poppy eradication best practices. The United States has provided more than $130 million in non-intrusive inspection equipment, maintenance, technical assistance, and capacity building to enhance the capabilities of Mexican officials at internal checkpoints and points of entry along Mexico's northern and southern border. INL is also working with the U.S. Drug Enforcement Administration (DEA) to provide training to augment Mexico's ability to identify, investigate, and interdict clandestine heroin labs, and better prepare Mexican officials to dismantle them.

This year, the Government of Mexico is expected to finalize its National Drug Control Policy Plan, and to lay out protocols for poppy eradication. Mexico is also working with the United Nations Office on Drugs and Crime (UNODC) on a yield study that will enable more accurate estimates of potential heroin production. Initial reports outlining baseline poppy cultivation estimates will be completed this year. These reports will provide a greater understanding of how Mexican eradication and interdiction responsibilities will be organized going forward, and will help shape the best areas for U.S. assistance. INL will continue to work closely with Mexico to increase efforts to combat heroin.

Question 7. How would you assess the assertion made by a group of experts from the Inter-American Commission on Human Rights, that there may have been another bus involved in the incident in which 43 students disappeared in Guerrero, Mexico, that was packed with heroin bound for the U.S.?

Answer. We strongly support the work of the Interdisciplinary Group of Independent Experts affiliated with the Inter-American Commission on Human Rights and commend the assistance they have provided to the Government of Mexico with respect to the investigation of the September 2014 disappearance of 43 students in Iguala, Mexico. We have encouraged Mexican authorities to incorporate the experts' findings into the ongoing official investigation.

In the reports released in September 2015 and April 2016, the experts noted the organized crime group alleged to be involved in the attack on the students and their disappearance is connected to drug trafficking to the United States and, specifically, to a case before a federal court in Chicago. The experts hypothesized that the extreme violence against the students and the alleged "missing" fifth bus might be related to this drug trafficking—i.e., that unknown to the students who seized several buses, one of those buses could have contained drugs or drug money, which in turn led to the violent attacks of September 26, 2014. The Department of State is not in a position to evaluate the merits of that hypothesis.

WITNESSES PREPARED STATEMENTS

Prepared Statement of Daniel L. Foote, Deputy Assistant Secretary, Bureau of International Narcotics and Law Enforcement Affairs

Chairman Rubio, Senator Boxer, and distinguished Members of the Subcommittee: thank you for the opportunity to appear before you to discuss U.S. government efforts to combat the production and trafficking of heroin and the violence and instability it brings to our communities, our citizens, and the world in which we live.

The flow of illicit narcotics across our shared border with Mexico threatens citizen security in both countries. Recognizing that we have a shared responsibility to address common challenges, in 2007, the United States forged a comprehensive security partnership with Mexico. Through the Merida Initiative, we work in partnership with Mexico to build the capacity of Mexican institutions to counter organized crime, uphold the rule of law, and protect our shared border from the movement of illicit drugs, money, and goods.

The need for effective collaboration is now more important than ever. Heroin and fentanyl-laced heroin is a public health crisis in the United States, and Mexican drug trafficking organizations are the primary suppliers of heroin to the United States. We must aggressively respond to this growing threat in concert with our broader work through the Merida Initiative to counter all illicit drugs and to end the impunity with which trafficking organizations are able to operate, putting their leaders in jail, seizing their weapons, drugs, and money, and dismantling their illicit businesses.

To date through the Merida Initiative, the United States government has provided nearly $1.5 billion worth of capacity building assistance to our Mexican partners. This includes training and equipment which complements the significant resources the Government of Mexico has dedicated to our shared security goals. Today there are more than $700 million in bilaterally agreed upon projects with the Peña Nieto administration, which fully support the Merida Initiative's strategic framework that underpins the basis of our security cooperation. Most of these projects fall into three priority areas: professionalizing and building the capacity of Mexican law enforcement agencies; supporting the Government of Mexico's efforts to strengthen border management and security; and helping advance reforms across Mexico's justice sector.

In partnership with the Department of Justice, INL is building the skills of prosecutors, investigators, and forensic experts in Mexico and preparing them for their responsibilities under the oral accusatory system, the transition to which is well underway throughout Mexico. This includes helping enhance the technical capacity of courtrooms throughout the country to host oral trials. We are also assisting in the training of the next generation of Mexican attorneys as they learn crucial oral trial skills in Mexican law schools.

Through Merida, INL is enhancing federal, state, and municipal policing capacity throughout Mexico. These programs provide a full range of professionalization activities including: the development of enforceable police standards; basic training and academy accreditation; continuing and leadership education programs; law enforcement vetting programs; and the development of effective internal affairs units. The continued professionalization of Mexican law enforcement will result in a greater observance of and accountability for civil and human rights, increasing trust in these institutions by the people of Mexico, and making them better partners for other law enforcement organizations both within Mexico and with the United States. This is vital to any effort to stem drug trafficking and reduce the capabilities and influence of drug trafficking organizations.

Strengthening border security capacity on Mexico's borders is a priority for both our nations. Our governments have committed to further enhancing Mexico's ability to interdict illicit narcotics, arms, and money. INL has provided more than $125 million in inspection equipment and more than 340 canine teams deployed at ports of entry, border crossings, and internal checkpoints throughout Mexico. In Mexico's northern border region, INL has provided equipment and technical assistance to improve communications between the Mexican Federal Police and U.S. Customs and Border Protection (CBP). We are working in conjunction with CBP to provide training to Mexico's Federal Police who will be deployed to the northern border region, advancing cooperation between our countries along our shared border.

Through Merida, we continue to make progress with Mexico in targeting heroin production and trafficking. We work with the U.S. Drug Enforcement Administration to provide training to augment Mexico's ability to identify, investigate, and interdict clandestine heroin labs, and better prepare Mexican authorities to dismantle them. We are improving information sharing between our governments on heroin and fentanyl, working together to better assess poppy cultivation and heroin production in Mexico, and with our interagency partners, continuing our high-level focus on exploring other avenues to enhance our bilateral cooperation when it comes to heroin.

At the last high level Security Cooperation Group held in Mexico City in October 2015, heroin was the group's highest priority. We agreed to continue working in partnership on a bilateral approach for combating the cultivation, production, and trafficking of heroin and to determine how U.S. assistance can best support Mexico's efforts in this area.

Building strong, effective justice sector institutions in Mexico capable of confronting organized crime and the violence and corruption for which it is responsible is a difficult, long-term challenge. Our work across numerous institutions and sectors must be sustained, for it is only with a concerted, committed effort that the capacity to deter the cultivation, production, and trafficking of heroin and other illicit drugs in Mexico will be strengthened. Past investments by the American people in this partnership have produced results, and with your continued support, our collaboration with Mexico on this important work will continue.

Prepared Statement of Kemp L. Chester, Associate Director for the National Heroin Coordination Group, Office of National Drug Policy

Chairman Rubio, Ranking Member Boxer, and members of the subcommittee, thank you for inviting me to discuss the public health and public safety issues resulting from heroin use; the Government of Mexico's efforts to reduce the availability of heroin in the United States; and the U.S.-Mexico cooperation to address heroin issues in both countries.

Background

In 2014, more than 47,000 Americans, or approximately 129 people each day, died from a drug overdose. Opioids—a category of drugs that includes heroin and prescription pain medicines like oxycodone, oxymorphone, hydrocodone, and fentanyl— are having a considerable impact on public health and safety in communities across the United States. Of the overdose deaths in 2014, 61 percent (28,647) involved an opioid, 44 percent (20,808) involved prescription pain medicines, and 22 percent (10,574) involved heroin.[1] The threat posed by heroin has continued to grow dramatically over the past several years. Since 2007, deaths involving heroin have risen 340 percent, from 2,402 in 2007 to 10,574 in 2014.[2]

There are several principal factors contributing to the current nationwide heroin crisis: the increased availability of heroin in the U.S. market,[3] the availability of purer forms of heroin that allow for non-intravenous use,[4] its relatively low price,[5] and a relatively small percentage of non-medical users of opioid prescription drugs transitioning to heroin.[6] The purity of retail-level heroin has increased since the 1990s while prices have remained low.[7] Further increases in purity since 2010 have enabled

---

[1] An opioid-related death may involve more than one type of opioid.

[2] Centers for Disease Control and Prevention, National Center for Health Statistics. Multiple Cause of Death, 1999-2014 on CDC WONDER Online Database, released 2015.

[3] Drug Enforcement Administration, El Paso Intelligence Center, National Seizure System, 2008-2014.

[4] Drug Enforcement Administration. Strategic Intelligence Section. 2015 National Heroin Threat Assessment. DEA-DCT-DIR-039-15.

[5] Drug Enforcement Administration. System to Retrieve Information from Drug Evidence (STRIDE), Price and Purity Data, 2015.

[6] Muhuri PK, Gfroerer, JC and Davies, MC. (2013). Associations of nonmedical pain reliever use and initiation of heroin use in the United States. Substance Abuse and Mental Health Services Administration.

[7] Drug Enforcement Administration. System to Retrieve Information from Drug Evidence (STRIDE), Price and Purity Data, 2015.

heroin use by a variety of means including snorting or smoking which broadens the drug's appeal to a large population that is disinclined to inject the drug intravenously. Heroin's relatively low price makes it a viable alternative to many prescription opioids which command higher prices on the street.[8] Heroin use has spread into suburban and rural communities and is growing among most socioeconomic classes, age groups, and races.[9]

The Administration recognizes that the heroin threat is a global issue; however, Mexico is currently the primary supplier of heroin to the United States, with Mexican drug traffickers cultivating opium poppy and producing heroin in Mexico, and smuggling the finished product into the United States.[10] Opium poppy cultivation in Mexico has increased substantially in recent years, rising from 17,000 hectares in 2014, with an estimated potential pure heroin production of 42 metric tons, to 28,000 hectares in 2015 with a potential production of 70 metric tons of pure heroin.[11]

The reemergence of illicit fentanyl, a powerful Schedule II synthetic opioid more potent than morphine or heroin, exacerbates the heroin crisis.[12] Illicit fentanyl is sometimes mixed with powder heroin to increase its effects or with diluents and sold as "synthetic heroin," with or without the buyers' knowledge.[13] Increasingly, illicit fentanyl is pressed into pill form and sold as counterfeit prescription opioid pills. Illicit fentanyl comes from several sources. The majority of the illicit fentanyl in the U.S. market is smuggled into the country after being clandestinely produced in Mexico or China.[14]

Illicit fentanyl is extremely dangerous and deadly. In 2014, there were more than 5,544 drug overdose deaths involving synthetic narcotics other than methadone, a category that includes fentanyl. This number has more than doubled from two years earlier (2,628 in 2012).[15] Moreover, overdose deaths involving opioids like illicit fentanyl are likely undercounted. Of deaths where drug overdose is cited as the underlying cause

---

[8] Drug Enforcement Administration. Strategic Intelligence Section. 2015 National Heroin Threat Assessment. DEA-DCT-DIR-039-15.

[9] Cicero, T., Ellis, MS, Surratt, HL, Kurtz, SP. (2014). The changing face of heroin in the United States: A retrospective analysis of the past 50 years. *JAMA Psychiatry*, 71(1): 821-826.

[10] Drug Enforcement Administration. Strategic Intelligence Section. 2015 National Heroin Threat Assessment. DEA-DCT-DIR-039-15.

[11] U.S. Department of State, Bureau of International Narcotics and Law Enforcement Affairs. International Narcotics Control Strategy Report—2015 [INCSR] (March 2015) for data from 2013–2014 and unpublished U.S. Government Estimates.

[12] Zuurmond WW, Meert TF, and Noorduin H. (2002). Partial versus full agonists for opioid- mediated analgesia--focus on fentanyl and buprenorphine. *Acta Anaesthesiol Belg*, 53(3):193- 201.

[13] Drug Enforcement Administration. Strategic Intelligence Section. 2015 National Heroin Threat Assessment. DEA-DCT-DIR-039-15.

[14] Drug Enforcement Administration. Strategic Intelligence Section. 2015 National Heroin Threat Assessment. DEA-DCT-DIR-039-15.

[15] Centers for Disease Control and Prevention, National Center for Health Statistics. Multiple Cause of Death 1999-2014 on CDC WONDER Online Database, released 2015. Data are from the Multiple Cause of Death Files, 1999-2014, as compiled from data provided by the 57 vital statistics jurisdictions through the Vital Statistics Cooperative Program.

of death, approximately one-fifth of the death certificates do not list the specific drug(s) involved in the fatal overdose.[16]

There are several reasons why it is important that we address concerns regarding heroin and illicit fentanyl in a single problem set. First, traffickers who add illicit fentanyl as an adulterant to boost the effect of their heroin, or mix it with diluents to sell as synthetic heroin, likely utilize the same supply chains and distribution mechanisms for both drugs. Moreover, both heroin and fentanyl belong to the same class of opioid drugs that have similar effects making their illicit user populations one and the same. Second, both heroin and clandestinely-produced fentanyl can be manufactured by the same drug trafficking organizations that can bring both drugs into the country using the same trafficking routes. And finally, addressing both illicit drugs together allows us to address the heroin crisis while avoiding unintended uptick in illicit fentanyl use. If we move too quickly in reducing the availability of heroin without simultaneously addressing illicit fentanyl availability, it could increase the price of heroin, and risk driving more people to use illicit fentanyl-thereby creating the prospect of an additional and potentially more deadly opioid drug threat.[17,18]

The dramatic increase in the availability and use of heroin and illicit fentanyl is a national security, law enforcement, and public health issue, and it has become the highest priority illicit drug threat to the Nation.[19] Addressing this complex problem demands significant effort, creativity, and interagency collaboration.

The Federal Response

The National Heroin Coordination Group

In November of 2015, the National Security Council (NSC) Transborder Security and Western Hemisphere Directorates Interagency Policy Committee (IPC) on Mexico Security Priorities directed the formation of the National Heroin Coordination Group (NHCG) within the Office of National Drug Control Policy (ONDCP). The NHCG is the hub of a network of interagency partners who leverage their home agency authorities and resources to synchronize interagency activities against the heroin and illicit fentanyl supply chains to the United States. I serve as the Director of the NHCG, which ensures that Federal counterdrug efforts focused on the heroin problem complement the NSC's ongoing work related to Mexico security priorities, and that the NHCG connects the

---

[16] Rudd, RA, Aleshire, N, Zibbell, JE, and Gladden, RM. Increases in Drug and Opioid Overdose Deaths—2000-2014. Centers for Disease Control and Prevention: *Mortality and Morbidity Weekly Report*. Jan. 1, 2016. 64(50);1378-82.

[17] National Institute for Health Development, Infectious Diseases and Drug Monitoring Centre. 2014 National Report to the EMCDDA by the REITOX National Focal Point. Tallinn, Estonia.

[18] European Monitoring Centre for Drugs and Drug Addiction. Fentanyl in Europe EMCDDA Trendspotter Study: Report from an EMCDDA expert meeting 9 to 10 October 2012. Lisbon, Portugal.

[19] The White House, Strategy to Combat Transnational Organized Crime, 25 July 2011.

actions taken on the front end of the supply chain with the effects on the domestic market and user population.

Bi-Lateral Engagement

U.S.-Mexico engagement regarding heroin has been robust. In October 2015, ONDCP Director Michael Botticelli participated in a U.S.- Mexico Security Cooperation Group dialogue that included heroin as the first security cooperation agenda topic. The importance of increased poppy eradication efforts by the Government of Mexico, as well as drug interdiction, clandestine laboratory destruction, and disruption of precursor chemical trafficking were all highlighted as crucial issues to be addressed.

Director Botticelli and I traveled to Mexico in early March 2016 with Ambassador William Brownfield, Assistant Secretary of State for International Narcotics and Law Enforcement Affairs (INL), to engage on heroin and illicit fentanyl issues specifically and to impress upon our Mexican partners the urgency with which the United States is addressing the heroin problem. We met with Mexican Attorney General Gómez and senior members of her staff, as well as with senior officers from the Mexican Army, the Mexican Navy, and the Secretariat of the Government. Attorney General Gómez announced her role as the synchronizer of Mexico's efforts to disrupt the production of heroin and illicit fentanyl including poppy eradication and the identification and neutralization of production laboratories.

Importantly, we agreed to conduct joint planning and to develop a simple and focused national strategy to direct and concentrate Mexico's efforts against heroin and illicit fentanyl. We expect this plan to delineate responsibilities, identify gaps, and help synchronize heroin and illicit fentanyl efforts across the Mexican government. This plan will be beneficial for both countries and we look forward to collaborating on its development. The country team at the U.S. Embassy in Mexico City has led efforts to foster partnerships within the Government of Mexico, and increased information sharing continues to enhance this relationship. The United States continues to work with the Government of Mexico on important efforts under the Merida Initiative, a joint effort to fight transnational criminal organizations and reduce associated violence. Building upon the Mexican Government's own investment in equipment and border security infrastructure, the Merida Initiative will continue to strengthen border security that facilitates the flow of legitimate commerce and travel, while reducing the movement of illicit narcotics, currency, weapons, explosives, black market goods, and undocumented migrants.

U.S. Federal law enforcement agencies are aggressively addressing the heroin and illicit fentanyl issue both here and abroad. The Drug Enforcement Administration and other agencies have co-located Special Agents with international partners in Mexico and throughout Latin America to assist in criminal investigations targeting drug trafficking organizations, and to help their international counterparts develop their capacity to conduct the full range of narcotics interdiction activities within their countries to target both heroin and illicit fentanyl. Our Federal law enforcement agencies, in conjunction with the Department of State, are working with the countries who supply illicit fentanyl and the precursor chemicals used in its manufacture to stem the flow of these dangerous chemicals to the Western Hemisphere.

Interagency Partnerships

Our ability to bring together, contextualize, and synchronize the strategies and partnerships currently taking place at the Federal, state, local, and tribal levels to reduce the availability of heroin in the United States is critical to our overall efforts. The urgent need to sustain progress toward addressing the heroin crisis, combined with the expanding and dynamic nature of the problem itself, requires increased collaboration among Federal agencies, and with our partners working at the state, local and tribal level where the crisis is felt most deeply and where there is an enormous amount of energy and innovation. This cooperation will allow for greater situational awareness to provide more comprehensive understanding of expected changes in the domestic environment related to interagency heroin/illicit fentanyl supply reduction efforts.

The ONDCP funded High Intensity Drug Trafficking Areas (HIDTA) Program is a locally-based program that responds to the drug trafficking issues facing specific areas of the country. Law enforcement agencies at all levels of government share information and implement coordinated enforcement activities; enhance intelligence sharing among Federal, state, local, and tribal law enforcement agencies; provide reliable intelligence to law enforcement agencies to develop effective enforcement strategies and operations; and support coordinated law enforcement strategies to maximize available resources and reduce the supply of illegal drugs in designated areas. In August 2015, ONDCP committed $2.5 million in HIDTA funds to develop a strategy to respond to the heroin crisis in the United States. This unprecedented project combines prevention, education, intelligence, and enforcement resources to address the heroin threat across 17 states and the District of Columbia. The effort is carried out through a unique partnership of seven regional HIDTAs—Appalachia, Michigan, New England, New York/New Jersey, Ohio, Philadelphia/Camden, and Washington/Baltimore. The HIDTA heroin response strategy will foster a collaborative network of public health-public safety partnerships, sharing best practices, innovative pilots, and identifying new opportunities to leverage resources.

Along our Southwest border, U.S. Customs and Border Protection (CBP) continues to detect and interdict illicit narcotics entering the United States. CBP reports seizing 1,121,411 kilograms of illegal drugs in 2015. Of that amount, CBP seized 2,745 kilograms of heroin, 25 percent more than CBP seized in 2014.

The Department of Justice's Organized Crime Drug Enforcement Task Forces (OCDETF) partnered with the Federal Bureau of Investigation, Homeland Security Investigations, and the Drug Enforcement Administration target, disrupt, and dismantle international drug trafficking organizations that manufacture, transport, and distribute heroin and illicit fentanyl destined for and distributed across the United States. In addition, OCDETF's National Heroin Initiative, launched in December 2014, seeks to coordinate innovative regional approaches that improve information sharing and data collection to support multi-agency, multi-jurisdictional enforcement actions.

Challenges

While we have worked tirelessly to address the heroin crisis and have laid a firm foundation for future efforts, much remains to be done. We have gaps in our capability to detect illicit fentanyl at our borders and in our air freight package locations, and our Mexican partners could certainly do more to strategically dismantle criminal organizations and conduct opium poppy eradication and clandestine laboratory identification and neutralization.

We are working to close information gaps. Although it is abundantly clear that the number of overdose deaths involving illicit fentanyl nationwide has increased dramatically, it is likely that the overdose numbers underreport the actual number of deaths due to heroin and illicit fentanyl. The ability to detect illicit fentanyl in overdose victims, and the standard inclusion of illicit fentanyl in overdose death toxicology screening, varies widely among localities. This likely results in the undercounting of heroin and illicit fentanyl-related deaths and actual numbers of heroin- related overdoses are probably much higher. In localities where detailed toxicology screening is performed, information suggests higher numbers of illicit fentanyl-related overdose.

We look forward to working with our Federal and state government partners, as well as our international counterparts, to address these problem areas.

Conclusion

We cannot forget that the epidemic of opioid use and overdose deaths is fundamentally a public health problem that is exploited by criminal organizations, and addressing it adequately requires substance use prevention and treatment strategies and recovery support services. Law enforcement officials are increasingly becoming public health partners, linking individuals with opioid use disorder to treatment.

For this reason, in the FY 2017 budget President Obama proposed $1 billion in new mandatory funding over two years to expand the availability of opioid use disorder services, target areas of highest need, and allow states to implement evidence- based strategies that best meet local needs, such as medication-assisted treatment and expansion of the availability of substance abuse treatment providers (through enhanced loan repayment for healthcare providers that offer medication-assisted treatment). Such efforts will help individuals seek treatment, successfully complete treatment, and sustain recovery.

ONDCP will continue to work with our Federal government departments and agencies, partners at the state, local and tribal levels, and international counterparts to reduce heroin and illicit fentanyl production and trafficking and to combat the profound effect these dangerous drugs are having in our communities.

Thank you for affording me the opportunity to testify today and for your commitment to this important issue.

Prepared Statement of Teresa Jacobs, Mayor of Orange County, Florida

Chairman Rubio, Ranking Member Boxer, members of the committee, thank you for calling this important hearing, and for allowing me to share a local perspective on the terrible threat that heroin poses for cities and counties throughout our country.

First a bit about Orange County: We're home to the City of Orlando and 12 other municipalities, with a population of 1.2 million people, a strong economy and an exceptional quality of life. In 2015, we shattered national tourism records, hosting more than 66 million visitors.

No doubt you know us as the vacation capital of the world, but tragically, like too many other states and communities, Orange County has seen an alarming increase in the number of heroin overdoses and related deaths. Last year, we lost 85 lives to heroin—a staggering 600% increase since 2011. Already this year we've had more than 90 heroin overdoses in the county, with about one-in-ten resulting in death.

Florida's fight against this current wave of opioid addiction began about five years ago, in the midst of our battle against the pill mills.

You may remember the shocking statistics from 2010, when it was discovered that Florida practitioners purchased more than 41 million oxycodone pills in the first six months of that year—more than the other 49 states of the union combined.

Like countless cities, towns and counties across the U.S., we worked to outlaw unauthorized pain clinics and provide resources for breaking opioid addiction.

In Florida, the pill mill 'legacy" has impacted us beyond measure. I can't prove it, but I think it's very likely that cartels took notice of what they perceived to be a ripe "marketplace." Today, predatory drug dealers are targeting us with heroin, as well as cheap and deadly strains of fentanyl. Unfortunately, it's nearly impossible to accurately assess the threat in Florida, since no statewide databases exist. Instead, numbers are captured by individual agencies and municipalities—there is simply no mechanism for synergy or sharing.

What we do know? We know that last year, approximately 2,000 heroin users moved through our Orange County jail. Many of those were arrested not for heroin possession, but for other offenses related to heroin addiction.

We know that in 2015, we housed 100 expectant mothers tragically addicted to opiates or heroin, as our Jail has become the treatment center of last resort for so many people.

For the good of our citizens and our community, we are fighting back.

Last summer I convened the Orange County Heroin Task Force, and asked our sheriff to Co-Chair the effort. Our joint work is having a positive impact, including passage in the 2016 Florida Legislature of a measure allowing Naloxone sales without an individual prescription.

We know there is no single solution, but there are some universally effective approaches:

- Enforcement is critical. In a world of increasingly sophisticated technology, our local efforts—no matter how highly leveraged and coordinated—are simply no match against organized traffickers.
- Equally important, and in keeping with what we learned with pill mills, we must be tireless in educating people that addiction is an illness. An illness that requires treatment and support not only for the addict, but also for the families who are ravaged by addiction.

In closing, I respectfully ask for your help:

- *Help to stop the influx of drugs* across the border. We've got our hands full at the local level, and are simply not equipped to fight the cartels. This is where we really need your help—to stop these deadly drugs before they cross our borders.
- *Help to treat more addicts.* With a regional population of 2.5 million, we have one Addictions Receiving Facility with 26 detox beds serving four counties for the uninsured.
- *Help to raise awareness* so more people will choose not to try this deadly drug in the first place.

To end this crisis and save lives, we all need to be engaged. Thank you for your attention to this critical issue and thank you for your leadership and your service.

Prepared Statement of Steven Dudley, Co-Director, Insight Crime

Chairman Rubio, Ranking Member Boxer, and members of the subcommittee: I am grateful for the opportunity to appear before you on behalf of InSight Crime and the Center for Latin American and Latino Studies at American University to discuss the criminal dynamics connected to the illegal opiate market, specifically the heroin market in the United States related to poppy production in Mexico.

Mexico's Increased Market Share

U.S. consumption of heroin has increased significantly in the last few years. The reasons for this are complex but have to do with the increase of prescription drugs in the United States, a rise in prices of these prescription drugs and their black market counterparts, and the subsequent safeguards on this prescription medicine market, specifically OxyContin.

The U.S. portion of the world heroin market is small by comparison in terms of users, but outsized in terms of potential earnings. The Rand Corporation estimated in 2014, that U.S. consumers spend as much as $27 billion on heroin each year, an increase from $20 billion per year in 2000.[20] Only the marijuana market is worth more in the U.S.[21]

Mexican, Guatemalan and Colombian criminal organizations have reacted to these changes by producing more heroin. Only a small percentage of the world's opium poppy is cultivated in this hemisphere, but after it is processed into heroin, almost all of it is sold in the United States where the number of consumers for the drug has more than doubled since the early 2000s.

Mexico accounts for the bulk of poppy production in the region. According to estimates by the Drug Enforcement Administration (DEA), the production of poppy, the raw ingredient for the production of heroin, increased from 10,500 hectares in 2012 to 17,000 hectares in 2014, giving the groups the potential to produce 42 metric tons, up from 26 metric tons in 2012.[22] By comparison, the DEA says Colombia produces only two metric tons per year.[23]

Seizure data of heroin along the southwest border also indicate that Mexican criminal groups are moving increasing amounts of heroin into the U.S. market. Mexican criminal organizations are also the key transporters of Colombian heroin to the United States, and they manage and purchase the heroin produced in Guatemala or buy the opium gum wholesale to process it into heroin themselves in Mexico.

Inside the U.S., the trend appears to be the same. The DEA says that Mexican groups are seeking an increasing amount of the market share in the distribution business itself, displacing other wholesalers. In sum, the picture is one of an increasingly lucrative, vertically integrated market, with large Mexican criminal organizations managing the product from the point of production to the point of sale and seeking a greater market share of these sales.

---

[20] Beau Kilmer, et al., "How Big is the U.S. Market for Illegal Drugs," *Rand Corporation* (2014).

[21] Ibid.

[22] Drug Enforcement Administration (DEA), "National Drug Threat Assessment 2015," p. 34

[23] The United Nations' most recent estimate for global heroin production is 526 tons. See: UNODC, "World Drug Report 2015," p. 41. Av.

The Reality of the Heroin Supply Chain

The reality of the supply chain is much more complex. While it helps us to use well-worn monikers when talking about these organizations, the truth is that they are not nearly as strong or monolithic as they once were. Names such as the Tijuana Cartel, the Juárez Cartel, the Zetas, or La Familia Michoacana may still evoke fear and sometimes awe, but they are not organizations as much as brand names. In many cases, the individual parts of the organization have as much contact with the bosses as a local Coca-Cola bottling plant manager might have with corporate headquarters.

Even the vaunted Sinaloa Cartel is more horizontally than vertically integrated. Take the recent case of the Flores brothers in Chicago. Before they were arrested, Pedro and Margarito Flores were said to be Sinaloa Cartel distributors in Chicago, one of the areas of greatest interest to this subcommittee. And they were. But as federal intercepts of their conversations with cartel leaders show, the two brothers negotiated independently with each of the top two members of the Sinaloa criminal organization, obtaining different prices with different leaders and managing shipments separately.[24] Even after a war started between the Sinaloa Cartel and the Beltra´n Leyva Organization, the Flores brothers continued to purchase drugs from portions of the Beltrán Leyva Organization and the Sinaloa Cartel.

The Flores case cuts at two different myths about the Sinaloa Cartel: 1) that this is one single organization; 2) that it is tightly controlled by a single leader or a single group of leaders. The point is that as shipments get further and further from Mexico's wholesale points, the loyalties become more disperse, and in some cases completely disappear. This is especially true in the U.S. market where violence is not a viable long-term option to ensure loyalty, win market share or become a monopoly.

The effectiveness of U.S. law enforcement has made violence terrible for business and made the distribution chain a more democratic, capitalist affair. This is evident in other ways as well. While the amount of seizures indicates that there is more heroin available in the United States, it is still moved in very small quantities. The median seizure for the Los Angeles Field Division of the DEA in 2014, for example, was a kilogram.[25] In Denver, a 10 to 12 pound shipment is considered large.[26]

The amount of profits reaped by these Mexican criminal organizations also raises questions about how much control they exert in the United States. The Rand Corporation estimated in 2010 that Mexican criminal groups earn in the range of $400 million per year from their heroin exports and possibly another $700 million for transporting Colombian heroin to the U.S. market.[27] While this has undoubtedly increased, there is

---

[24] Michelle Garcia, "Court Docs Raise Questions about Mexico Sinaloa Cartel Narrative," 12 November 2013.

[25] DEA, op. cit., p. 37.

[26] Ibid.

[27] Kilmer, et al., "Reducing Drug Trafficking Revenues and Violence in Mexico: Would Legalizing Marijuana in California Help?" *Rand Corporation* (2010), p. 30.

still the question of where the rest of the over $20 billion spent on heroin in the U.S. annually goes.

The case of the Laredo brothers, recently indicted in the Eastern District of Pennsylvania, is indicative of these trends. The Laredo brothers are charged with moving one ton of heroin over a six-year period. This is about 14 kilos per month. The organization was so subtle and, as one Mexican analyst put it, "mom-and-pop," the Mexican authorities did not even know it existed.[28]

This brings us to Mexico. First, it is important to note that, unlike the cocaine market, Mexico is not dependent on other countries for its product. It is home grown. Second, the horizontal nature of the distribution chain makes it a difficult law enforcement problem in that country as well. As noted, the once monolithic criminal organizations are shells of what they once were. This is in part due to in- fighting of the type mentioned earlier but also Mexican law enforcement efforts. Many of the fragmented pieces have formed their own criminal operations and brand names.

The most well-known is arguably the Guerreros Unidos, the criminal group held responsible for the disappearance of the 43 students in Mexico in 2014. The Guerreros Unidos used to be under the umbrella of the Beltra´n Leyva Organization. When the Beltra´n Leyva Organization fell to pieces during their war with the Sinaloa Cartel, the Guerreros Unidos became independent, as did several other criminal groups in the embattled state of Guerrero, which is one of the centers of opium cultivation, heroin production, wholesale and transport. Indeed, the mystery of what happened to those students, may hinge on whether the Guerreros Unidos were using commercial buses to move heroin to Chicago.[29] The upshot is that the chain of production in Mexico is broken into numerous pieces, including small and large producers of opium poppy plants, the opium gum producers, the processors, the wholesale purchasers, and the transporters. Production, transport and distribution may all be different organizations. The Laredo brothers, for example, were purchasing opium gum from an independent broker then processing it themselves and distributing it in those small quantities in the U.S. for years without running into trouble with the large, supposedly all-controlling Sinaloa Cartel.

To be sure, violence is still a viable option in Mexico, so the pendulum may swing back towards more monolithic criminal organizations. But for the moment, the reality is that there are literally dozens of small criminal organizations involved in this trade from the point of production to the point of sale.

Impact on Law Enforcement Efforts

In sum, while the level of control that the Mexican production and transport groups exert over the supply chain is clear, we are not talking about one or two criminal groups, but dozens of interlocking organizations whose alliances are constantly shifting. The

[28] Alejandro Hope, "The Laredo DTO and what it says about the heroin trade," 19 April 2016.

[29] Elyssa Pachico, "Four Questions about the '5th Bus' in Case of Mexico's Missing 43," 27 April 2016.

heroin supply chain appears to be a largely horizontal, diversified operation with multiple actors, and one that is obedient to market forces rather than one or two single vertically integrated distributors. The result is that law enforcement efforts are largely muted. Whether you debilitate the Sinaloa Cartel or the Laredo brothers, you are hindering a small part of the overall production and distribution chain. Even if you did slow the heroin from Mexico, you would face an insurmountable task: stopping the flow from other countries, which would undoubtedly fill the void and account for the bulk of world-wide production. Canada already gets up to 90 percent of its heroin from Afghanistan.[30]

And the United States once got all of its heroin from the Asian markets that supply the rest of the world. Thank you for your time and attention. I look forward to your questions.

Statement for the Record Submitted by Jack Riley, Acting Deputy Administrator, Drug Enforcement Administration

Introduction

Chairman Rubio, Ranking Member Boxer, and members of the subcommittee, on behalf of the approximately 9,000 employees of the Drug Enforcement Administration (DEA), thank you for the opportunity to discuss the issue of Cartels, the U.S. heroin epidemic, and DEA's response to combating the drug violence and public health crisis.

Today, Mexican Transnational Criminal Organizations (TCOs) remain the greatest criminal drug threat to the United States; no other group can challenge them in the near term. These Mexican poly-drug organizations traffic heroin, illicit fentanyl, methamphetamine, cocaine, and marijuana throughout the United States, using established transportation routes and distribution networks. They control drug trafficking across the Southwest border (SWB) and are moving to expand their share of U.S. illicit drug markets, particularly heroin markets.

National-level gangs and neighborhood gangs continue to form and expand relationships with Mexican TCOs. Many gangs rely on Mexican TCOs as their primary drug supply source, and Mexican TCOs depend on street-level gangs, many of which already have a customer base, for drug distribution. Additionally, gangs profit through drug transportation activities, enforcement of drug payments, and by securing drug transportation corridors from use by rival gangs.

Mexican TCOs exploit a user population struggling with the disease of addiction. Drug overdoses are the leading cause of injury-related death in the United States, eclipsing deaths from motor vehicle crashes or firearms.[31] There were over 47,000

---

30 UNODC, op. cit., p. 46.

31 Centers for Disease Control and Prevention, Web-based Injury Statistics Query and Reporting System (WISQARS) [online], (2014).

overdose deaths in 2014, or approximately 129 per day, over half (61 percent) of which involved either a prescription opioid or heroin.[32] These are our family members, friends, neighbors, and colleagues.

The DEA's focus is targeting the most significant, sophisticated, and violent trafficking organizations that profit from exploiting persons with substance use disorders. DEA's strategic priorities include targeting Mexican Consolidated Priority Organization Targets (CPOTs) and Priority Target Organizations (PTOs), which are the most significant international and domestic drug trafficking and money laundering organizations.

Current Assessment of the Threat

Based on active law enforcement cases, the following Mexican TCOs are operating in the United States: the Sinaloa Cartel, Beltrán-Leyva Organization (BLO), New Generation Jalisco Cartel (Cartel de Jalisco Nueva Generación or CJNG), Los Cuinis, Gulf Cartel (Cartel del Golfo or CDG), Juarez Cartel Michoacán Family (La Familia Michoacána or LFM), Knights Templar (Los Caballeros Templarios or LCT), and Los Zetas. While all of these Mexican TCOs transport wholesale quantities of illicit drugs into the United States, the Sinaloa Cartel remains the most active supplier. The Sinaloa Cartel leverages its expansive resources and organizational structure in Mexico to facilitate the smuggling and transportation of drugs throughout the United States.

Mexican TCO operations in the United States typically take the form of a supply chain system that relies on compartmentalized operators who are only aware of their own specific function, and remain largely unaware of other operational aspects. In most instances, transporters for the drug shipments are independent third parties who work for more than one Mexican TCO. Since operators in the supply chain are insulated from one another, if a transporter is arrested the transporter is easily replaced and unable to reveal the rest of the network to law enforcement.

Mexican TCOs in the United States utilize a network of extended family and friends to conduct their operations. Families affiliated with various Mexican TCOs in Mexico vouch for U.S.-based relatives or friends that are deemed trustworthy to run various aspects of the drug trafficking operations in the United States. Actual members of Mexican TCOs are usually sent to important U.S. hub cities to manage stash houses containing drug shipments and bulk cash drug proceeds. While operating in the United States, Mexican TCOs actively seek to maintain low profiles and avoid violent confrontations between rival TCOs or U.S. law enforcement.

Mexican TCOs transport illicit drugs over the SWB through ports of entry using passenger vehicles or tractor trailers. Illicit drugs are typically secreted in hidden compartments when transported in passenger vehicles or comingled with legitimate

[32] Rose A. Rudd, Noah Aleshire, Jon E. Zibbell, R. Matthew Gladden. Increases in Drug and Opioid Overdose Deaths—United States, *2000–2014 Morbidity and Mortality Weekly Report*, 2016;64:1378–1382.

goods when transported in tractor trailers. Once across the SWB, Mexican TCOs will initially utilize stash houses in a number of hub cities to include Dallas, Houston, Los Angeles, Atlanta, and Phoenix. The illicit products will then be transported via these same conveyances to distribution groups in the Midwest and on the East Coast. Mexican TCOs also smuggle illicit drugs across the SWB using other methods including tunnels, maritime conveyances, and aircraft.

Heroin Availability to the U.S. Market

There are four major heroin-producing areas in the world, but heroin bound for the U.S. market originates predominantly from Mexico and, to a lesser extent, Colombia. The heroin market in the United States has been historically divided along the Mississippi River, with western markets using Mexican black tar and brown powder heroin, and eastern markets using white powder, which over the last two decades has been sourced primarily from Colombia. The largest, most lucrative heroin markets in the United States are the white powder markets in major East Coast cities: New York City and the surrounding metropolitan areas, Philadelphia, Boston and its surrounding cities, Washington, D.C., Baltimore, as well as Chicago. Given the growing number of individuals with an opioid use disorder in the United States, Mexican TCOs have seized upon a business opportunity to increase their profits. Mexican TCOs are now competing for the East Coast and Mid-Atlantic markets by introducing Mexican brown/black tar heroin, as well as by developing new techniques to produce highly refined white powder heroin.

Poppy cultivation in Mexico increased 160 percent between 2013 and 2015, resulting in an estimated 70 metric tons of potential heroin. Cultivation in Mexico is located primarily in the state of Guerrero and the Mexican 'Golden Triangle" which includes the states of Chihuahua, Sinaloa, and Durango. The increased cultivation and trafficking from Mexico to the United States impacts both of our nations by supporting the escalation of heroin use in the United States, as well as the instability and violence associated with drug trafficking in Mexico.

The majority of Mexican and Colombian heroin bound for the United States is smuggled into the United States via the SWB, and heroin seizures at the border have more than doubled, from 1,016 kilograms in 2010 to 2,524 kilograms in 2015.[33] During this time, the average seizure at the Border also increased from 2.0 kilograms to 3.5 kilograms. Most heroin smuggled across the border is transported in privately-owned vehicles, usually through California, as well as through south Texas. In 2014, more than half of U.S. Customs and Border Protection (CBP) heroin seizures at the SWB were in the southern California corridors of San Diego and El Centro. The distribution cells, and the Mexican and South American traffickers who supply them, are the main sources of

---

[33] Drug Enforcement Administration, Unclassified Summary, 2015 National Drug Threat Assessment, Pg. 35.

heroin in the United States today. In Mexico, the threat of these organizations is magnified by the high level of violence associated with their attempts to control and expand drug distribution operations.

DEA has become increasingly alarmed over the addition of fentanyl into heroin sold on the streets as well as the use of fentanyl analogues such as acetyl fentanyl. The more potent opioids like fentanyl[34] present a serious risk of overdose death for a user. In addition, this drug can be absorbed by the skin or inhaled, which makes it particularly dangerous for law enforcement, public safety, or health care personnel who encounter the substance during the course of their daily operations. On March 18, 2015, DEA issued a nationwide alert to all U.S. law enforcement officials about the dangers of illicit fentanyl and fentanyl analogues and related compounds. In addition, due to a recent spike in overdose deaths related to the use of acetyl fentanyl, on July 17, 2015, DEA used its emergency scheduling authority to place acetyl fentanyl in Schedule I of the CSA.

DEA Response to the Heroin Threat

DEA'S 360 Strategy

DEA is rolling out the 360 Strategy to address the opioid, heroin, and violent crime crisis. The strategy leverages existing federal, state, and local partnerships to address the problem on three different fronts: law enforcement, diversion control, and community relations. The strategy is founded upon our continued enforcement activities directed at the violent street gangs responsible for feeding the heroin and prescription drug abuse epidemic in our communities.

While law enforcement plays a central role in the 360 Strategy, enforcement actions alone are not enough to make lasting changes in our communities. The 360 Strategy, therefore, also focuses on preventing diversion by providing education and training within the pharmaceutical community and to pursue those practitioners who are operating outside of the law. The final component of the strategy is a community effort designed to maximize all available resources to help communities turn around the recurring problems that have historically allowed the drug and violent crime problems to resurface after enforcement operations.

Additional Resources in Fiscal Year 2017

DEA plays an important part in the U.S. government's drug control strategy that includes enforcement, treatment, and prevention. While there are complex issues affecting spikes in heroin use and overdoses, including prescription drug abuse, the same significant poly-drug trafficking organizations responsible for other illicit drug threats are

---

[34] Centers for Disease Control, Emergency Response Safety and Health Database, FENTANYL: Incapacitating Agent, accessed March 19, 2015; U.S. Department of Justice, Drug Enforcement Administration, Office of Diversion Control, Drug & Chemical Evaluation Section, Fentanyl, March 2015.

also responsible for the vast majority of the heroin supply. Additionally, drug trafficking has a proven linkage to gangs and other violent criminal organizations. The FY 2017 President's Budget request provides $12.5 million and 42 positions, including 32 special agents, to create new enforcement groups in DEA domestic field divisions.

Heroin Task Force

As directed by Congress, the Department of Justice joined with the Office of National Drug Control Policy (ONDCP) to develop strategies to confront the heroin problem and curtail the escalating overdose epidemic and death rates. DEA and more than 28 Federal agencies and their components participated in this initiative. The task force provided its Report to Congress on December 31, 2015.

International Enforcement: Sensitive Investigative Units

DEA's Sensitive Investigative Units (SIU) program, nine of which are in the Western Hemisphere, helps build effective and vetted host nation units capable of conducting complex investigations targeting major TCOs. DEA, with funding support from the Department of State, currently mentors and supports 13 SIUs, which are staffed by over 900 foreign counterparts. The success of this program has enhanced DEA's ability to fight drug trafficking on a global scale.

International Enforcement: Bilateral Investigations Units

Bilateral Investigations Units (BIUs) are one of DEA's most important tools for targeting, disrupting, and dismantling significant TCOs. The BIUs have used extraterritorial authorities to infiltrate, indict, arrest, and convict previously "untouchable" TCO leaders involved in drug trafficking.

Special Operations Division

Established in 1994, the Special Operations Division (SOD) is a DEA-led multi-agency operations coordination center with participation from Federal law enforcement agencies, the Department of Defense, the Intelligence Community, and international law enforcement partners. SOD's mission is to establish strategies and operations to dismantle national and international trafficking organizations by attacking their command and control communications. Special emphasis is placed on those major drug trafficking and narco-terrorism organizations that operate across jurisdictional boundaries on a regional, national, and international level.

El Paso Intelligence Center

The El Paso Intelligence Center (EPIC) is a national intelligence center focused on supporting law enforcement efforts in the Western Hemisphere with a significant emphasis on the SWB. Through its 24-hour watch function, EPIC provides law enforcement officers, investigators, and analysts immediate access to participating agencies' databases. This function is critical in the dissemination of relevant information in support of tactical and investigative agencies, deconfliction, and officer safety. EPIC also provides significant tactical, operational, and strategic intelligence support to state and local law enforcement agencies, especially in the areas of clandestine laboratory investigations and highway interdiction.

Cooperation with Mexico

The DEA's presence in Mexico represents our largest international footprint. The ability to have DEA Special Agents assigned to 11 different offices throughout Mexico is a reflection of the level of cooperation that we continue to enjoy with our Mexican counterparts. DEA supports bi-lateral investigations with the Government of Mexico by providing information and intelligence to develop investigations that target leaders of TCOs throughout Mexico.

We view our working relationship with the Mexican Authorities as strong, and getting stronger. In 2014, Mexican law enforcement officials arrested cartel leaders Hector Beltra´n-Leyva, Servando Gomez-Martinez, and Omar Trevino Morales. These actions represent significant successes for both the United States and Mexico in our shared struggle against TCOs. The arrests struck at the heart of the leadership structure of the Knights Templar Cartel, the Beltrán-Leyva Organization, and the Los Zetas Cartel; and highlight the continuing cooperation between Mexican and U.S. law enforcement. The United States and Mexico have established a strong and successful security partnership in the last decade and, to that end, the U.S. government stands ready to work with our Mexican partners to provide any assistance, as requested, to build upon these successes.

Conclusion

Mexican TCOs remain the greatest criminal drug threat to the United States. These Mexican poly-drug organizations traffic heroin, methamphetamine, cocaine, and marijuana throughout the United States, using established transportation routes and distribution networks. They control drug trafficking across the SWB and are moving to expand their share of U.S. illicit drug markets. Their influence up and down the supply chain, their ability to enter into new markets, and associations with domestic gangs are of particular concern for the DEA. DEA will continue to address this threat domestically and abroad by attacking the crime and violence perpetrated by the Mexican-based TCOs which inflict tremendous harm to our communities.

In: Battling the Opioid Epidemic
Editor: Vincent Hardy

ISBN: 978-1-53615-548-8

Chapter 4

HEROIN TRAFFICKING IN THE UNITED STATES*

Kristin Finklea

ABSTRACT

Over the past several years, the nation has seen an uptick in the use and abuse of opioids—both prescription opioids and non-prescription opioids such as heroin. In 2016, there were an estimated 948,000 individuals (0.4% of the 12 and older population) who reported using heroin within the past year—up from 0.2% to 0.3% of this population reporting use in the previous decade. In addition to an increase in heroin use over the past several years, there has been a simultaneous increase in its availability in the United States. The increase in availability has been fueled by a number of factors, including increased production and trafficking of heroin—principally by Mexican criminal networks.

Mexican transnational criminal organizations are the major suppliers and key producers of most illegal drugs smuggled into the United States. They have been increasing their share of the U.S. drug market—particularly with respect to heroin—even though the United States still receives some heroin from South America and, to a lesser extent, Southwest Asia. To facilitate the distribution and sale of drugs in the United States, Mexican drug traffickers have formed relationships with U.S. gangs.

Heroin seizures across the country, as well as those at the Southwest border, have generally increased over the past decade. Nationwide heroin seizures reached 7,979 kg in 2017, with 3,090 kg (39%) seized at the Southwest border. This is up from about 2,000 kg seized at the Southwest border a decade prior. Further, there has been an increase in federal arrests and sentences for heroin-related crimes. For instance, the Drug Enforcement Administration made 5,408 heroin-related arrests in 2017—up from about 2,500 a decade prior. In addition, U.S. Sentencing Commission data indicate that from 2007 to 2017, there was a general increase in the number of individuals sentenced for heroin trafficking offenses in U.S. District Courts.

* This is an edited, reformatted and augmented version of Congressional Research Service, Publication No. R44599, dated February 14, 2019.

The federal government—specifically, law enforcement—relies on a number of tools and initiatives to counter heroin trafficking. Many of these efforts focus on drug trafficking broadly and prioritize the greatest drug trafficking threats in a given area, whether those threats come from trafficking heroin or other illicit drugs or substances.

Going forward, there are a number of issues policymakers may consider as they address heroin trafficking. For instance, what is known about drug trafficking is contingent on data surrounding poppy cultivation, heroin production, and product inflows into the United States. Given that these are often based on snapshots of knowledge from disparate sources, Congress may question how these data are collected and their adequacy. In addition, Congress may examine current law enforcement efforts to dismantle heroin trafficking networks and prosecute their leaders. Policymakers may also look at existing federal strategies on drug control and transnational crime to evaluate whether they are able to target the heroin trafficking threat effectively.

INTRODUCTION

In the midst of ongoing concerns about illicit drug use and abuse, there has been heightened attention to the issue of opioid abuse—including both prescription opioids and nonprescription opioids such as heroin.[1] The increased attention to opioid abuse and addiction first centered on the abuse of prescription painkillers. According to the Substance Abuse and Mental Health Services Administration (SAMHSA), about 3.3 million individuals were current (at least once in the past month) nonmedical users of prescription pain relievers such as OxyContin in 2016.[2] Mirroring the nation's concern about prescription drug abuse, there has been corresponding unease regarding the rise in heroin abuse.

According to the 2016 National Survey on Drug Use and Health, there were an estimated 948,000 individuals (0.4% of the 12 and older population) who reported using heroin within the past year—up from 0.2% to 0.3% of this population reporting use in the previous decade.[3] In addition, about 626,000 individuals (0.2% of the 12 and older population) had a heroin use disorder in 2016.[4] While this is similar to the proportion of

---

[1] Heroin is listed as a Schedule I controlled substance under the Controlled Substances Act (CSA, P.L. 91-513), meaning the federal government has deemed heroin as having a high potential for abuse, no currently accepted medical use in treatment, and a lack of accepted safety for its use under medical supervision. Under the CSA, there are five schedules under which substances may be classified—Schedule I being the most restrictive. For more information on the CSA, see CRS Report R45164, *Legal Authorities Under the Controlled Substances Act to Combat the Opioid Crisis*; and CRS Report RL30722, *Drug Offenses: Maximum Fines and Terms of Imprisonment for Violation of the Federal Controlled Substances Act and Related Laws*.

[2] Substance Abuse and Mental Health Services Administration, Key Substance Use and Mental Health Indicators in the United States: Results from the 2016 National Survey on Drug Use and Health, September 2017. For more information on prescription drug abuse, see CRS Report R44987, *The Opioid Epidemic and Federal Efforts to Address It: Frequently Asked Questions*.

[3] Substance Abuse and Mental Health Services Administration, *Key Substance Use and Mental Health Indicators in the United States: Results from the 2016 National Survey on Drug Use and Health*, September 2017.

[4] Ibid. The National Survey on Drug Use and Health (NSDUH) notes that "[h]eroin use disorder occurs when someone experiences clinically significant impairment caused by the recurrent use of heroin, including health problems, physical withdrawal, persistent or increasing use, and failure to meet major responsibilities at work, school, or home. NSDUH respondents who used heroin in the past 12 months were categorized as having a

the 12 and older population with a heroin use disorder from 2011 to 2015, it is significantly greater than the proportion from 2002 to 2010. Further, heroin overdose deaths increased by about 20% nationally between 2015 and 2016,[5] and the Midwest and Northeast regions have been highlighted as areas of particular concern.[6]

In addition to increases in heroin use and abuse, there has been a simultaneous increase in its availability in the United States over the past decade.[7] This has been fueled by a number of factors, including increased production and trafficking of heroin—principally by Mexican criminal networks. Mexican drug traffickers have been expanding their control of the U.S. heroin market, though the United States still receives some heroin from South America and Southwest Asia as well.[8] Notably, while the majority of the world's opium is produced in Afghanistan,[9] only a small proportion of that feeds the U.S. heroin market.

Policymakers may want to examine U.S. efforts to counter heroin trafficking as a means of addressing opioid abuse in the United States. This report provides an overview of heroin trafficking into and within the United States. It includes a discussion of links between the trafficking of heroin and the illicit movement of related substances such as controlled prescription opioids and synthetic substances like fentanyl. The report also outlines existing U.S. efforts to counter heroin trafficking and possible congressional considerations going forward.[10]

HEROIN TRAFFICKERS

Mexican transnational criminal organizations (TCOs) "remain the greatest criminal drug threat to the United States; no other group is currently positioned to challenge them."[11] They are the major suppliers and key producers of most illegal drugs smuggled into the United States, and they have been increasing their share of the U.S. drug market—particularly with respect to heroin.[12] The Drug Enforcement Administration

---

heroin use disorder if they met the DSM-IV criteria for either dependence or abuse for heroin." DSM-IV is the Diagnostic and Statistical Manual of Mental Disorders, 4th Edition.

5 Centers for Disease Control and Prevention, *Heroin Overdose Data*, https://www.cdc.gov/drugoverdose/data/heroin.html.

6 Drug Enforcement Administration, *2017 National Drug Threat Assessment Summary*, October 2017, p. 51.

7 Drug Enforcement Administration, *2018 National Drug Threat Assessment Summary*, October 2018.

8 Ibid.

9 United Nations Office on Drugs and Crime, *World Drug Report 2018*, June 2018.

10 Discussions of the overarching U.S. drug policy and of heroin abuse, prevention, and treatment are outside the scope of this report. For more information on these issues, see CRS Report R43749, *Drug Enforcement in the United States: History, Policy, and Trends*; and CRS In Focus IF10741, *Naloxone for Opioid Overdose: Regulation and Policy Options*.

11 Drug Enforcement Administration, *2018 National Drug Threat Assessment*, October 2018, p. vi.

12 Drug Enforcement Administration, 2017 National Drug Threat Assessment, October 2017, p. 1. For more information on Mexican TCOs, see CRS Report R41576, *Mexico: Organized Crime and Drug Trafficking Organizations*.

(DEA) notes that the Southwest border "remains the primary entry point for heroin into the United States."[13] Mexican TCOs control the flow of heroin across the border, the majority of which "is through [privately owned vehicles] entering the United States at legal ports of entry, followed by tractor-trailers, where the heroin is co-mingled with legal goods."[14]

Mexican criminal networks have not always featured so prominently (or broadly) in the U.S. heroin market. Historically, Colombian criminal organizations controlled heroin markets in the Midwest and on the East Coast.[15] Now, supply for these markets also comes directly from Mexican traffickers. The DEA indicates that "[s]ince 2015 most of the heroin sold in the U.S. is from Mexico."[16] Mexican poppy cultivation reportedly increased by 35% from 2016 to 2017; officials project that the estimated 44,100 hectares cultivated in 2017 allowed for about 111 metric tons of pure heroin production.[17]

The DEA has observed that "[t]he increased role of Mexican traffickers is affecting heroin trafficking patterns."[18] Historically, Mexican-produced black tar and brown powder heroin have been consumed in markets west of the Mississippi River, while markets east of the Mississippi have consumed more white powder heroin from South America. However, as the Mexican traffickers have taken on a larger role in the U.S. heroin market and have developed techniques to produce white powder heroin, they have moved their white powder heroin into both eastern and western U.S. markets.[19]

Heroin Production

Created from the morphine molecule of the opium poppy, heroin can be produced in a number of purity grades (white powder heroin being the most pure and black tar heroin being the least) and can be administered through a number of means (e.g., smoking, snorting, or injecting). In the process of creating heroin, "white heroin is made by isolating morphine from opium and then synthesizing heroin from morphine."[20] Producing black tar heroin, however, "skips the intermediate step of morphine isolation and synthesizes heroin straight from the opium."[21] As such, producing black tar heroin is faster and less costly than producing white heroin and thus it may be a cheaper high for opioid abusers.

To facilitate the distribution and local sale of drugs in the United States, Mexican drug traffickers have sometimes formed relationships with U.S. gangs.[22] Trafficking and

[13] Drug Enforcement Administration, *2018 National Drug Threat Assessment*, October 2018, p. 18.
[14] Ibid., p. 19.
[15] Drug Enforcement Administration, *2017 National Drug Threat Assessment*, October 2017, p. 11.
[16] Drug Enforcement Administration, *2018 National Drug Threat Assessment*, October 2018, p. 13.
[17] Ibid., p. 18.
[18] Drug Enforcement Administration, *National Heroin Threat Assessment Summary*, June 2016, p. 5.
[19] Drug Enforcement Administration, *National Drug Threat Assessment Summary 2017*, October 2017.
[20] Stratfor, *Criminal Commodities Series: Black Tar Heroin*, March 9, 2012.
[21] Ibid.
[22] Drug Enforcement Administration, *2018 National Drug Threat Assessment*, October 2018, p. 97.

distribution of illicit drugs is a primary source of revenue for these gangs[23] and among the most common of their criminal activities.[24] Gangs may work with a variety of drug trafficking organizations, and are often involved in selling multiple types of drugs besides heroin or other opioids.[25]

Heroin Seizures

The majority of heroin making its way to the United States originates in Mexico and, to a lesser degree, Colombia.[26] The amount of heroin seized across the United States, including at the Southwest border, has generally increased over the past decade, as illustrated in Figure 1. Nationwide heroin seizures reached 7,979 kg in 2017, with 3,090 kg (39%) seized at the Southwest border.[27]

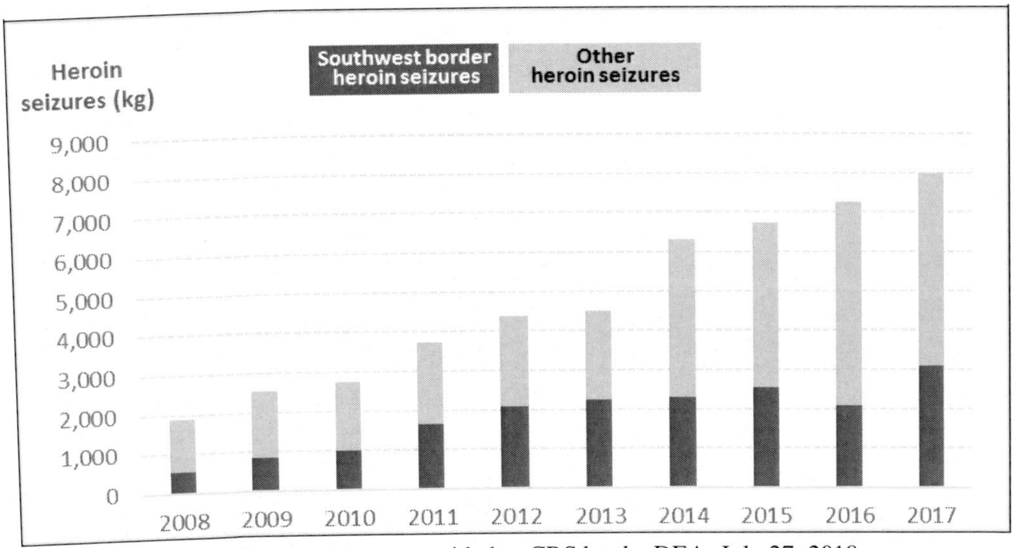

Source: National Seizure System data, as provided to CRS by the DEA, July 27, 2018.

Figure 1. Heroin Seized in the United States; 2008–2017.

The United Nations Office on Drugs and Crime (UNODC) has outlined how seizure data can be used in combination with data on drug prices and purity to help serve as a drug market indicator. The UNODC notes that "[f]alling seizures in combination with rising drug prices and falling purity levels may suggest a decline in overall drug supply,

---

23 Ibid., p.107.
24 National Gang Intelligence Center, *2015 National Gang Report*.
25 Drug Enforcement Administration, *2018 National Drug Threat Assessment*, October 2018.
26 Ibid.
27 Data provided to CRS by DEA Congressional Affairs, July 27, 2018.

while rising seizures in combination with falling drug prices and rising purity levels are usually considered a good indicator of an increase in drug supply."[28]

The UNODC's model can be applied to heroin seizure data to help assess the scope of the heroin market in the United States. Notably, heroin seizures have generally been increasing, as illustrated in Figure 1. In addition, the average purity of retail-level heroin has been between 31% and 39% from 2012 to 2016;[29] while the purity has fluctuated somewhat, it has remained elevated relative to levels in the 1980s.[30] And while the retail-level price per gram has vacillated over the past couple of decades, it has remained lower than prices in the 1980s.[31] This combination of seizures, purity, and price could indicate that there is an increased heroin supply for the U.S. market. Experts have noted an increase in Mexican heroin production, which is primarily destined for the United States.

The increase in seizures, however, may reflect more than just increases in the heroin supply and demand in the U.S. market. This could also be driven by factors such as enhanced U.S. law enforcement efforts to interdict and seize the contraband and/or by less stringent efforts by traffickers and buyers to conceal the drugs.

Arrests and Prosecutions

Data from the DEA indicate that many of their heroin-related arrests are for trafficking-related offenses. In 2017, the DEA made 5,408 heroin-related arrests. The bulk of these were made for conspiracy (35%), distribution (24%), possession with intent[32] (23%), and simple possession (11%). Other offense categories for which a much smaller proportion of arrests were made include importation, manufacture, RICO (Racketeer Influenced and Corrupt Organization), and CCE (continuing criminal enterprise).[33] In other words, more of these heroin-related arrests were for offenses that may be considered to fall under the umbrella of trafficking rather than simple possession.[34] DEA heroin arrest data indicate that since remaining relatively flat in the

---

[28] United Nations Office on Drugs and Crime, *World Drug Report 2015*, May 2015, p. 37.

[29] Data from 2002 are from the Office of National Drug Control Policy, *National Drug Control Strategy, Data Supplement 2015*, p. 89. 2013-2016 data are from the Drug Enforcement Administration, *2018 National Drug Threat Assessment*, October 2018, p. 12.

[30] For comparison, the average retail-level purity in 1981 was 10%. Drug Enforcement Administration, *National Heroin Threat Assessment Summary*, June 2016, p. 6.

[31] In 1980, the average retail-level price per gram of pure heroin was $3,260 (in 2012 dollars). Recent data indicate that between 2012 and 2016, this price fluctuated between $465 and $1,020. Historical data and 2012 data are from the Drug Enforcement Administration, *National Heroin Threat Assessment Summary*, June 2016. Data from 2013 to 2016 are from the Drug Enforcement Administration, *2018 National Drug Threat Assessment*, October 2018.

[32] In this category, the intention is to manufacture, distribute, or dispense a controlled substance—heroin.

[33] Data provided by the DEA to CRS, July 27, 2018.

[34] Trafficking offenses are generally considered those involving unlawful distribution, possession with intent to distribute, manufacture, importation and exportation, etc. For more information on trafficking offenses and associated penalties (as well as other drug offenses and penalties), see CRS Report RL30722, *Drug Offenses:*

mid-2000s, overall heroin arrests generally increased through 2015 before declining through 2017 (see Figure 2).[35]

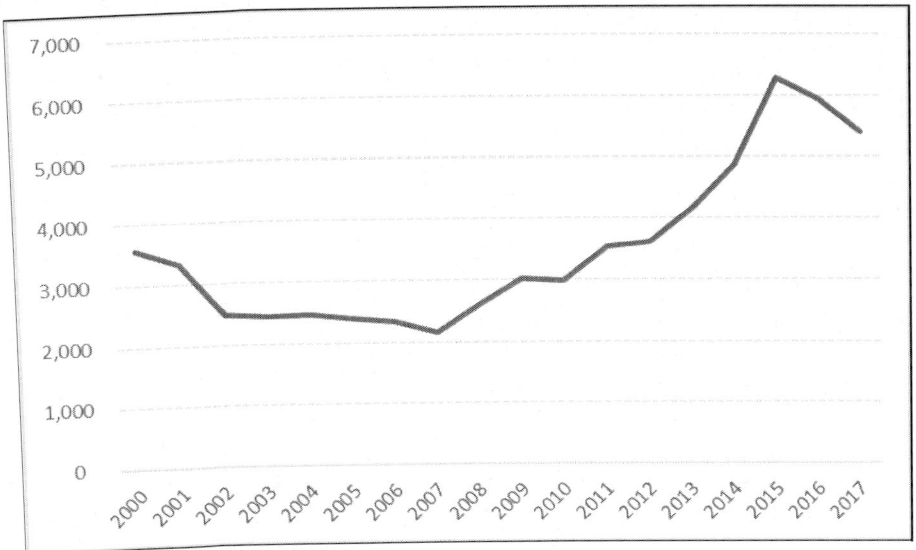

Source: Data provided to CRS by the DEA, July 27, 2018.

Figure 2. DEA Heroin Arrests; 2000–2017.

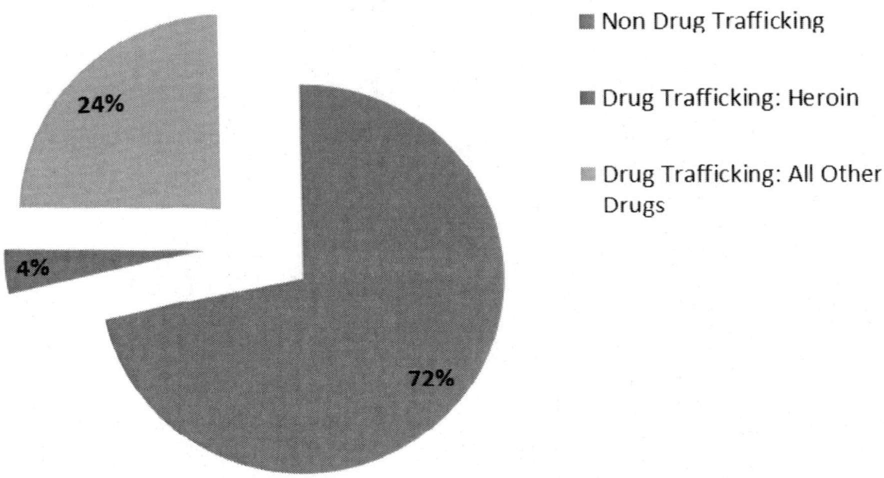

Source: U.S. Sentencing Commission, *Quick Facts: Drug Trafficking Offenses*, July 2018.

Notes: Numbers depicted reflect the overall percentage of cases sentenced. There were 66,873 offenders sentenced in FY2017.

Figure 3. Cases Sentenced in U.S. District Court; FY2017.

Maximum Fines and Terms of Imprisonment for Violation of the Federal Controlled Substances Act and Related Laws.

[35] Data provided by the DEA to CRS, July 27, 2018.

The U.S. Sentencing Commission reports that 2,658 individuals were sentenced for heroin trafficking offenses in U.S. District Courts in FY2017.[36] While this was a decrease from FY2016, the number of individuals sentenced for heroin trafficking has generally moved upward over the past decade.[37] FY2017 data indicate that of the 19,240 cases involving individuals sentenced for drug trafficking offenses, 2,658 (13.8%) involved individuals who were sentenced for heroin trafficking.[38] That amounts to 4% of all cases sentenced in U.S. District Courts. (See Figure 3.)

Links to Related Substances

Prescription Opioids

Some have theorized that prescription opioid abuse may lead to, or be a "gateway" for, abuse of nonprescription opioids such as heroin. Results from one SAMHSA study indicate that the "recent (12 months preceding interview) heroin incidence rate was 19 times higher among those who reported prior nonmedical pain reliever (NMPR) use than among those who did not (0.39% vs. 0.02%)."[39] However, while "four out of five recent heroin initiates (79.5%) previously used NMPR ... the vast majority of NMPR users have not progressed to heroin use."[40] The *2016 National Heroin Threat Assessment Summary* notes that about 4% of individuals who abuse prescription drugs will go on to use heroin.[41]

One factor that may sway opioid abusers' shifts from prescription opioids to heroin may be the cost. If users cannot afford prescription opioids, they may switch to heroin as a lower-cost alternative. While estimates vary, some have noted that an 80 mg pill of OxyContin (a prescription opioid containing oxycodone) can cost $80 on the street; a bag of heroin can cost $5- $10.[42] The DEA reported that drug trafficking organizations have

---

[36] U.S. Sentencing Commission, *Quick Facts: Heroin Trafficking Offenses*, July 2018.

[37] U.S. Sentencing Commission, Quick Facts: Drug Trafficking Offenses, July 2018.

[38] Ibid. Among drug trafficking cases, 36.9% were for methamphetamine offenses, 20.3% were for powder cocaine (and 8.2% were for crack cocaine), 14.1% were for marijuana, 2.8% were for oxycodone, and 3.9% were for other drug offenses.

[39] Pradip K. Muhuri, Joseph C. Gfroerer, and M. Christine Davies, *Associations of Nonmedical Pain Reliever Use and Initiation of Heroin Use in the United States*, Substance Abuse and Mental Health Services Administration, Center for Behavioral Health Statistics and Quality, August 2013, p. 1.

[40] Ibid. Other studies have had similar findings. For instance, 2016 research published in The New England Journal of Medicine notes that "although the majority of current heroin users report having used prescription opioids nonmedically before they initiated heroin use, heroin use among people who use prescription opioids for nonmedical reasons is rare, and the transition to heroin use appears to occur at a low rate." Wilson M. Compton, Christopher M. Jones, and Grant T. Baldwin, "Relationship between Nonmedical Prescription-Opioid Use and Heroin Use," *The New England Journal of Medicine*, January 14, 2016.

[41] Drug Enforcement Administration, *National Heroin Threat Assessment Summary 2016*, June 2016.

[42] Drug Enforcement Administration, *DEA Trends & Update*, San Juan, Puerto Rico Pharmacy Diversion Awareness Conference, March 26, 2017.

responded to the demand for lower cost opioids by sometimes shifting heroin trafficking operations to areas with higher prevalence of nonmedical prescription drug use.[43]

Fentanyl

Fentanyl is a synthetic opioid that is approximately 50 times stronger than heroin and 100 times more potent than morphine. There are both legal and illegal forms of fentanyl. Legal fentanyl has pharmaceutical uses for treating post-operative pain and chronic pain associated with late stage cancer, and illicit fentanyl is sold on the black market and used/abused in similar ways as other opioid drugs.

Most cases of fentanyl-related overdoses are associated with non-pharmaceutical, illegal fentanyl[44]; non-pharmaceutical fentanyl is often mixed with heroin and/or other drugs, sometimes without the consumer's knowledge. Some have purported that fentanyl is easier to mix with white powder heroin than with the black tar variety.[45] As such, there have reportedly been more fentanyl-related overdose deaths in U.S. markets fueled by white powder heroin than those dominated by the black tar form. However, this could change as distributors are finding ways to incorporate fentanyl into the black tar heroin.[46]

Non-pharmaceutical fentanyl found in the United States is manufactured in China and Mexico.[47] It is trafficked into the United States across the Southwest border or delivered through mail couriers directly from China, or from China through Canada.[48] In addition, fentanyl-related substances—substances that are in the fentanyl chemical family but have minor variations in chemical structure—may be attractive to traffickers because the analogs are often unscheduled or unregulated.[49] Like fentanyl, they can be sold as, or mixed in with, heroin or pressed into counterfeit pills.

The DEA indicates that the majority of seized fentanyl samples analyzed involved fentanyl in powder form.[50] However, law enforcement is concerned about the risks from fentanyl being pressed into counterfeit pills, in part, because there are more abusers of prescription pain pills than of heroin. As such, fentanyl pressed into counterfeit pills could ultimately affect a larger population of individuals.[51]

---

43 Drug Enforcement Administration, *FY2017 Performance Budget Congressional Submission*, p. DEA-86.

44 Centers for Disease Control and Prevention (CDC), Synthetic Opioid Overdose Data, December 16, 2016; see also CRS Insight IN10914, *Increase in Illicit Fentanyl Overdose Deaths*.

45 See, for example, Margot Sanger-Katz, "Bleak New Estimates in Drug Epidemic: A Record 72,000 Overdose Deaths in 2017," *The New York Times*, August 15, 2018.

46 Ibid.

47 Drug Enforcement Administration, *2018 National Drug Threat Assessment*, October 2018.

48 Ibid. See also CRS In Focus IF10890, *Illicit Fentanyl, China's Role, and U.S. Foreign Policy Options*.

49 Drug Enforcement Administration, *2018 National Drug Threat Assessment*, October 2018.

50 Ibid.

51 Ibid.

U.S. Heroin Trafficking Enforcement Efforts

The United States confronts the drug problem through a combination of efforts targeting both the supply of and demand for drugs. As such, the Administration has directed resources into the areas of law enforcement initiatives, prevention, and treatment. In targeting one element of the drug problem—trafficking—U.S. efforts have centered on law enforcement initiatives.

There are a number of federal law enforcement activities aimed specifically at (or which may be tailored to) curbing heroin trafficking. This section contains a snapshot of some of these efforts.

DEA 360 Strategy

The DEA has developed a 360 Strategy aimed at "tackling the cycle of violence and addiction generated by the link between drug cartels, violent gangs, and the rising problem of prescription opioid and heroin abuse."[52] The strategy was launched in November 2015 as a pilot program in Pittsburgh, PA, and has since expanded to other cities.[53] It leverages federal, state, and local law enforcement, diversion control, and community outreach organizations. As the program is relatively new, there have only been anecdotal reports of the operations that fall under the 360 Strategy framework, and an outcome evaluation of the strategy has not been conducted.

Heroin and Fentanyl Signature Programs

The DEA operates a heroin signature program (HSP) and a heroin domestic monitor program (HDMP), with the goal of identifying the geographic source of heroin found in the United States. The HSP analyzes wholesale-level samples of "heroin seized at U.S. ports of entry (POEs), all non-POE heroin exhibits weighing more than one kilogram, randomly chosen samples, and special requests for analysis."[54] Chemical analysis of a given heroin sample can identify its "signature," which indicates a particular heroin production process that has been linked to a specific geographic source region. The HDMP assesses the signature source of retail-level heroin seized in the United States. This program samples retail-level heroin seized in 27 cities across the country and provides data on the price, purity, and geographic source of the heroin.[55] The results from the HSP and HDMP can be used to help understand trafficking and distribution patterns throughout the country. The HSP started in 1977, and the HDMP began in 1979.

---

[52] Drug Enforcement Administration, *DEA 360 Strategy: Working Together to Break the Cycle of Drug Trafficking, Drug Violence, and Drug Abuse*, p. 1.

[53] See, for example, the expansion to Baltimore, MD. Jessica Anderson, "DEA Launches '360 Strategy' to Combat Heroin and Prescription Drug Abuse Epidemic in Baltimore," *The Baltimore Sun*, September 26, 2018.

[54] Drug Enforcement Administration, *The 2016 Heroin Signature Program Report*, October 2018, p. 2.

[55] Drug Enforcement Administration, *FY 2019 Performance Budget Congressional Submission*.

The HSP tests about 600-900 heroin samples annually.[56] In 2016, the HSP tested 744 samples from seizures totaling 1,632 kg—slightly more than 22% of the total heroin seized that year.[57] Of the heroin analyzed in the HSP in 2016, 86% was identified as originating from Mexico, 10% was inconclusive,[58] 4% was from South America, and less than 1% was from Southwest Asia. Wholesale-level Mexican white powder heroin produced with South American techniques had an average purity of 82%.[59] Data from the HDMP indicate that retail-level Mexican white powder heroin produced with South American techniques had an average purity of 39.7% in 2016.[60]

The DEA has also started a Fentanyl Signature Profiling Program (FSPP), analyzing samples from fentanyl seizures to help "identify the international and domestic trafficking networks responsible for many of the drugs fueling the opioid crisis."[61] In 2017, the FSPP analyzed 520 fentanyl powder samples from seizures totaling 960 kg of fentanyl. While the average purity was 5%, the DEA has indicated that fentanyl shipped directly from China often has purity levels above 90%, while fentanyl trafficked over the Southwest border from Mexico often has purity levels below 10%.[62]

HIDTA

The High Intensity Drug Trafficking Areas (HIDTA) program provides assistance to law enforcement agencies—at the federal, state, local, and tribal levels—that are operating in regions of the United States that have been deemed critical drug trafficking areas. There are 29 designated HIDTAs throughout the United States and its territories.[63] Administered by the Office of National Drug Control Policy (ONDCP), the program aims to reduce drug production and trafficking through four means:

- promoting coordination and information sharing between federal, state, local, and tribal law enforcement;
- bolstering intelligence sharing between federal, state, local, and tribal law enforcement;
- providing reliable intelligence to law enforcement agencies such that they may be better equipped to design effective enforcement operations and strategies; and

---

56 Drug Enforcement Administration, *FY2018 Performance Budget Congressional Submission,* p. 40.

57 Drug Enforcement Administration, *2018 National Drug Threat Assessment*, October 2018. Percentage calculated by CRS based on total seizure data reported by the Drug Enforcement Administration, as illustrated in Figure 1.

58 These 10% were samples of "white powder heroin processed using the South American method but unable to be sourced to Mexico or Colombia." Ibid., p. 12.

59 Ibid., p. 13.

60 Ibid., p. 14.

61 Drug Enforcement Administration, *FY 2019 Performance Budget Congressional Submission*, p. 47.

62 Drug Enforcement Administration, *2018 National Drug Threat Assessment*, October 2018, p. 24.

63 CRS Report R45188, *High Intensity Drug Trafficking Areas (HIDTA) Program*. See also Executive Office of the President, Office of National Drug Control Policy, *High Intensity Drug Trafficking Areas (HIDTA) Program*, https://obamawhitehouse.archives.gov/ondcp/high-intensity-drug-trafficking-areas-program.

- promoting coordinated law enforcement strategies that rely upon available resources to reduce illegal drug supplies not only in a given area, but throughout the country.[64]

The HIDTA program does not mandate that all regional HIDTAs focus on the same drug threat— such as heroin trafficking; rather, funds can be used to support the most pressing drug threats in the region. As such, when heroin trafficking is found to be a top priority in a HIDTA region, funds may be used to support initiatives targeting it.

In 2015, ONDCP launched the Heroin Response Strategy (HRS), "a multi-HIDTA, cross-disciplinary approach that develops partnerships among public safety and public health agencies at the Federal, state and local levels to reduce drug overdose fatalities and disrupt trafficking in illicit opioids."[65] Within the HRS, a Public Health and Public Safety Network coordinates teams of drug intelligence officers and public health analysts in each state. The HRS not only provides information to these participating entities on drug trafficking and use, but it has "developed and disseminated prevention activities, including a parent helpline and online materials."[66]

Organized Crime Drug Enforcement Task Forces (OCDETF)

The OCDETF program targets—with the intent to disrupt and dismantle—major drug trafficking and money laundering organizations. Federal agencies that participate in the OCDETF program include the DEA; Federal Bureau of Investigation (FBI); Bureau of Alcohol, Tobacco, Firearms, and Explosives (ATF); U.S. Marshals; Internal Revenue Service (IRS); U.S. Immigration and Customs Enforcement (ICE); U.S. Coast Guard (USCG); Offices of the U.S. Attorneys; and the Department of Justice's (DOJ's) Criminal Division. These federal agencies also collaborate with state and local law enforcement on task forces.[67] There are 14 OCDETF strike forces around the country and an OCDETF Fusion Center that gathers and analyzes intelligence and information to support OCDETF operations. The OCDETFs target those organizations that have been identified on the Consolidated Priority Organization Targets (CPOT) List, the "most wanted" list for leaders of drug trafficking and money laundering organizations. During FY2017, 20% (932) of active OCDETF investigations were linked to valid CPOTs.[68] Notably, 50% of the FY2017 CPOT investigations involved heroin trafficking.[69]

---

[64] 21 U.S.C. §1706(a)(2).

[65] Executive Office of the President, Office of National Drug Control Policy, *Heroin Response Strategy, Annual Program Report for 2016*, May 2, 2017, p. 1.

[66] Ibid.

[67] U.S. Department of Justice, *FY2019 Interagency Crime and Drug Enforcement, Congressional Budget Submission.*

[68] Ibid., p. 26.

[69] Ibid., p. 27.

COPS Anti-Heroin Task Force Program

Within DOJ, the Community Oriented Policing Services (COPS) Office's Anti-Heroin Task Force (AHTF) Program provides funding assistance to state law enforcement agencies to investigate illicit activities related to the trafficking or distribution of heroin or diverted prescription opioids. While the AHTF program is not a federal enforcement program, it is a federal grant program that exclusively provides money targeted specifically for heroin trafficking enforcement efforts.[70] Funds cannot be used for treatment or other purposes because the program focuses on trafficking and distribution. Further, the program focuses its funding on state law enforcement agencies with multi -jurisdictional reach and interdisciplinary team structures—such as task forces.[71] For FY2017, grants were awarded to entities in eight states.[72]

GOING FORWARD

Adequacy of Data on Heroin Flows

What is known about heroin trafficking flows is contingent on a number of factors surrounding the collection and reporting of these data, which are both multifaceted and incomplete. Data on various elements (e.g., production, price, purity, seizures, etc.) can help provide insight into the landscape of heroin trafficking, though these data are sometimes imprecise.

For example, as the bulk of heroin consumed in the United States has been traced to Mexico, one central piece of data in understanding trafficking flows to the United States is the total potential production in the source countries. The United Nations Office on Drugs and Crime has noted, however, that "[o]nly partial information about the extent of opium poppy cultivation and heroin production in the Americas is available."[73] The DEA's *2018 National Drug Threat Assessment* estimates that Mexico may have cultivated 44,100 hectares of opium poppy in 2017, potentially yielding 111 metric tons of pure heroin.[74] This is 38% higher than the estimated production in 2016. In the past, officials have noted that crop yield data are unreliable,[75] and it is unclear whether the newer data are more reliable. Even with these questions about the data's reliability, U.S.

---

70 There are a number of grant programs that may allow money to be used, in part, to support heroin trafficking enforcement efforts; those grant programs are beyond the scope of this report. The AHTF program is highlighted for its sole focus on countering heroin trafficking.

71 U.S. Department of Justice, Community Oriented Policing Services, *Fact Sheet: 2018 COPS Anti-Heroin Task Force Program*.

72 For FY2017, police agencies in Kentucky, Maine, Maryland, Minnesota, New Hampshire, New Jersey, New York, and Vermont received AHTF awards. U.S. Department of Justice, *FY2017 COPS Anti Heroin Task Force Awards*.

73 United Nations Office on Drugs and Crime, *World Drug Report 2015*, 2015, p. 41.

74 Drug Enforcement Administration, *2018 National Drug Threat Assessment*, October 2018, p. 18.

75 See, for example, Drug Enforcement Administration, *2015 National Drug Threat Assessment*, November 2015.

officials state that production of heroin in Mexico has increased. While much of Mexican-produced heroin is reportedly destined for the United States, that proportion is unknown.

In addition, it is unknown how much pure heroin is making its way into the United States. Data on seizures are available, but these reflect an unknown portion of total drugs traversing U.S. borders. In addition, as noted, officials have estimated heroin availability in the United States based, in part, on estimated production, known seizures, and the price and purity of select samples of wholesale and retail-level heroin, but these numbers collectively represent an imprecise picture of heroin trafficking. Policymakers may, in their oversight of efforts to counter the flow of heroin into the country, assess means to bolster the accuracy and completeness of data.

Prioritizing Heroin Trafficking Enforcement

Over the past few years, officials have repeatedly referred to heroin as a top drug threat in the United States. The *2018 National Drug Threat Assessment* notes that heroin is one of the most significant drug threats.[76] This is largely based on the health risks—overdose and death—posed by these substances. Nationally, however, federal law enforcement seizures of heroin have generally increased in the past several years, as illustrated in Figure 1. Policymakers may question whether federal enforcement efforts prioritize curbing heroin trafficking to an extent commensurate with the reported threat of the drug. While seizures have generally increased both along the Southwest border and throughout the country, it is unclear whether enforcement efforts should, or are able to, increasingly target heroin trafficking networks.

In addition, law enforcement data indicate that there have been changes in heroin trafficking patterns along the Southwest border. For instance, from 2016 to 2017 heroin trafficking, by weight, increased 238% in the El Centro corridor, 174% in the Del Rio corridor, and 104% in the Yuma corridor, while it declined in other areas such as the Rio Grande Valley (by 24%).[77] Policymakers may ask if heroin enforcement efforts are nimble and able to respond (and if so, how) to shifts in heroin trafficking patterns and maximize seizures in the areas where heroin flows are increasing.

ONDCP has noted that the "responsibility for curbing heroin production and trafficking lies primarily with the source countries."[78] Policymakers may examine the

---

[76] Drug Enforcement Administration, *2018 National Drug Threat Assessment*, October 2018. It also notes other opioids (including controlled prescription drugs and fentanyl) as being among the significant drug threats.

[77] Drug Enforcement Administration, *2018 National Drug Threat Assessment*, October 2018, p. 19. For more information on these and other sectors, see https://www.cbp.gov/border-security/along-us-borders/border-patrolsectors.

[78] Office of National Drug Control Policy, *The International Heroin Market*, https://obamawhitehouse.archives.gov/ondcp/global-heroin-market.

balance of resources targeted toward domestic efforts to reduce drug trafficking through interdiction and prosecution relative to resources dedicated to eradication, alternative economic development, and other options abroad.[79]

Evaluating Goals and Outcomes of U.S. Strategies

The United States has a number of strategies and initiatives targeting illicit drugs. While they do not all focus on drug *trafficking* per se—or even more specifically, heroin trafficking—their goals include reducing drug trafficking. Policymakers may evaluate whether these strategies and initiatives are sufficient to effectively respond to the threat of heroin trafficking in the United States as well as to the role heroin trafficking may play in the opioid epidemic. If not, how might a strategy look that focuses specifically on heroin/opioid trafficking, and would such a strategy be nimble enough to counter the constantly evolving drug trafficking threats facing the United States? Examples of existing efforts are outlined here.

National Drug Control Strategy

ONDCP is charged with coordinating federal drug control policy.[80] In doing so, ONDCP is responsible for producing the annual *National Drug Control Strategy* (strategy), the purpose of which is to outline a plan to reduce illicit drug consumption in the United States and the consequences of such use.[81] The most recent strategy was released in 2016.[82] The 2016 strategy prioritizes seven approaches to reduce both illicit drug use and its consequences:

- preventing drug use in U.S. communities;
- seeking early intervention opportunities in health care;
- increasing access to treatment and supporting recovery;
- reforming the criminal justice system to better address substance use disorders;
- disrupting domestic drug trafficking and production;
- bolstering international partnerships; and
- improving information systems for analysis, assessment, and management.[83]

Each of these approaches is based on several principles and fosters certain federal drug control activities.[84] While these approaches and principles are not necessarily

---

[79] International options are beyond the scope of this report. For more information, see CRS In Focus IF10400, *Transnational Crime Issues: Heroin Production, Fentanyl Trafficking, and U.S.-Mexico Security Cooperation.*
[80] CRS Insight IN10912, *The Role of the Office of National Drug Control Policy (ONDCP).*
[81] 21 U.S.C. §1705(a)(1).
[82] The Trump Administration has not released a strategy for 2017 or 2018.
[83] Office of National Drug Control Policy, *National Drug Control Strategy, 2016.*

directed at countering *heroin* trafficking, they focus on confronting the top drug threats, which have in recent years involved heroin trafficking and its role in the opioid epidemic. Notably, the 2016 strategy identified the greatest drug threat to the United States as "the continuing opioid epidemic, which began with the overprescribing of powerful long-acting, time-released opioid medications ... [and] was further complicated by a sharp increase in the supply and subsequent use of high purity, low cost heroin produced in Mexico and Colombia and the trafficking of illicitly produced fentanyl."[85] It is unclear whether the Trump Administration will release a strategy or how prominently countering heroin trafficking as it contributes to the opioid epidemic may feature in that strategy.

National Southwest Border Counternarcotics Strategy

The *National Southwest Border Counternarcotics Strategy* (NSBCS) was first launched in 2009, and it outlines domestic and transnational efforts to reduce the flow of illegal drugs, money, and contraband across the Southwest border. It has a number of strategic objectives:

- enhance intelligence and information sharing capabilities and processes;
- reduce the flow of drugs, drug proceeds, and associated instruments of crime that cross the Southwest border;
- develop strong, resilient communities that resist criminal activity and promote healthy lifestyles;
- disrupt and dismantle TCOs operating along the Southwest border;
- stem the flow of illicit proceeds across the Southwest border; and
- enhance U.S.-Mexican-Central American cooperation on joint counterdrug efforts.[86]

The 2016 NSBCS focuses on drug trafficking broadly, noting that the Southwest border is the primary entry point for many illegal drugs arriving in the United States. Nonetheless, it mentions that "the threat posed by heroin in the United States is serious and continues to intensify."[87] The objectives and action items, however, target the broader array of drug and criminal threats at the border. It is unclear whether the Trump Administration will use the NSBCS, modify it, or develop other measures and strategies to counter the threats—including those posed by heroin trafficking—at the Southwest border.

---

[84] For instance, the action items associated with disrupting domestic drug trafficking and production are coordinating federal enforcement initiatives with state, local, and tribal partners; securing U.S. borders; and focusing national efforts on specific drug problems.

[85] Office of National Drug Control Policy, *National Drug Control Strategy, 2016*, pp. 1-2.

[86] Office of National Drug Control Policy, *National Southwest Border Counternarcotics Strategy*, May 2016.

[87] Ibid., p. 1.

National Strategy to Combat Transnational Organized Crime

In July 2011, the Obama Administration released the *Strategy to Combat Transnational Organized Crime: Addressing Converging Threats to National Security*.[88] The strategy provided the federal government's first broad conceptualization of "transnational organized crime," highlighting it as a national security concern.[89] It highlights 10 primary categories of threats posed by transnational organized crime, one of which is the expansion of drug trafficking. Additionally, the strategy outlines six key priority actions to counter threats posed by transnational organized crime:

- taking shared responsibility and identifying what actions the United States can take to protect against the threat and impact of transnational organized crime;
- enhancing intelligence and information sharing;
- protecting the financial system and strategic markets;
- strengthening interdiction, investigations, and prosecutions;
- disrupting drug trafficking and its facilitation of other transnational threats; and
- building international capacity, cooperation, and partnerships.

While this strategy is not tailored solely to drug trafficking (or more specifically, heroin trafficking) activities of criminal networks, it includes a discussion of the threat. Additionally, the strategy notes that a number of the threats outlined in the strategy may be facilitated by drug trafficking and the proceeds generated by those activities. For instance, the illicit drugs trade is at times linked to crimes such as weapons trafficking or human trafficking. Similar to the case with the NSBCS, it is unclear whether the Trump Administration will rely upon this strategy either broadly or more specifically to counter heroin trafficking.

Executive Orders

The Trump Administration has issued executive orders that could affect federal efforts to counter heroin trafficking, though they do not focus solely on them. For instance, the executive order *Enforcing Federal Law with Respect to Transnational Criminal Organizations and Preventing International Trafficking*,[90] issued in February 2017, relies in part on the Threat Mitigation Working Group—which was established as part of the Strategy to Combat Transnational Organized Crime—to, among other things, support and bolster U.S. efforts to counter criminal organizations. However, the executive order does not speak to the larger strategy or specific efforts to counter heroin

---

88 The White House, *Strategy To Combat Transnational Organized Crime: Addressing Converging Threats to National Security*, July 2011.

89 For a discussion of organized crime and this strategy, see CRS Report R41547, *Organized Crime: An Evolving Challenge for U.S. Law Enforcement*.

90 Executive Order 13773, "Enforcing Federal Law With Respect to Transnational Criminal Organizations and Preventing International Trafficking," 82 *Federal Register* 10691-10693, February 14, 2017.

trafficking. In addition, President Trump issued the executive order *Establishing the President's Commission on Combating Drug Addiction and the Opioid Crisis*[91] in March 2017. The commission's final report recommended a number of actions, including providing enhanced penalties for the trafficking of fentanyl and its analogues as well as bolstering tools and technologies to detect fentanyl before it enters the United States.[92]

National Heroin Task Force

The National Heroin Task Force was convened by DOJ and ONDCP in March 2015 pursuant to P.L. 113-235. The task force examined the Administration's efforts to tackle the heroin epidemic from various angles including criminal enforcement, prevention, and substance use disorder treatment and recovery services, and it developed a set of recommendations to "curtail the escalating overdose epidemic and death rates."[93] The report's recommendations target the public safety and public health aspects of the opioid epidemic, and several specifically address countering heroin trafficking.

The task force suggested, for instance, that the federal government prioritize prosecutions of heroin distributors and enhance investigation and prosecution techniques to target the heroin supply chain—particularly when the drug caused a death. The report noted that identifying the source of particularly potent heroin and cutting off the flow of heroin from the source may ultimately save lives. It also noted that prominent prosecutions of distributors and traffickers can help serve as a deterrent to other potential drug dealers.[94]

The task force also recommended using coordinated, real time data sharing to disrupt drug supply and to focus prevention, treatment, and intervention resources on the areas that need them most. It highlights the HIDTA program and the OCDETF program as examples of task forces that can be leveraged for information sharing purposes;[95] while these programs have information sharing capacities, it is unclear how rapidly this sharing could be executed to fulfill the task force's recommendation of striving for "real time" information sharing.

---

[91] Executive Order 13784, "Establishing the President's Commission on Combating Drug Addiction and the Opioid Crisis," 82 *Federal Register* 16283-16285, March 29, 2017.

[92] The President's Commission on Combating Drug Addiction and the Opioid Crisis, *Final Report Draft*, November 1, 2017.

[93] National Heroin Task Force, *Final Report and Recommendations*, December 31, 2015.

[94] Ibid., p. 12.

[95] Ibid., p. 10.

In: Battling the Opioid Epidemic
Editor: Vincent Hardy

ISBN: 978-1-53615-548-8

Chapter 5

DRUG CONTROL: DOD SHOULD IMPROVE ITS OVERSIGHT OF THE NATIONAL GUARD COUNTERDRUG PROGRAM*

United States Government Accountability Office

ABBREVIATIONS

ASD (HD&GS)	Assistant Secretary of Defense for Homeland Defense and Global Security
CR	Continuing Resolution
DASD (CN&GT)	Deputy Assistant Secretary of Defense for Counternarcotics and Global Threats
DOD	Department of Defense
OMB	Office of Management and Budget
OUSD (C)	Office of the Undersecretary of Defense, Comptroller

WHY GAO DID THIS STUDY

Since 1989, DOD has received billions of dollars to fund the National Guard's participation in a counterdrug program focused on domestic drug interdiction activities.

* This is an edited, reformatted and augmented version of United States Government Accountability Office; Report to Congressional Committees, Publication No. GAO-19-27, dated January 2019.

DOD received $261 million for this program in fiscal year 2018. This program provides military support to assist state, local, and tribal law enforcement organizations with counterdrug activities and operates in 54 states and territories across the United States.

Senate Report 115-125 included a provision for GAO to evaluate the National Guard counterdrug program. This report (1) evaluates the extent to which DOD has strategy and implementing guidance for the National Guard counterdrug program, and (2) assesses DOD's processes to approve states' counterdrug plans and distribute funding to the program, among other things. GAO reviewed DOD's counterdrug strategy and guidance; DOD funding and personnel data; and its processes to distribute funding.

WHAT GAO RECOMMENDS

GAO is making a total of five recommendations, including, among others, that DOD issue a strategic framework that addresses current drug threats, the National Guard issue guidance with detailed procedures on how states should administer the program, DOD assess the revised process for approving state plans, and the National Guard incorporate DOD's strategic counternarcotics priorities into its funding distribution process. DOD concurred with GAO's recommendations.

WHAT GAO FOUND

The Department of Defense (DOD) lacks current strategy and guidance to implement the National Guard counterdrug program. Although a number of key national-level strategies, such as the National Drug Control Strategy, have been updated since 2011 to address changing drug threats, GAO found that DOD's 2011 Counternarcotics and Global Threats Strategy has not been updated to reflect these changes. In addition, the National Guard lacks detailed procedures and processes for the states to implement the National Guard counterdrug program, such as how to conduct cross-state aerial reconnaissance. Without current strategy or guidance, it will be difficult for the National Guard to operate its counterdrug program effectively.

DOD's processes to approve state counterdrug plans and distribute funding to the state-level counterdrug programs could be improved. Since at least 2009, DOD has provided funding to the states without first approving state plans for counterdrug activities, as required by statute. GAO found that the delay in approval of state counterdrug plans has worsened since fiscal year 2009; in fiscal year 2018, approval took over 9 months (283 days); see figure below. In 2018, DOD took some steps to address the timely review of state plans, but GAO found that those steps did not rectify the problem.

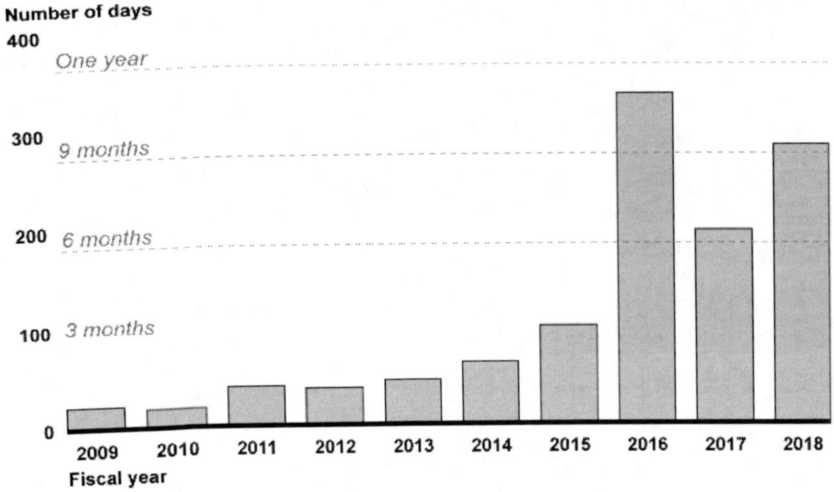

Source: GAO analysis of Department of Defense data. | GAO-19-27.

Number of Days Between the Beginning of the Fiscal Year and when DOD Approved All State Counterdrug Plans, Fiscal Years 2009 through 2018.

GAO also found that the process used by the National Guard to distribute funding to the states within the program does not incorporate DOD's strategic counternarcotics priorities, such as the U.S. southwest and northern border areas. GAO's work on results-oriented management states that strategy should inform program activities and resourcing. Until National Guard's process to distribute funding to state counterdrug programs is improved, it risks directing funding toward lower priority counterdrug activities at the expense of higher priority activities.

January 17, 2019
The Honorable James M. Inhofe
Chairman

The Honorable Jack Reed
Ranking Member
Committee on Armed Services United States Senate

The Honorable Adam Smith
Chairman

The Honorable Mac Thornberry
Ranking Member

Committee on Armed Services
House of Representatives

Since 1989, Congress has provided billions of dollars to the Department of Defense (DOD) to fund the National Guard's participation in domestic drug interdiction and counterdrug activities. The type of military support provided by the National Guard can range from reconnaissance to analytical support, but it generally reflects the drug interdiction priorities of the Governors of the 50 states, the District of Columbia, and three U.S. territories; the capabilities of each state's National Guard; and the needs of interagency partners. These interagency partners include state, local, and tribal law enforcement organizations, as well as several federal agencies— including the Departments of Justice, Homeland Security, and Treasury—all of which are involved in efforts to disrupt and dismantle the infrastructure of major drug-trafficking organizations. According to the National Guard Bureau, in fiscal year 2017, the National Guard counterdrug program employed over 3,700 personnel who supported law enforcement's efforts to remove over 3.3 million pounds, or nearly $11.2 billion, in illicit drugs from U.S. communities.[1] In addition to providing support to law enforcement partners, the National Guard Bureau operates five counterdrug schools that provide training in drug interdiction and counterdrug activities.[2] According to the National Guard Bureau, these schools trained over 41,400 law enforcement officers, community based organization members, and military personnel in fiscal year 2017.[3]

Senate Report 115-125 accompanying a bill for the National Defense Authorization Act for Fiscal Year 2018 contained a provision that we evaluate the National Guard counterdrug program and its approach to resource allocation.[4] This report: (1) evaluates the extent to which DOD has strategy and implementing guidance for the National Guard counterdrug program, (2) describes the actions taken by the National Guard Bureau to improve the availability of funds when operating under continuing resolutions, and (3) assesses DOD's processes to approve states' counterdrug plans and distribute funding to the program.

To address our objectives, we reviewed documentation and interviewed officials from the Office of the Deputy Assistant Secretary of Defense for Counternarcotics and Global Threats; the National Guard Bureau; select state counterdrug programs; Office of the Under Secretary of Defense, Comptroller; and Army and Air National Guard Budget Execution Offices. Our analysis of the National Guard counterdrug program focused on

---

[1] Department of Defense, *2019 National Guard Bureau Posture Statement Focused on Readiness*.

[2] The five counterdrug schools are: 1) Multi-jurisdictional Counterdrug Task Force Training, Starke, Florida; 2) Midwest Counterdrug Training Center, Johnston, Iowa; 3) Regional Counterdrug Training Academy, Meridian, Mississippi; 4) Northeast Counterdrug Training Center, Fort Indiantown Gap, Pennsylvania; and 5) Western Regional Counterdrug Training Center, Tacoma, Washington.

[3] Department of Defense, *2019 National Guard Bureau Posture Statement Focused on Readiness*. According to DOD officials, these figures include law enforcement officers, community-based organization members, and military personnel trained on-site and by mobile training teams. Officials from the Office of the Deputy Assistant Secretary of Defense for Counternarcotics and Global Threats stated that they are concerned that a high percentage of the instruction hours provided by the National Guard counterdrug schools have been for commonly expected law enforcement training contracted at the state level to non-government civilian instructors to provide training not organic to the DOD.

[4] S. Rep. No. 115-125, at 247 (2017).

Title 32 state activities, which includes five specific projects: 1) state plans, 2) counterdrug schools, 3) counterthreat finance, 4) linguist support, and 5) linguist and data analysis.[5]

In addition, we used a non-generalizable sample of 9 of the 54 participating states, territories, and the District of Columbia as case studies and interviewed officials in those states to get their perspectives on strategy, policy, guidance, and funding for the program. The nine states we included in our review were: Alaska, California, Maine, Mississippi, Missouri, New Mexico, New York, Tennessee, and Texas. To select these case studies for our sample, we relied on five criteria. First, we selected states from each of the four counterdrug program regions: Northeast, Northwest, Southeast, and Southwest. Second, we selected both low and high drug threat level states from each region, as determined by the National Guard Bureau's funding distribution model known as the threat-based resource model in 2018. Third, we selected states that experienced large fluctuations in their threat level between fiscal years 2016 and 2018 as a consequence of changes to the National Guard Bureau's threat-based resource model for fiscal year 2018, such as the expansion in the number of drug threat variables in the model and the institution of seizure thresholds to better distinguish which drug seizures would be considered within the model. Fourth, we selected states that received what National Guard Bureau officials referred to as a "functional" level of funding for fiscal year 2018, meaning that funding was provided at a level necessary to support two counterdrug missions in that state or territory, regardless of its threat level. Finally, we selected from states that have an international border and that border international waters.

To address our first objective, we reviewed DOD's 2011 Counternarcotics and Global Threats Strategy and other executive branch strategy documents, including the Office of National Drug Control Policy's National Drug Control Strategy and geographic drug control strategies. We evaluated DOD's strategy to determine the extent to which it aligned with current national-level strategies and drug threats. We also reviewed a DOD Inspector General assessment of the National Guard counterdrug program that addresses the counternarcotics and global threats strategy. In addition, we reviewed whether the National Guard Bureau has issued guidance on counterdrug support in accordance with Chief National Guard Bureau policy that assigns responsibility for the issuance of supporting guidance for the National Guard counterdrug program.

To address our second objective, we analyzed DOD's budget requests and congressionally-directed increases for fiscal years 2004 through 2018.[6] We also analyzed the National Guard counterdrug program's total budget authority and obligation amounts by project code and calculated overall obligation rates for fiscal years 2010 through

---

[5] See Appendix I for a description of the five projects that make up the National Guard counterdrug program's Title 32 activities.

[6] Throughout this report, we refer to the funds Congress has appropriated above budget request levels for the National Guard counterdrug program as congressionally-directed increases.

2017.[7] Further, we examined the number of personnel on-orders by month supporting National Guard counterdrug program activities for October 2012 through August 2018. Finally, we reviewed DOD's process to distribute funds to the National Guard counterdrug program and funding received under each appropriation period—including continuing resolutions and final appropriations—for fiscal years 2014 and 2018, including the timing and amount of funds received.

To address our third objective, we reviewed DOD's process for approving state drug interdiction and counterdrug activities plan submissions and distributing funding to state counterdrug programs for fiscal years 2009 through 2018.[8] We compared DOD's process for approving state plan submissions to the law governing the use of funds for state counterdrug activities and to DOD policy. Finally, we examined the National Guard Bureau's threat-based resource model and its process to distribute funding to the program and assessed it based on GAO's work on results-oriented management.

We assessed the reliability of the following types of data on the National Guard counterdrug program: DOD's budget requests and congressionally-directed increases for fiscal years 2004 through 2018; total budget authority and obligations amounts for fiscal years 2010 through 2017; program personnel on orders by month for October 2012 through August 2018; threat-based resource model percentages for fiscal years 2015 through 2018 and planned funding levels by state or territory program for fiscal years 2012 through 2018; and state plans approval dates for fiscal years 2009 through 2018.[9] We assessed the reliability of all sources of data by examining them for missing values, outliers, and obvious errors as well as by interviewing knowledgeable agency officials regarding their accuracy and completeness. For data on DOD's budget requests, congressionally-directed increases, total budget authority, and obligation amounts, we examined other sources that provide the same types of data to ensure consistency. In addition, we also assessed data on DOD's budget requests and congressionally-directed increases by comparing them to amounts presented in a prior GAO report.[10] We determined that all the data we report on were sufficiently reliable for the purposes of our review.

We conducted this performance audit from August 2017 to January 2019 in accordance with generally accepted government auditing standards. Those standards require that we plan and perform the audit to obtain sufficient, appropriate evidence to provide a reasonable basis for our findings and conclusions based on our audit objectives. We believe that the evidence obtained provides a reasonable basis for our findings and conclusions based on our audit objectives.

---

[7] Total budget authority is the authority to incur obligations and pay expenses.

[8] Throughout this report, we refer to state drug interdiction and counterdrug activities plans as state plans.

[9] We analyzed National Guard counterdrug program data based on the availability of complete and reliable data from DOD.

[10] GAO, *Drug Control: Additional Performance Information Is Needed to Oversee the National Guard's State Counterdrug Program,* GAO-16-133 (Washington, D.C.: Oct. 21, 2015).

BACKGROUND

National Guard Counterdrug Program

The National Guard counterdrug program is part of DOD's broader counterdrug mission, which focuses on supporting local, state, federal, and foreign government agencies in addressing the illegal drug trade and narcotics-related terrorism.[11] The program was originally conceived as a reconnaissance support mission largely focused on marijuana eradication efforts. In 1977, the Hawaii National Guard became the first state National Guard to assist law enforcement agencies in counterdrug missions. Hawaii law enforcement officials sought Hawaii National Guard helicopter transport to support Operation Green Harvest, a marijuana eradication mission. By 1984, four additional states' National Guards were supporting state law enforcement agencies with counterdrug efforts. That number grew to 32 states in 1988. However, this assistance was limited in scope and generally conducted as Guard units performed normal training activities, and costs associated with this assistance were paid for by the states.

The National Defense Authorization Act, Fiscal Year 1989 tasked DOD with the mission to ensure the availability of military support to law enforcement agencies nationwide.[12] This law established DOD as the single lead agency of the federal government for the detection and monitoring of aerial and maritime transit of illegal drugs into the United States,[13] and it amplified the National Guard's role as a support agency for state law enforcement in counterdrug support missions under the Governor of each state, territory, and the District of Columbia. By 1994, the program was in operation in 54 states and territories across the United States.

As of fiscal year 2018, National Guard Bureau policy allows state counterdrug programs to perform 15 support activities grouped into five broad mission categories—(1) technical support (including linguist and translator, operational and investigative case and criminal analyst, and counterthreat finance support), (2) general support (including domestic cannabis suppression and eradication operations and transportation support), (3) reconnaissance and observation (including ground and aerial reconnaissance), (4) civil operations and coalition development, and (5) counterdrug training.[14]

---

[11] According to DOD officials, DOD conducts its counterdrug mission in two primary areas: detecting and monitoring drug trafficking into the United States and sharing information on illegal drugs with U.S. and foreign government agencies.

[12] Pub. L. No. 100-456, § 1104 (1988).

[13] *Id.* at § 1102(a), repealed by Pub. L. No. 101-189, § 1202 (1989) (codifying this provision at 10 U.S.C. § 124).

[14] Chief National Guard Bureau Instruction 3100.01A, *National Guard Counterdrug Support* (June 22, 2015). The Office of the Deputy Assistant Secretary of Defense for Counternarcotics and Global Threats recategorized counterthreat finance activities in fiscal year 2018 and beyond to, according to DOD officials, more accurately reflect the type of National Guard investigative case analysis support provided to law enforcement. The program also includes a mission category for internal program management. Since this mission category does not provide support to interagency partners, we did not include it in our analysis. For an overview of approved counterdrug support activities, see appendix II.

Legal Authorities of the National Guard Counterdrug Program

The National Guard counterdrug program conducts activities under the authority of two titles in the United States Code—Title 32 and Title 10. Section 502 of title 32 allows a member of the National Guard to be ordered to full-time National Guard duty status under regulations prescribed by the Secretary of the Army or Secretary of the Air Force. In addition, Section 112 of title 32 authorizes personnel of the National Guard of a State, under regulations prescribed by the Secretary of Defense, to be ordered to perform full-time National Guard duty under section 502 for the purposes of carrying out drug interdiction and counterdrug activities in accordance with state plans.[15] Section 112 also authorizes the Secretary of Defense to provide funds to support the approved drug interdiction and counter-drug activities plan of state governors.

In addition, Title 10 allows the Secretary of the Army or Air Force to order a member of the National Guard, under the Secretary's jurisdiction, to active duty with the consent of the member and the governor of that state.[16] Under Section 284 of title 10, DOD provides support to a number of partners, such as federal agencies, in their counterdrug activities, at times using National Guard personnel on active duty. Table 1 provides a summary of the Title 32 and Title 10 authorities.

Table 1. Summary of Title 32 and Title 10 Authorities for Use of the National Guard

	Title 32	Title 10
Command and control	State governor	President
Duty status	Full-time National Guard duty	Active duty in Reserves ofArmy and Air Force
Where duty is performed	Within the United States, U.S. territories and possessions, and the District of Columbia	Worldwide and within the U.S.

Source: GAO analysis of National Guard statutory authorities. | GAO-19-27.

Funding for the National Guard Counterdrug Program

To fund DOD's counterdrug mission, Congress appropriates amounts to DOD's Drug Interdiction and Counterdrug Activities, Defense account.[17] The categories of activities funded by the account include: detection and monitoring; international support;

[15] Governors and the Commanding General of the National Guard of the District of Columbia each submit a state drug interdiction and counter-drug activities plan that, among other things, specifies how National Guard personnel within their state are to be used in drug interdiction and counter-drug activities and includes a certification that those operations are to be conducted at a time when the personnel involved are not in Federal service.

[16] 10 U.S.C. § 12301(d).

[17] This account, originally called Drug Interdiction, Defense, was established by the Department of Defense Appropriations Act, 1989.

intelligence, technology, and other; domestic support, which includes the National Guard counterdrug program; and drug demand reduction.[18] Of all the activities, the domestic support activity, which includes the National Guard counterdrug program, receives the largest amount of funding from DOD's Drug Interdiction and Counterdrug Activities account. In fiscal year 2018, Congress appropriated about $934.8 million to the Drug Interdiction and Counterdrug Activities, Defense account,[19] of which about $261.4 million, or 28 percent, was appropriated for the National Guard counterdrug program.[20] Figure 1 shows the program funding in DOD's Drug Interdiction and Counterdrug Activities Account for fiscal year 2018.

DOD's budget request to the President for the National Guard counterdrug program was generally steady from fiscal year 2004 through fiscal year 2012, but was reduced significantly in fiscal year 2013.[21] Since then, congressionally-directed increases have generally accounted for 50 percent or more of the program's total funding, as shown in Figure 2 below.[22]

In fiscal year 2018, the Senate Committee on Appropriations expressed concerns that DOD reduced overall funding for the National Guard counterdrug program from the fiscal year 2017 enacted levels and failed to include an individual budget line in its budget request for the National Guard counterdrug schools program.[23] DOD's budget request for fiscal year 2018 was about $116.4 million, while the final appropriation designated $261.4 million for the program—approximately a 125 percent increase.

---

[18] For fiscal year 2018, the National Guard counterdrug program is comprised of five projects: state plans, counterdrug schools, counterthreat finance, and two projects that provide linguist support to law enforcement partners. Throughout this report, we refer to these projects collectively as the National Guard counterdrug program.

[19] The $934.8 million appropriated amount does not include any Overseas Contingency Operations funding.

[20] About $236.4 million was appropriated for the state-level National Guard counterdrug programs, and $25 million was appropriated for the National Guard counterdrug schools program.

[21] From fiscal years 2013 to 2016, DOD reduced its budget request for domestic counterdrug efforts such as those supported by the National Guard counterdrug program. DOD officials stated that to address spending limits required by the Budget Control Act of 2011, some programs had to be reduced in order to maintain support for higher priority U.S. programs aimed at supporting Afghanistan operations and to address drug cartel violence in Mexico and Central America that were destabilizing the region and threatened to spill over into the United States. The Budget Control Act of 2011, Pub. L. No. 112-25 (2011), amends the Balanced Budget and Emergency Deficit Control Act of 1985, Pub. L. No. 99-177 (1985), codified at 2 U.S.C. § 901, and provides that new budget authority may not exceed the discretionary spending limits for a fiscal year. Subsequent amendments have revised the discretionary spending limits and extended the sequestration of direct spending through fiscal year 2027. *See* Bipartisan Budget Act of 2018, Pub. L. No. 115-123, § 30101 (2018); Bipartisan Budget Act of 2015, Pub. L. No. 114-74, § 101 (2015); Bipartisan Budget Act of 2013, Pub. L. No. 113-67, § 101 (2013).

[22] Appendix I provides additional information on DOD's budget requests and congressionally-directed increases for the National Guard counterdrug program and counterdrug schools program.

[23] S. Comm. on Appropriations, 115th Cong., Explanatory Statement for the Department of Defense Appropriations Bill, 2018 (2017) (accompanying the recommendations of the Chairman of the Senate Appropriations Committee). According to DOD officials, DOD requested funding for the counterdrug schools program in fiscal year 2018; however, Congress desired greater visibility for the program in the form of a separate budget line item. DOD officials stated that Congress's request for greater visibility was partially addressed in the fiscal year 2019 budget request and has now been fully implemented for the fiscal year 2020 budget request.

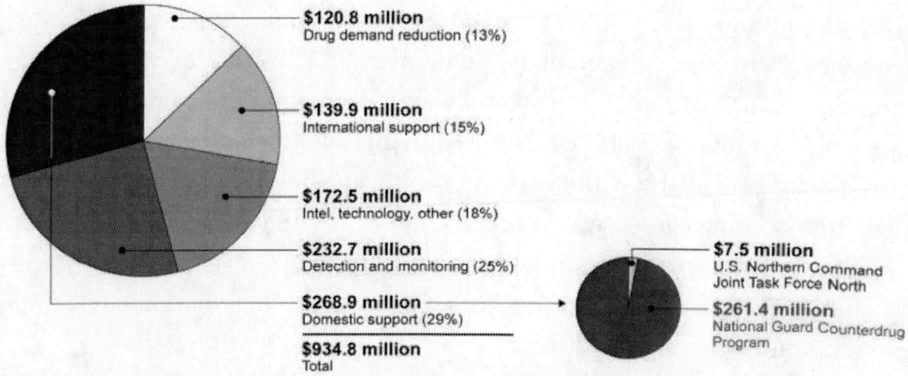

Source: GAO analysis of Department of Defense data. | GAO-19-27.

Note: Overseas Contingency Operations funding is not included in this analysis.

Figure 1. Program Funding in DOD's Drug Interdiction and Counterdrug Activities, Defense Account in Fiscal Year 2018.

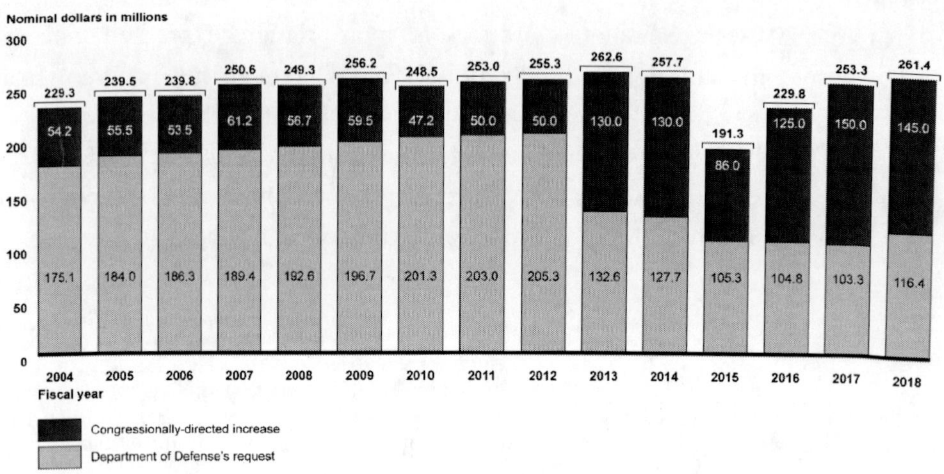

Source: GAO analysis of Department of Defense data. | GAO-19-27.

Figure 2. DOD's Budget Requests and Congressionally-Directed Increases for the National Guard Counterdrug Program, Fiscal Years 2004 through 2018.

Roles and Responsibilities

On July 31, 2002, the Deputy Secretary of Defense issued a memorandum that, among other things, assigned responsibility for DOD's counternarcotics program to the Deputy Assistant Secretary of Defense for Counternarcotics.[24] The responsibilities include developing and implementing DOD's counternarcotics policy, conducting analyses, making recommendations, and issuing guidance regarding DOD's

[24] Deputy Secretary of Defense Memorandum, *Department of Defense Counternarcotics Policy* (July 31, 2002). Today, the official is named the Deputy Assistant Secretary of Defense for Counternarcotics and Global Threats.

counternarcotics plans and programs. In addition, the office is responsible for coordinating and monitoring DOD's counternarcotics plans and programs to ensure adherence to this policy.

Chief National Guard Bureau Instruction 3100.01A, *National Guard Counterdrug Support*, establishes policy and assigns responsibilities for the National Guard counterdrug program.[25] The instruction assigns the Director of the National Guard Domestic Operations and Force Development as the proponent for the program. The Director's responsibilities include publishing supporting documents for the instruction, verifying that the plans outlining each state's proposed activities are consistent with annual instructions published by the Office of the Deputy Assistant Secretary of Defense for Counternarcotics and Global Threats and are processed efficiently and on-time, and conducting periodic evaluations of program operations at the state level.

DOD LACKS A CURRENT STRATEGY AND GUIDANCE FOR THE NATIONAL GUARD COUNTERDRUG PROGRAM

DOD Counternarcotics and Global Threats Strategy Is Outdated

DOD's 2011 Counternarcotics and Global Threats Strategy, the governing strategy for the National Guard counterdrug program, is outdated and does not reflect current drug threats outlined in more recent executive branch strategies.[26] While the 2011 Counternarcotics and Global Threats Strategy shares common themes with the updated executive branch strategies, such as the importance of combatting transnational criminal organizations involved in drug trafficking, it has not been updated to reflect changes in the drug threats faced by the United States that are outlined by the more recent executive branch strategies. Table 2 provides details on national-level strategies that have been released since 2011.

The Office of National Drug Control Policy released a new National Drug Control Strategy each year between 2011 and 2016.[27] Each update discussed the threat posed by opioids, which the 2016 update labeled as the greatest drug threat facing the nation.[28] The

---

25 Chief National Guard Bureau Instruction 3100.01A, *National Guard Counterdrug Support* (June 22, 2015). This instruction applies to National Guard personnel when not in federal service.

26 *Department of Defense Counternarcotics and Global Threats Strategy* (Apr. 27, 2011).

27 The Office of National Drug Control Policy is a component of the Executive Office of the President. This office is responsible for, among other things, overseeing and coordinating implementation of national drug control policy and responding to emerging threats related to illicit drug use. 21 U.S.C. § 1702(a).

28 The United States has experienced a recent rise in opioid use involving the abuse of prescription drugs and more traditional illicit opioids, such as heroin. Coinciding with this increase, there has been a significant increase in the use of man-made (synthetic) opioids, such as fentanyl and fentanyl analogues, which are a main contributor to the spikes in overdose deaths. To respond to the rise in opioid use, the President directed the Acting Secretary of Health and Human Services to declare the drug demand and opioid crisis to be a public health emergency on October 26, 2017. That day, the Acting Health and Human Services Secretary declared

2017 National Security Strategy also addressed opioids by emphasizing the need to dismantle transnational criminal organizations that feed the illicit opioid epidemic.[29] However, DOD's 2011 Counternarcotics and Global Threats Strategy does not address the domestic opioid epidemic. In addition, the 2016 National Southwest Border Counternarcotics Strategy states that the increased role of Mexican heroin manufacturers and traffickers is altering previously established trafficking patterns. While the 2011 Counternarcotics and Global Threats Strategy considers the illicit trafficking of cocaine from the Southwest border, it does not consider changes in the heroin threat.[30] Further, because DOD's Counternarcotics and Global Threats Strategy has not been updated, it does not take into consideration other strategies that have since been issued, such as the 2015 Caribbean Border Counternarcotics Strategy.[31] According to officials from the National Guard Bureau, DOD's 2011 counternarcotics strategy only addresses the National Guard counterdrug program in a limited capacity and therefore they are challenged to provide strategic direction to the state counterdrug programs.

Table 2. Executive Branch Strategies Addressing U.S. Drug Threats, 2012 through 2018

Strategy	Source	Releases since 2011	Purpose
National Drug Control Strategy	Office of National Drug Control Policy	2012, 2013, 2014, 2015, and 2016	Outlines the President's drug policy to reduce illicit drug use and its consequences in the United States
National Security Strategy	President	2015 and 2017	Describes international interests, goals, and objectives of the United States that are vital to national security and plans for achieving them
National Defense Strategy	Secretary of Defense	2012 and 2018	Outlines the President's strategic direction and priorities for the Department of Defense
National Southwest Border Counternarcotics Strategy	Office of National Drug Control Policy	2013 and 2016	Outlines the Federal, State, local, tribal and international actions that will reduce the flow of illicit drugs, cash, and weapons across the southwest border of the United States
National Northern Border Counternarcotics Strategy	Office of National Drug Control Policy	2012 and 2014	Outlines plans for preventing the illegal trafficking of drugs across the northern border of the United States
Caribbean Border Counternarcotics Strategy	Office of National Drug Control Policy	2015	Outlines the United States' framework for reducing the threats associated with drugs at the Caribbean border

Source: GAO analysis of national-level strategies. | GAO-19-27.

the public health emergency under the Public Health Service Act, 42 U.S.C. § 247d. GAO, *Illicit Opioids: While Greater Attention Given to Combating Synthetic Opioids, Agencies Need to Better Assess their Efforts*, GAO-18-205 (Washington, D.C.: Mar. 29, 2018).

[29] The White House, *National Security Strategy of the United States of America* (December 2017).

[30] Office of National Drug Control Policy, *National Southwest Border Counternarcotics Strategy* (May 2016).

[31] Office of National Drug Control Policy, *Caribbean Border Counternarcotics Strategy* (January 2015).

DOD's 2011 Counternarcotics and Global Threats Strategy states that officials will ensure that the strategy remains consistent with and integrates key DOD and executive branch strategies, such as National Drug Control Strategy. It also states that, given the dynamic environment within which the challenges related to the flow and impact of illegal drugs exist, the strategy is meant to be a living document, to be modified regularly. However, officials from the Office of the Deputy Assistant Secretary of Defense for Counternarcotics and Global Threats acknowledged that they have not regularly modified the strategy and that the security environment has changed. These officials stated that they have been in the process of developing an updated Counternarcotics and Global Threats Strategy with revised strategic goals and objectives since 2013, but the document has not been signed and released by the Secretary of Defense. DOD officials stated that after the 2018 National Defense Strategy was issued, they delayed the release of an updated Counternarcotics and Global Threats Strategy in order to ensure alignment between the two documents. However, according to DOD officials, the 2018 National Defense Strategy, which was issued in January 2018, did not address DOD counternarcotics efforts as they had anticipated, requiring them to reconsider their approach.

Officials from the Office of the Deputy Assistant Secretary of Defense for Counternarcotics and Global Threats stated that they now plan to issue a strategic framework, which would allow them to respond to changes in the security environment more quickly because updates to the framework would not require Secretary of Defense approval, as is the case with a DOD strategy. However, they stated that they are now waiting for the release of a new National Drug Control Strategy before issuing the framework.[32] Officials with the Office of National Drug Control Policy stated that, while they have drafted a new National Drug Control Strategy, they have not committed to an issuance date and are waiting for their new director to be confirmed by the Senate before proceeding with reviewing and issuing the draft.[33] However, a substantial amount of time has lapsed since DOD's counternarcotics strategy was last issued—over 7 years— and there have been significant developments during that time in the nature of the drug threats facing the United States. DOD officials acknowledged that because the process to update its strategic framework requires less review than a full strategy, DOD could quickly update it, if necessary, to ensure that it aligns with a new National Drug Control Strategy once one is released. Without a DOD counternarcotics and global threats strategic framework that reflects DOD's current strategic priorities and drug threats, the National

---

[32] The Office of National Drug Control Policy is required to develop a comprehensive annual National Drug Control Strategy that sets forth a plan to reduce illicit drug use and the consequences of such illicit drug use in the United States by limiting the availability of, and reducing the demand for, illegal drugs. As of January 2019, a new strategy has not been issued.

[33] Current and former members of the House Oversight and Government Reform Committee have expressed concern regarding the lack of a current National Drug Control Strategy. GAO has ongoing work related to the programs and strategy of Office of National Drug Control Policy, which is planned for release in 2019.

Guard counterdrug program risks focusing activities and resources in areas that are less imperative to address than others and that do not counter current drug threats.

The National Guard Bureau Does Not Have Guidance for Operating and Administering the Counterdrug Program

The National Guard Bureau had guidance—National Guard Regulation 500-2—that prescribed policies, procedures, and responsibilities for the National Guard counterdrug program, but it was rescinded in September 2014 by Chief National Guard Bureau Instruction 3100.01 to conform with new National Guard publications guidance, according to National Guard Bureau officials. Chief National Guard Bureau Instruction 3100.01A, which replaced Chief National Guard Bureau Instruction 3100.01 in June 2015, establishes policies and assigns responsibilities for the National Guard counterdrug program, but it does not provide detailed procedures and processes that states can use to implement these policies. For example, National Guard Regulation 500-2 provided information on how states should operate and administer the National Guard counterdrug program, including how to perform counterdrug financial management, acquisition and logistics management, personnel and administration, records and reports, and operate the counterdrug schools. Chief National Guard Bureau Instruction 3100.01A does not provide these types of instructions. State counterdrug program officials we interviewed stated that without the detailed procedures and processes included in National Guard Regulation 500-2, they have no administrative guidance regarding hiring, retirement, budgeting, and planning for their counterdrug programs. Additionally, National Guard Bureau officials stated that they do not have procedures and processes instructing states on how to provide cross-state support. For example, there are currently no guidelines on how a state that can perform aerial reconnaissance activities could provide these resources to another state upon request. National Guard Bureau officials told us they should have guidelines to facilitate cross-state support.[34] Table 3 provides an overview of National Guard Bureau publications.

To help implement policy established by Chief National Guard Bureau instructions, the National Guard Bureau can issue more detailed guidance on the corresponding procedures and processes in the form of a Chief National Guard Bureau Manual.[35] Additionally, Chief National Guard Bureau Instruction 3100.01A, *National Guard Counterdrug Support*, assigns the Director of National Guard Domestic Operations and Force Development the responsibility to publish supporting documents to implement the

[34] National Guard Bureau officials stated that states seeking cross-state support must maintain an approved state plan that authorizes the performance of the activity for which they are requesting support.

[35] Chief National Guard Bureau Instruction 5000.01A, *Chief of the National Guard Bureau Issuances* (Apr. 26, 2017).

instruction and counterdrug program when required. However, the National Guard Bureau officials acknowledge that they have not issued a manual that provides detailed procedures and processes to implement National Guard counterdrug program policies since the prior operating guidance in the National Guard regulation was rescinded in September 2014.

Table 3. National Guard Bureau Publications

Issuance	Purpose	Status
National Guard Regulation 500-2/ Air National Guard Instruction 10-801	Prescribes policies, procedures, and responsibilities governing the utilization of National Guard and Department of Defense resources in the National Guard counterdrug program and the National Guard counterdrug schools.	Replaced by Chief National Guard Bureau Instruction 3100.01
Chief National Guard Bureau Instruction 3100.01A	Establishes policies and assigns responsibilities for the National Guard counterdrug program	Current (last updated June 22, 2015)
Chief National Guard Bureau Manual	Provide detailed procedures and processes to implement policy established by Chief National Guard Bureau Instruction 3100.01A	Not issued

Source: GAO analysis of National Guard Bureau publications. | GAO-19-27.

National Guard Bureau officials stated that they intended to publish a Chief National Guard Bureau Manual in September 2014, concurrent with Chief National Guard Bureau Instruction 3100.01, which would have provided additional operating guidance for administering and operating the counterdrug program. However, according to National Guard officials, issuance of the manual was delayed because of disagreements among National Guard Bureau officials about its content. Specifically, some National Guard Bureau officials stated that the draft manual was too focused on support for Title 10 activities and did not adequately address Title 32 support, which reflects the bulk of the activities conducted by the program. National Guard Bureau officials stated that they intended to reissue National Guard Regulation 500-2 as interim guidance until they completed the Chief National Guard Bureau Manual; however, they have yet to do so because they have been focused on other efforts. National Guard Bureau officials stated that they have now worked with state counterdrug program officials to more adequately address Title 32 support activities and intend to publish a Chief National Guard Bureau Manual in June 2019.

The draft manual is in the beginning of the review process. However, the National Guard Bureau will not have guidance to operate the counterdrug program until at least June 2019. Without interim guidance that provides detailed procedures and processes for the National Guard counterdrug program, such as reissuing National Guard Regulation 500-2, states will continue to be left without clear instructions on how to operate and administer the program, such as how and when to provide support across state lines and to interagency partners.

THE NATIONAL GUARD BUREAU HAS TAKEN STEPS TO IMPROVE THE AVAILABILITY OF FUNDS WHEN OPERATING UNDER CONTINUING RESOLUTIONS

The federal government has operated under a continuing resolution for 36 of the last 40 years. National Guard counterdrug program officials stated that they have experienced program disruptions during these periods. The disruptions described by the officials are similar to the problems that other programs experience during continuing resolutions.[36] For example, National Guard Bureau officials stated that continuing resolutions have created challenges for the National Guard counterdrug program in fully obligating its funds. DOD data show that the program obligated 84 and 82 percent of total budget authority amounts in fiscal year 2011 and 2013 respectively, although the gap between total budget authority amounts and obligations has decreased since then. According to National Guard officials, the differences over the years between the amounts obligated and total budget authority amounts were partly due to the timing and amount of funding received by the program. Specifically, they stated that it is difficult to fully obligate funds when DOD provides them with a significant portion of their funding close to the end of the fiscal year. Remaining unobligated amounts are transferred back to DOD's Drug Interdiction and Counterdrug Activities, Defense account.[37] Figure 3 details the counterdrug program's obligations from fiscal years 2010 through 2017.[38]

State counterdrug program officials stated that the timing of DOD's distribution of funds also creates program execution challenges. For example, state counterdrug program officials stated that prior to fiscal year 2017, they began each year with a minimal number of personnel performing state drug interdiction and counterdrug activities until DOD provided more funding to the program after the enactment of the appropriation for the remainder of the fiscal year. Thereafter, state program officials stated that they increased the number of National Guard personnel supporting National Guard counterdrug program activities. However, state program officials said that after the appropriation expired at the end of each fiscal year, they were once again forced to reduce the number of personnel performing state drug interdiction and counterdrug activities until the enactment of another final appropriation was passed. Figure 4 provides a summary of the number of

---

[36] In 2009, we examined the effect of continuing resolutions on selected case study agency operations. We found that all six case study agencies reported that operating within the limitations of the continuing resolutions resulted in inefficiencies, including delays to certain activities such as hiring, and repetitive work, including issuing multiple grants or contracts. GAO, *Continuing Resolutions: Uncertainty Limited Management Options and Increased Workload in Selected Agencies*, GAO-09-879 (Washington, D.C.: Sept. 24, 2009).

[37] Funds transferred from the Drug Interdiction and Counterdrug Activities, Defense account to various other programs, including the National Guard program, can be transferred back to the account upon a determination that all or part of the funds are not necessary and remain unobligated. For an overview of DOD's process to fund the National Guard counterdrug program, see appendix III.

[38] See appendix I for additional information on the National Guard counterdrug program's total budget authority and obligation amounts for fiscal years 2010 through 2017.

National Guard personnel performing state drug interdiction and counterdrug activities by month during fiscal years 2012 through 2017.

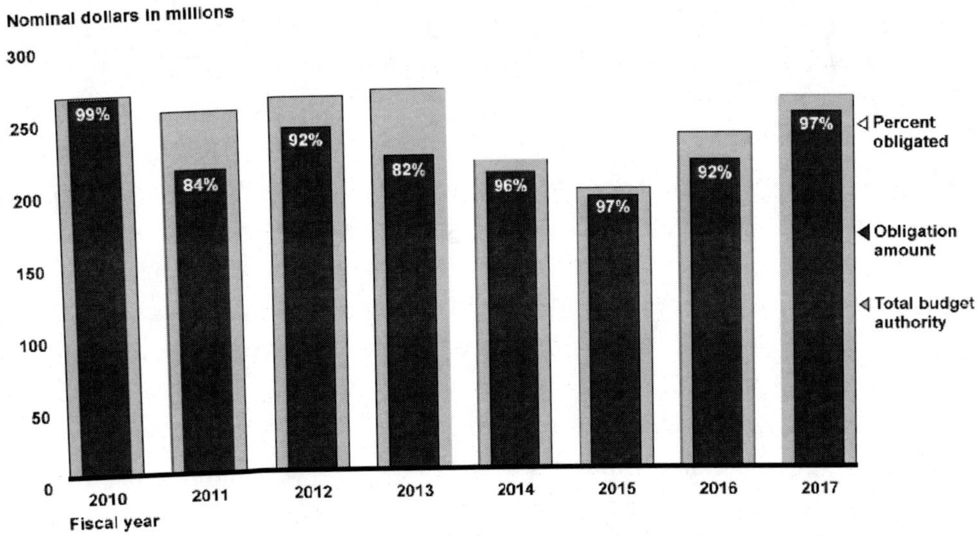

Source: GAO analysis of Department of Defense data. | GAO-19-27.

Note: The National Guard counterdrug program's obligations may be above or below the congressionally-directed program level which does not equal total budget authority available for the National Guard's counterdrug program in a given year. In no year did programmatic obligations exceed actual budget authority.

Figure 3. National Guard Counterdrug Program Obligation Amounts and Total Budget Authority Amounts, Fiscal Years 2010 through 2017.

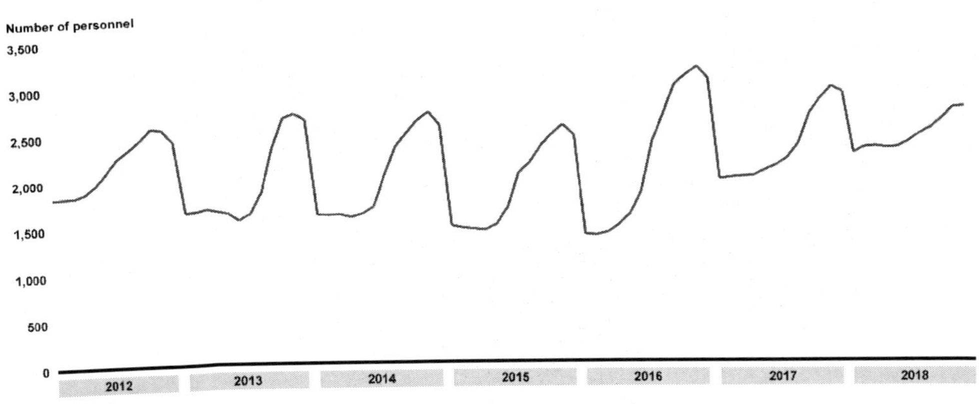

Source: GAO analysis of National Guard Bureau data. | GAO-19-27.

Note: This figure does not include personnel in a Title 10 active duty status, such as those supporting some counterthreat finance activities or personnel supporting international counterdrug efforts.

Figure 4. Number of National Guard Personnel Performing State Drug Interdiction and Counterdrug Activities by Month, Fiscal Years 2012 through 2018.

According to state counterdrug program officials, the majority of funds provided after a final appropriation is passed fund temporary personnel and seasonal work, rather than analysis support activities deemed a priority for the National Guard counterdrug program by the Office of the Deputy Assistant Secretary of Defense for Counternarcotics and Global Threats. State counterdrug program officials stated that this is because they cannot hire, train, and integrate personnel on a full-time basis and that law enforcement agencies are looking more for long-term, rather than temporary support. State counterdrug officials told us that as a result of the funding uncertainty they experience significant fluctuations in the number of personnel performing state drug interdiction and counterdrug activities and that they are challenged in obtaining and retaining highly qualified National Guard personnel. Additionally, state counterdrug program officials stated that withdrawing National Guard personnel from partner organizations after appropriations expire can severely affect their operations and diminish trust between counterdrug programs and law enforcement partners.

According to National Guard Bureau officials, the National Guard Bureau revised its process for funding the National Guard counterdrug program in fiscal year 2017 to try to mitigate the effects of DOD's process for providing funds under continuing resolutions on the program. Specifically, the National Guard Bureau worked with the Army and Air National Guard budget execution offices to establish a process to expedite funding made available to the state-level counterdrug programs. Under the revised process, the Army and Air National Guard budget execution offices reprogram available amounts from other programmatic activities, such as funds for annual training, to the counterdrug program earlier in the fiscal year. According to Army and Air National Guard budget execution officials, amounts provided through reprogramming are based on a number of factors, including prior years' appropriations for the program, execution levels, current-year appropriations and congressional directions, and an assessment of risk to the other activities.[39]

The National Guard Bureau and state counterdrug program officials stated that this revised funding process has helped mitigate challenges arising from uncertainty of when and how much funding would be provided to the states.[40] For example, state counterdrug program officials said that in fiscal year 2017, the funding process enabled them to retain more personnel on orders and decrease the amount of funds that went unspent. The total number of personnel assigned to the National Guard counterdrug program at the beginning of fiscal year 2018 was approximately 2,250. Conversely, the program began fiscal year 2016 with approximately 1,350 personnel on orders. In addition, program

---

[39] Officials from the National Guard Bureau and Army and Air National Guard budget execution offices stated that the amounts provided to the National Guard counterdrug program from other programs' available funding is replenished when the National Guard counterdrug program receives program funding from the Office of the Deputy Assistant Secretary of Defense for Counternarcotics and Global Threats.

[40] Appendix IV provides an overview of amounts received by the National Guard counterdrug program during each appropriations period for fiscal years 2014 through 2018.

officials stated that the process to provide funding earlier in the fiscal year helped them to obligate almost 97 percent of the total budget authority in fiscal year 2017, a higher percentage compared to many of the previous fiscal years. National Guard officials stated that while reprogramming amounts from other programmatic activities has helped to address the fiscal challenges of the National Guard counterdrug program, they cannot provide assurance that this funding process will continue from year to year. However, National Guard Bureau officials have assessed the risks and believe this is the best solution available for funding the program during a continuing resolution until the enactment of the final appropriation.

DOD Could Improve Its Processes for Approving and Distributing Funds to State Counterdrug Programs

DOD Has Provided Funding to State Counterdrug Programs without Approved Plans

DOD has established a process for development and review of the state plans—an annual plan of each state's counterdrug activities—to ensure that state counterdrug program activities reflect DOD's counternarcotics strategic priorities. However, since at least 2009 DOD has not met the statutory requirement to examine the adequacy of state plans prior to distributing funding to state counterdrug programs.[41]

To develop the state plans, counterdrug coordinators in each state counterdrug program use guidance in annual memorandums issued by DOD.[42] According to the guidance, the plans should identify the state's counterdrug priorities and how each state counterdrug program intends to obligate its available funds. Counterdrug coordinators then work with their state's Adjutant General, Attorney General, and Governor, who each review and sign them, before the plans are sent to the National Guard Bureau for further review. Once the National Guard Bureau reviews the plans, they are forwarded to the Office of the Deputy Assistant Secretary of Defense for Counternarcotics and Global Threats. Officials from that office review the plans and make recommendations to the Secretary of Defense to approve or disapprove the plans. Based on these recommendations, the Secretary of Defense reviews the plans for adequacy, and when

---

[41] 32 U.S.C. § 112(d)(1).

[42] DOD has provided the National Guard counterdrug program with annual state plans development memorandums that list specific activities on which state counterdrug programs should focus their efforts and provide instructions programs should use when developing their state plans.

satisfied, signs a memorandum of agreement approving the plans.[43] Figure 5 provides an outline of the process to approve state plans for their counterdrug activities.

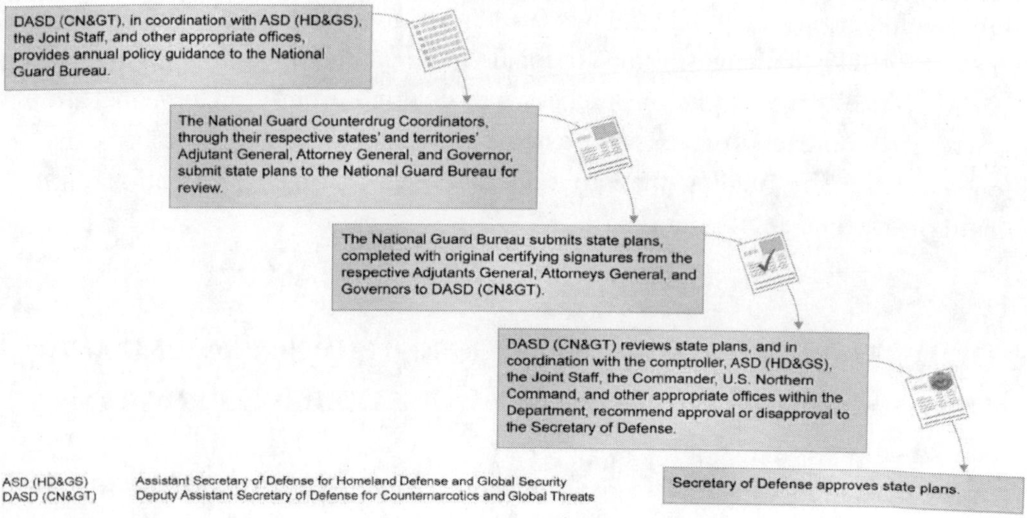

Source: GAO analysis of Department of Defense policy. | GAO-19-27.

Figure 5. Department of Defense's Process for Approving State Drug Interdiction and Counterdrug Activities Plans.

However, since at least 2009, DOD has provided funding to the state counterdrug programs prior to the Secretary of Defense approving states' plans for their counterdrug activities, according to National Guard Bureau officials. This is inconsistent with section 112 of title 32 of the United States Code, which requires that before funds are provided to the Governor of a state for counterdrug activities and before members of the National Guard of that State are ordered to full-time National Guard duty, the Secretary of Defense must examine the adequacy of the plan submitted by the Governor. We found that that the delay in approval of states' plans for their counterdrug activities has worsened since 2009, and in fiscal year 2018, approval took over 9 months (283 days) after funding was provided at the beginning of the fiscal year.[44] Figure 6 provides information on the

---

[43] Section 112(c) of title 32 requires that state plans shall: (1) specify how personnel of the National Guard of that State are to be used in drug interdiction and counter-drug activities; (2) certify that those operations are to be conducted at a time when the personnel involved are not in Federal service; (3) certify that participation by National Guard personnel in those operations is service in addition to training required under section 502 of title 32; (4) certify that any engineer-type activities (as defined by the Secretary of Defense) under the plan will be performed only by units and members of the National Guard; (5) include a certification by the Attorney General of the State (or, in the case of a State with no position of Attorney General, a civilian official of the State equivalent to a State attorney general) that the use of the National Guard of the State for the activities proposed under the plan is authorized by, and is consistent with, State law; and (6) certify that the Governor of the State or a civilian law enforcement official of the State designated by the Governor has determined that any activities included in the plan that are carried out in conjunction with Federal law enforcement agencies serve a State law enforcement purpose.

[44] According to officials from the Office of the Deputy Assistant Secretary of Defense for Counternarcotics and Global Threats, in fiscal year 2018, all but one of the state plans were approved on or before May 17, 2018. Officials stated that the final state plan was returned to the state for a revision, and was ultimately approved on

number of days between the beginning of the fiscal year, when states received funding, and when all plans were approved in fiscal years 2009 through 2018.

Officials from the Office of the Deputy Assistant Secretary of Defense for Counternarcotics and Global Threats and the National Guard Bureau stated that several factors have contributed to delays in the state plan approval process. First, officials stated that, prior to fiscal year 2016, the National Guard Bureau submitted state plans to the Office of the Deputy Assistant Secretary of Defense for Counternarcotics and Global Threats signed by the Division Chief of the National Guard counterdrug program, a colonel in the Army or the Air Force.

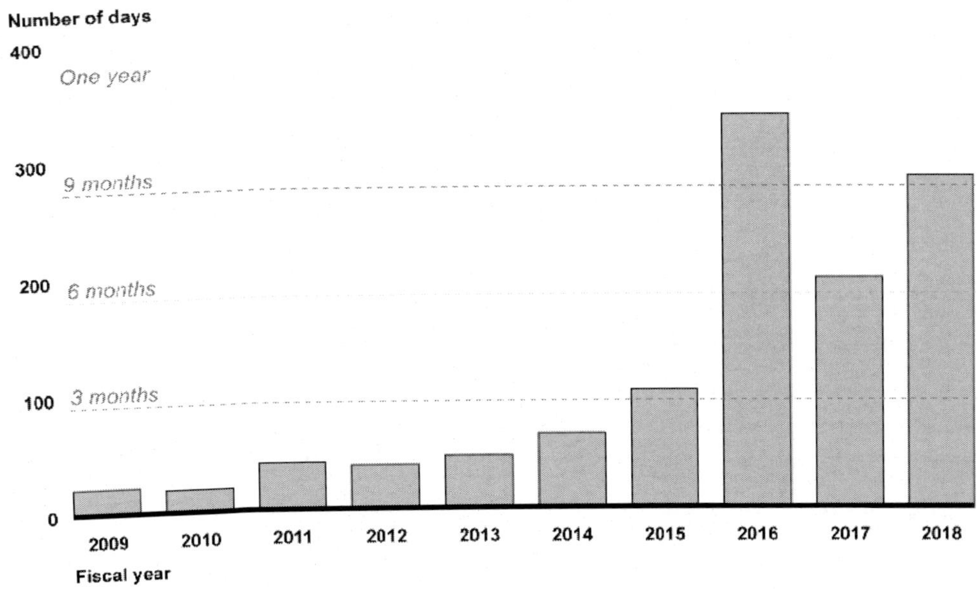

Source: GAO analysis of Department of Defense data. | GAO-19-27.

Note: The start of the fiscal year begins on October 1. According to officials from the Office of the Deputy Assistant Secretary of Defense for Counternarcotics and Global Threats, in fiscal year 2018, all states' drug interdiction and counterdrug activities plans were approved on May 17, 2018, except for Michigan's plan, which was returned for revision. The Michigan plan was subsequently approved on July 10, 2018.

Figure 6. Number of Days Between the Beginning of the Fiscal Year and when the Department of Defense Approved All State Drug Interdiction and Counterdrug Activities Plans, Fiscal Years 2009 through 2018.

However, in fiscal year 2016, officials from the Office of the Secretary of Defense found the Counterdrug Program Division Chief's review and approval of the state plans to be insufficient because the approving official did not have the appropriate rank to approve state plans on behalf of the National Guard Bureau. As a result, officials from

---

July 10, 2018. However DOD had provided funds to all the state counterdrug programs at the beginning of the fiscal year prior to approving state plans.

the National Guard Bureau elevated the level of approval within the National Guard Bureau to the National Guard Bureau Joint Staff Director of Domestic Operations and Force Development, a Major General in the Army National Guard or Air National Guard. Officials from the Office of the Deputy Assistant Secretary of Defense for Counternarcotics and Global Threats stated that this resulted in an increase in the number of days that it took the National Guard Bureau to provide reviewed state plans. Officials stated that they are working to develop an updated timeline to address delays created by the approval process. Specifically, officials stated that they are working to submit the plans for review earlier in order to allow enough time to ensure that state plans are approved before funds are provided to state counterdrug programs.

Second, officials from the Office of the Deputy Assistant Secretary of Defense for Counternarcotics and Global Threats stated that their office required state plans to include information, such as narratives detailing states' planned activities that were not critical to determining plans' alignment with DOD priorities. In addition, officials stated that, over time, states had expanded the narratives in their plans, which increased the length of each submission. As a result of this required information, officials stated that the department's review of state plans took longer than had the extra information not been included. Officials from the Office of the Deputy Assistant Secretary of Defense for Counternarcotics and Global Threats stated they have reviewed the statutory requirements for the plans to identify which components are necessary and streamlined the format of the plans for use in fiscal year 2019.

Third, officials from the Office of the Deputy Assistant Secretary of Defense for Counternarcotics and Global Threats stated that in the past the Office of the Secretary of Defense would not accept state plans from the National Guard Bureau in batches, but instead insisted on receiving and reviewing them altogether, delaying the review process. These officials noted that they have since begun accepting state plans from National Guard Bureau in batches in order to speed up the approval process.

On June 7, 2018, the Office of the Deputy Assistant Secretary of Defense for Counternarcotics and Global Threats issued a memorandum to the Chief of the National Guard Bureau that required all states and territories to submit their plans, through National Guard Bureau and the Joint Staff, to his office no later than August 31, 2018. According to officials from the Office of the Deputy Assistant Secretary of Defense for Counternarcotics and Global Threats, the state plans were to detail fiscal year 2019 National Guard counterdrug program activities and provide the Office of the Deputy Assistant Secretary of Defense for Counternarcotics and Global Threats additional time to review state plans prior to the beginning of the fiscal year.

However, in October 2018, officials from the National Guard Bureau and the Office of the Deputy Assistant Secretary of Defense for Counternarcotics and Global Threats told us that none of the fiscal year 2019 plans had been approved prior to the beginning of the fiscal year, and that DOD had provided state counterdrug programs with funding for fiscal year 2019. As of mid-November, officials from the Office of the Deputy Assistant Secretary of Defense for Counternarcotics and Global Threats told us that 39 of the 54 state plans had been approved. DOD has not assessed why the steps it took to improve the state plan review process did not result in timely approval of the state plans. GAO's *Standards for Internal Control in the Federal Government* note that management should monitor activities and evaluate the results of programmatic changes.[45] Assessing the revised process for reviewing states' plans would enable DOD to determine what additional actions are needed to ensure the plans are approved by the Secretary of Defense before funding is provided to state counterdrug programs, as statutorily required by section 112 of title 32.

National Guard Bureau's Funding Distribution Process Does Not Incorporate DOD Strategic Counternarcotics Priorities

We found that the National Guard Bureau's funding distribution process does not consider DOD's strategic counternarcotics priorities. For example, while DOD's 2011 Counternarcotics and Global Threats Strategy prioritizes efforts on the southwest and northern borders, the National Guard Bureau's funding distribution process does not specifically account for this. Rather than taking into account established DOD counternarcotics priorities to inform funding distribution, the National Guard Bureau uses survey results and statistics on drugs from a number of national-level databases to develop a distribution percentage for each state within its threat-based resource model that reflects its relative drug threat.[46] Each state's threat-based resource model percentage is then applied to the funding transferred to the National Guard Bureau from the Drug Interdiction and Counterdrug Activities, Defense account and disbursed to the 54 state programs.[47] For example, Arizona's threat percentage was determined to be 6.25 percent based on existing drug threats; as a result, Arizona received about $11.8 million in funding for state plans in fiscal year 2018.[48]

---

45 GAO, *Standards for Internal Control in the Federal Government,* GAO-14-704G (Washington, D.C.: Sept. 10, 2014).

46 An assumption of the threat-based resource model is that each state and territory has unique drug challenges, or threats, that continue to change, adapt, and emerge over time. In order to determine each state counterdrug program's funding distribution percentage, the National Guard Bureau administers a survey to subject matter experts in each state. Various drug-related variables are weighted against each other based on which variable poses a higher perceived challenge or threat level. After determining the relative weights of each variable in threat-based resource model, the National Guard Bureau establishes a funding distribution percentage for each state by multiplying the weighted variables against raw data on each variable for each state from national-level databases.

47 See appendix V for more information on the National Guard Bureau's threat-based resource model.

48 States' actual funding distribution percentages may not align with the overall amount of funding they received in a fiscal year because the National Guard Bureau provides additional funding to smaller states to ensure each state has a functional counterdrug program.

National Guard Bureau officials stated that while the threat-based resource model's variables and the data that feed the model relate to DOD strategic counternarcotics priorities, they do not adjust the process to reflect these priorities when distributing funding. When we asked National Guard Bureau officials why its funding distribution process does not consider DOD's strategic counternarcotics priorities, National Guard Bureau officials stated that they were focused on identifying variables and data sources within the threat-based resource model to reflect relative drug threats and did not consider incorporating DOD's strategic counternarcotics priorities as part of the funding distribution process.

Our work on results-oriented management states that strategy should inform program activities and resourcing.[49] In addition, the National Guard Bureau reported that the goal of the threat- based resource model is to prioritize the most pressing threats from a national perspective, informed by current national and DOD counternarcotics strategies. Both the Office of the Deputy Assistant Secretary of Defense for Counternarcotics and Global Threats and National Guard Bureau officials stated that incorporating DOD's strategic counternarcotics priorities into the National Guard Bureau's funding distribution process would help ensure that DOD priorities are resourced. National Guard Bureau officials stated that they are considering how to align the funding distribution process with DOD's strategic counternarcotics priorities. They added that the next time they could make changes to their funding distribution process would be for use in fiscal year 2020. Until the National Guard Bureau incorporates DOD's strategic counternarcotics priorities into the funding distribution process, the National Guard Bureau risks directing funding toward lower priority counterdrug activities at the expense of higher priority activities.

CONCLUSION

The National Guard counterdrug program was established nearly 30 years ago to assist efforts of the Governors of the 50 states, District of Columbia, and three U.S. territories in addressing illicit drug production, trade, and consumption. The drug threats facing the nation are complex and continue to evolve over time, and efforts to combat those threats will require continued support from DOD, to include the National Guard counterdrug program.

DOD lacks current strategy and guidance for the National Guard counterdrug program. Although DOD has a counternarcotics and global threats strategy from 2011, it is outdated and does not reflect current drug threats or changes in national-level

[49] GAO, *Managing For Results: Enhancing Agency Use of Performance Information for Management Decision Making*, GAO-05-927, (Washington, D.C.: Sept. 9, 2005).

strategies, which are critical for informing DOD's strategic counternarcotics priorities. Issuing a strategic framework will ensure that DOD's counterdrug priorities are aligned with the priorities of other agencies involved in counternarcotics efforts, provide direction for DOD's counternarcotics activities, and ensure that the National Guard counterdrug program addresses current drug threats. Further, the National Guard Bureau guidance to operate and administer the program was rescinded and has not been replaced, leaving state counterdrug programs officials without clear instructions on how to operate and administer program activities. Issuing interim guidance would provide detailed processes and procedures that states could use to operate their counterdrug programs. Without current strategy or guidance for the National Guard counterdrug program, it will be difficult for the program to operate effectively.

In addition, it is important to ensure that funding is distributed to the state-level programs in support of DOD's strategic counternarcotics priorities. Although the Secretary of Defense is statutorily responsible for reviewing the adequacy of states' plans prior to providing funds to the states, these reviews have not occurred before state counterdrug programs received funding. Also, the National Guard Bureau has not incorporated DOD's strategic counternarcotics priorities into its funding distribution process, which is instead wholly reliant on survey responses and drug data. While these are important factors to consider when distributing funding, incorporating DOD strategic counternarcotics priorities into the National Guard Bureau's funding distribution process would better inform such decisions. Until DOD's process to approve state plans and the National Guard Bureau's process to distribute funding are improved, DOD may not be able to ensure that resources are applied to its strategic counternarcotics priorities.

Taken together these actions should improve the Department's oversight of the National Guard counterdrug program and help ensure that the program uses resources effectively and achieves positive results.

RECOMMENDATIONS FOR EXECUTIVE ACTION

We are making five recommendations to DOD.

The Secretary of Defense should ensure that the Office of the Deputy Assistant Secretary of Defense for Counternarcotics and Global Threats issues its counternarcotics and global threats strategic framework that incorporates relevant national-level strategies and reflects current drug threats, and update it, as appropriate, upon issuance of the new National Drug Control Strategy. (Recommendation 1)

The Secretary of Defense should ensure that the Chief of the National Guard Bureau issues interim guidance that provides detailed procedures and processes on how to operate and administer the National Guard counterdrug program. (Recommendation 2)

The Secretary of Defense should ensure that the Chief of the National Guard Bureau take steps to ensure it issues a manual to accompany Chief National Guard Bureau Instruction 3100.01A, *National Guard Counterdrug Support*, by June 2019. (Recommendation 3)

The Secretary of Defense should ensure that the Office of the Deputy Assistant Secretary of Defense for Counternarcotics and Global Threats, in coordination with the Chief of the National Guard Bureau, assess the revised process for reviewing states' plans for their counterdrug activities, and take actions based on the assessment to ensure the plans are approved by the Secretary of Defense before funding is provided to state counterdrug programs, as statutorily required. (Recommendation 4)

The Secretary of Defense should ensure that the Chief of the National Guard Bureau incorporate the strategic counternarcotics priorities, to be outlined in DOD's counternarcotics and global threats strategic framework, into the National Guard Bureau's funding distribution process. (Recommendation 5)

AGENCY COMMENTS AND OUR EVALUATION

In written comments on a draft of this report, DOD concurred with all five of our recommendations and identified actions it plans to take to improve its oversight of the National Guard counterdrug program. DOD's comments are reprinted in their entirety in appendix VI. DOD also provided technical comments on a draft of this report, which we incorporated as appropriate. For example, we adjusted the wording of our fifth recommendation, replacing threat-based resource model with funding distribution process, to reflect the department's technical comment that it is unlikely that the National Guard Bureau would change the threat-based resource model, but rather add strategic priorities to the funding distribution process to meet the intent of our recommendation.

We are sending copies of this report to appropriate congressional committees, the Acting Secretary of Defense, the Assistant Secretary of Defense for Special Operations/Low-Intensity Conflict, and the Chief of the National Guard Bureau.

Elizabeth A. Field, Acting Director
Defense Capabilities and Management

APPENDIX I: NATIONAL GUARD COUNTERDRUG PROGRAM FUNDING BY PROJECT CODE

Department of Defense (DOD) budgets for National Guard counterdrug program activities using 5 projects codes:

7403—State Plans—funds DOD support to U.S. State Governors in accordance with State requests in the form of drug interdiction and counter-drug activities plans submitted in accordance with 32 U.S.C. § 112(c).

7415—Counterdrug Schools—funds five National Guard Counterdrug Schools as authorized by §901 of the Office of National Drug Control Policy Reauthorization Act of 2006, as amended, and as identified in plans submitted by host State Governors to the Secretary of Defense in accordance with 32 U.S.C. § 112(c).

9301—Counterthreat Finance—funded reserve military pay and associated support costs for National Guard personnel in support of State, Federal, and Combatant Command efforts to identify, target, and disrupt illicit financial systems that enable drug trafficking, and when vital to U.S. national security interests—terrorism and transnational organized crime.[50]

1295—Linguist and Data Analysis—funds DOD support for combatant command and interagency law enforcement efforts to detect and disrupt transnational criminal organizations' operations using linguistic and analytical skills of National Guard personnel.

9498—Linguist Support—funds language transcription, translation, and data analysis support to the U.S. Department of Justice and Drug Enforcement Administration using Utah National Guard personnel.

DOD's budget request for the National Guard counterdrug program increased steadily from fiscal year 2004 through fiscal year 2012, peaking at just more than $205 million. However, in fiscal year 2013 DOD's budget request for the program decreased substantially and continued to decline through fiscal year 2017. The decrease in requested funding amounts for the program is primarily in the State Plans and Counterdrug Schools project codes. In fiscal year 2018, the budget request for the program increased slightly and included additional funding amounts within the State Plans and Counterdrug Schools project codes. Table 4 provides a summary of DOD's budget request for the National Guard counterdrug program, by project code, in fiscal years 2004 through 2018.

---

50 The Office of the Deputy Assistant Secretary of Defense for Counternarcotics and Global Threats recategorized counterthreat finance activities in fiscal year 2018 and beyond to more accurately reflect the type of National Guard investigative case analysis support provided to law enforcement. Based on guidance provided by the Office of the Deputy Assistant Secretary of Defense for Counternarcotics and Global Threats, funds previously provided to the National Guard Bureau under project code 9301 were to be rolled into project code 7403, state plans, for disbursement in fiscal year 2019.

Table 4. Department of Defense's (DOD) Budget Request for the National Guard Counterdrug Program, Fiscal Years 2004 through 2018 (Nominal Dollars in Thousands by Fiscal Year)

Project Code	2004	2005	2006	2007	2008	2009	2010	2011	2012	2013	2014	2015	2016	2017	2018
7403—State Plans	160,309	164,746	166,696	166,496	169,148	172,171	176,365	177,691	179,718	105,853	104,688	86,698	80,075	79,077	88,307
7415— Counterdrug Schools	4,747	4,799	4,855	8,921	9,126	9,809	9,989	10,151	10,286	8,622	4,909	N/A	5,000	4,877	5,182
9301— Counterthreat Finance	N/A	N/A	N/A	N/A	N/A	N/A	N/A	N/A	N/A	2,526	2,525	2,767	2,823	2,981	3,289
1295— Linguist and Data Analysis	3,936	7,672	7,777	6,885	7,025	7,178	7,300	7,379	7,460	7,588	7,590	7,759	8,704	8,378	10,781
9498— Linguist Support	6,102	6,733	6,920	7,111	7,334	7,567	7,673	7,737	7,825	7,971	7,945	8,073	8,227	7,979	8,794
Total	175,094	183,950	186,248	189,413	192,633	196,725	201,327	202,958	205,289	132,560	127,657	105,297	104,829	103,292	116,353

Source: GAO Analysis of Department of Defense (DOD) data. I GAO-19-27.

Note: DOD's budget request for the Counterthreat Finance project code did not begin until 2013. Therefore no requested funding amount is recorded in this project code from fiscal years 2004 through 2012. In addition, DOD did not request funding for the National Guard counterdrug schools in fiscal year 2015 because, according to officials from the Office of the Deputy Assistant Secretary of Defense for Counternarcotics and Global Threats, they did not have a full understanding of the counterdrug schools' activities and wanted to assess the schools' training efforts before requesting a specific amount for this project code.

Table 5. Congressionally-Directed Increases for the National Guard Counterdrug Program, Fiscal Years 2004 through 2018 (Nominal Dollars in Thousands by Fiscal Year)

Project Code	2004	2005	2006	2007	2008	2009	2010	2011	2012	2013	2014	2015	2016	2017	2018
7403—State Plans	40,160	43,625	42,205	47,560	42,504	46,000	31,400	40,170	40,000	118,912	125,049	76,000	110,000	134,877	125,182
7415— Counterdrug Schools	14,035	11,900	11,325	13,660	14,160	13,500	15,800	9,830	10,000	11,088	4,951	10,000	15,000	15,123	19,818
9301— Counterthreat Finance	N/A	N/A	N/A	N/A	N/A	N/A	N/A	N/A	N/A	N/A	N/A	N/A	N/A	N/A	N/A
1295— Linguist and Data Analysis	N/A	N/A	N/A	N/A	N/A	N/A	N/A	N/A	N/A	N/A	N/A	N/A	N/A	N/A	N/A
9498— Linguist Support	N/A	N/A	N/A	N/A	N/A	N/A	N/A	N/A	N/A	N/A	N/A	N/A	N/A	N/A	N/A
Total	54,195	55,525	53,530	61,220	56,664	59,500	47,200	50,000	50,000	130,000	130,000	86,000	125,000	150,000	145,000

Source: GAO Analysis of Department of Defense (DOD) data. I GAO-19-27.

Note: Project codes 9301, 1295, and 9498 did not receive funds from congressionally-directed increases. Unless otherwise stated, total amounts reflect congressionally-directed increases as written in joint explanatory statements or conference reports accompanying the appropriations. There were no joint explanatory statements or conference reports in fiscal year 2011. Amounts for project codes 7403 and 7415 as shown above reflect DOD's reprogramming in response to congressional direction.

Table 6. Total Budget Authority for the National Guard Counterdrug Program, Fiscal Years 2010 through 2017 (Nominal Dollars in Thousands by Fiscal Year)

Project Code	2010	2011	2012	2013	2014	2015	2016	2017
7403—State Plans	219,814	212,493	214,029	221,652	179,322[a]	162,335	187,078	214,170
7415—Counterdrug Schools	27,361	21,335	23,621	19,961	8,693	10,130	21,820	20,007
9301—Counterthreat Finance	N/A	N/A	2,500	2,549	2,279	2,977	3,674	4,031
1295—Linguist and Data Analysis	7,469	9,191	9,427	8,797	11,887	9,719	10,475	8,761
9498—Linguist Support	7,705	7,803	8,795	9,601	10,760	8,110	8,336	7,713
Total	262,349	250,822	258,372	262,560	212,941	193,271	231,383	254,682

Source: GAO analysis of Department of Defense (DOD) data. | GAO-19-27.

[a]Fiscal year 2014 reflects a reduction of $41 million by DOD to 7403—State Plans project code—to address a congressional reduction to the DOD Drug Interdiction and Counterdrug Activities, Defense account of $50 million for prior-year under-execution. According to officials from the Office of the Deputy Assistant Secretary of Defense for Counternarcotics and Global Threats the prior year under-execution was primarily in 7403—State Plans.

Note: DOD did not request funding for the Counterthreat Finance project code in its budget until fiscal year 2013; however, DOD provided funding for the Counterthreat Finance project code in fiscal year 2012 through an execution year program adjustment. Therefore no funding is recorded in this project code for fiscal years 2010 and 2011.

Table 7. Obligation Amounts for the National Guard Counterdrug Program, Fiscal Years 2010 through 2017 (Nominal Dollars in Thousands by Fiscal Year)

Project Code	2010	2011	2012	2013	2014	2015	2016	2017
7403—State Plans	219,081	174,631	196,055	176,526	172,780	158,217	174,270	204,912
7415—Counterdrug Schools	27,341	19,997	22,323	19,452	7,043	9,781	17,185	18,622
9301—Counterthreat Finance	N/A	N/A	1,510	2,255	2,179	2,340	2,844	4,252
1295—Linguist and Data Analysis	7,370	9,171	8,629	8,721	11,759	9,716	9,857	9,361
9498—Linguist Support	7,219	6,438	8,763	9,597	10,543	8,108	8,205	8,644
Total	261,011	210,237	237,280	216,551	204,304	188,162	212,361	245,791

Source: GAO Analysis of Department of Defense (DOD) data. | GAO-19-27.

Note: DOD did not request funding for the Counterthreat Finance project code in its budget until fiscal year 2013; however, DOD provided funding for the Counterthreat Finance project code in fiscal year 2012 through an execution year program adjustment. Therefore no funding is recorded in this project code for fiscal years 2010 and 2011.

Since at least 2004, Congress has directed increases above DOD's budget request level for the activities of the National Guard counterdrug program. Congressionally-directed increases have been directed to the State Plans and Counterdrug Schools project codes. Beginning in fiscal year 2013, congressionally-directed increases have generally made up half or more of the total funding appropriated to the National Guard counterdrug program. Table 5 provides a summary of congressionally-directed increases for the National Guard counterdrug program, by project code, in fiscal years 2004 through 2018.

According to DOD's data, total budget authority for the National Guard counterdrug program varied from fiscal year 2010 through fiscal year 2017. Total budget authority may be above or below congressionally-enacted amounts because DOD can transfer or reprogram amounts into other authorized accounts and activities based on program requirements. Table 6 provides a summary of total budget authority for the National Guard counterdrug program, by project code, in fiscal years 2010 through 2017.

According to DOD's data, obligation amounts for the National Guard counterdrug program varied from fiscal year 2010 through fiscal year 2017. According to National Guard officials, variation was partly due to the timing and amount of allocations received by the program. Funds transferred from the Drug Interdiction and Counterdrug Activities, Defense account to various other DOD drug interdiction accounts or programs, including the National Guard program, can be transferred back to the account upon a determination that all or part of the funds are not necessary and remain unobligated. Once funds are returned to the Drug Interdiction and Counterdrug Activities, Defense account, they are available for transfer to other DOD counterdrug programs for obligation. Table 7 details the counterdrug program's obligations from fiscal years 2010 through 2017.

APPENDIX II: OVERVIEW OF STATE COUNTERDRUG PROGRAM PLANNED SUPPORT ACTIVITIES, FISCAL YEAR 2018

As of fiscal year 2018, National Guard Bureau policy allows state counterdrug programs to perform 15 approved support activities grouped into five broad mission categories.[51] The five mission categories are technical support (including linguist and translator, operational and investigative case and criminal analyst, and counterthreat finance support), general support (including domestic cannabis suppression and eradication operations and transportation support), reconnaissance and observation (including ground and aerial reconnaissance), civil operations and coalition development, and counterdrug training.[52]

Of the 15 approved support activities, the investigative case and analyst support activity was the most frequently provided activity; it accounted for 42 percent of all support provided in fiscal years 2011 to 2014. Among all of the supported organizations from fiscal year 2011 to fiscal year 2014, law enforcement agencies received about 38 percent of all support provided by the National Guard counterdrug program. Table 8 lists the fiscal year 2018 approved state plan mission categories and support activities.

---

[51] Chief National Guard Bureau Instruction 3100.01A, *National Guard Counterdrug Support* (June 22, 2015).

[52] In fiscal year 2011, the National Guard counterdrug program expanded its list of approved missions states could undertake to include the counterthreat finance mission. This mission aids in investigations to deny, disrupt, destroy or defeat finance systems and networks that negatively affect U.S. interests.

Table 8. State Plans' Mission Categories and Support Activities

Technical support
a. Linguist and translator support
b. Operationaland investigative case and criminal analyst support
c. Illicit narcotics detection support
d. Communications support
e. Engineer support
f. Subsurface and diver support
g. Counterthreat finance analyst supporta
h. Imagery and mapping support
General support
a. Domestic cannabis suppression and eradication operations
b. Transportation support
Reconnaissance and observation
a. Ground reconnaissance
b. Aerial reconnaissance
Civil operations and coalition development
a. Educational programs
b. Military unique tactics to community strategies
c. Civil operations support to coalitions
Counterdrug-related training

Source: GAO analysis of National Guard counterdrug missions and activities. I GAO-19-27.

Note: The program also includes a mission category for internal program management. Since this mission category does not provide support to interagency partners, we did not include it in this table.

[a]DOD's fiscal year 2019 guidance for the National Guard counterdrug program states that the counterthreat finance activity and its corresponding funding are not approved under section 112, title 32 authorities. The guidance further states that funds previously provided to the National Guard Bureau for counterthreat finance will be rolled into the state plan's project code for disbursement. DOD officials stated the counterthreat finance activity was recategorized to more accurately reflect the type of National Guard operational and investigative case and criminal analyst support provided to law enforcement.

APPENDIX III: PROCESS TO FUND THE NATIONAL GUARD COUNTERDRUG PROGRAM

After Congress appropriates amounts to the Drug Interdiction and Counterdrug Activities, Defense account, there are multiple steps performed by various organizations before counterdrug funds are provided to each individual state program.[53] To begin the process to distribute funding, the Department of Defense (DOD) Counternarcotics and Global Threats program officials prepare and submit to the Office of the Under Secretary of Defense (Comptroller) a reprogramming action (DD1415-3), which details the allocation of funds by appropriation or budget activity account for each program

[53] If no defense appropriations act has been passed and DOD is operating under a continuing resolution, amounts transferred are based on a rate-per-day formula developed by OMB.

they manage.[54] DOD Comptroller officials review and approve the DD1415-3 and forward it to the Office of Management and Budget.[55] Once approved by the Office of Management and Budget, the DOD Comptroller issues a funding authorization document to transfer funds to the military services appropriation accounts (such as military personnel or operation and maintenance). The military services then transfer funds to appropriation accounts managed by Army National Guard and Air National Guard, which, in turn, distribute the funds onto each state National Guard participating in the program. The National Guard Bureau's Counterdrug Program office coordinates the process involving the Office of the Deputy Assistant Secretary of Defense for Counternarcotics and Global Threats, the Army and Air National Guard budget and financial management offices, and the individual state counterdrug programs. According to officials from the Office of the Deputy Assistant Secretary of Defense for Counternarcotics and Global Threats, the process to complete the DD1415-3 takes 3 full weeks and then an additional 8 weeks, on average, for the funding to become available for state counterdrug programs. Figure 7 outlines the process to fund the National Guard counterdrug program.

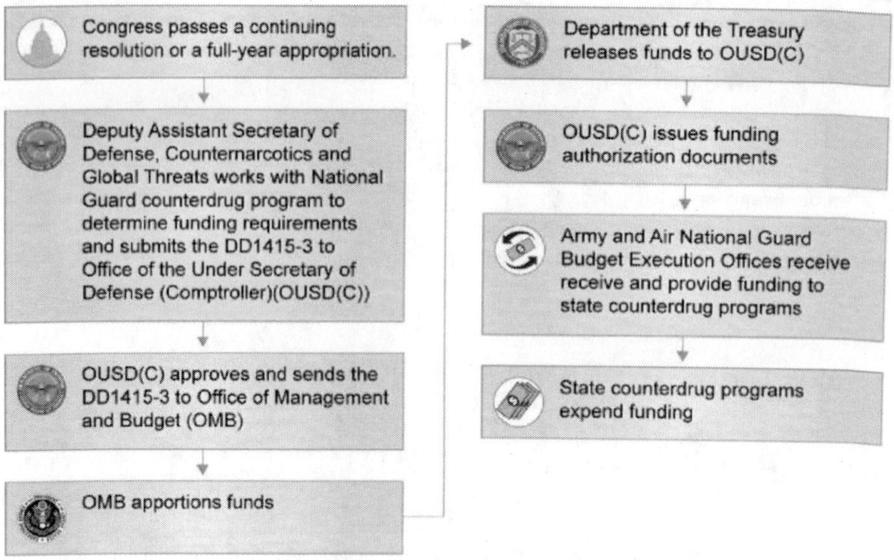

Source: GAO analysis of Department of Defense funding allocation process. | GAO-19-27.

Figure 7. Steps in the Process to Fund the National Guard Counterdrug Program.

---

[54] According to officials from the Office of the Deputy Assistant Secretary of Defense for Counternarcotics and Global Threats they did not submit a DD1414—baseline for reprogramming action—for fiscal year 2018 because the Consolidated Appropriations Act, 2018 included a provision that provided an exemption for the Drug Interdiction and Counterdrug Activities, Defense account.

[55] Office of Management and Budget (OMB) manages and approves apportionments at the Treasury appropriation fund level. Apportionment is part of the government-wide system for the administrative control of funds. Unless exempted by statute or automatically apportioned, all DOD appropriated resources require OMB approval through the apportionment process before they are available for distribution and legal obligation.

APPENDIX IV: FUNDING PROVIDED BY THE DEPARTMENT OF DEFENSE UNDER CONGRESSIONAL APPROPRIATIONS

Table 9. Funding Provided by the Department of Defense (DOD) for the National Guard Counterdrug Program under Congressional Appropriations in Fiscal Years 2014 through 2018 (Nominal Dollars in Millions)

Fiscal Year 2014 Appropriations	DOD provided funding	Amount provided	Date Received
Public Law 113-46 (CR)	✓	66.2	December, 2, 2013
Public Law 113-73 (CR)	✗	—	—
Public Law 113-76	✓	151.8	May 14, 2014
Fiscal Year 2015 Appropriations			
Public Law 113-164 (CR)	✓	26.1	October 21, 2014
Public Law 113-202 (CR)	✗	—	—
Public Law 113-203 (CR)	✗	—	—
Public Law 113-235	✓	166.1	March 24, 2015
Fiscal Year 2016 Appropriations			
Public Law 114-53 (CR)	✓	38.2	November 17, 2015
Public Law 114-96 (CR)	✗	—	—
Public Law 114-100 (CR)	✗	—	—
Public Law 114-113	✓	193.0	April 08, 2016
Fiscal Year 2017 Appropriations			
Public Law 114-223 (CR)	✓	49.7	November 5, 2016
Public Law 114-254(CR)	✓	85.2	March 15, 2017
Public Law 115-30 (CR)	✗	—	—
Public Law 115-31	✓	117.9	September 14, 2017
Fiscal Year 2018 Appropriations			
Public Law 115-56 (CR)	✓	47.0	January 18, 2018
Public Law 115-90 (CR)	✗	—	—
Public Law 115-96 (CR)	✗	—	—
Public Law 115-120 (CR)	✗	—	—
Public Law 115-123 (CR)	✗	—	—
Public Law 115-141	✓	214.3	July 3, 2018

Legend: CR = continuing resolution. ✓ = yes. ✗ = no. — = Not Applicable. Source: GAO analysis of public laws. | GAO-19-27.

APPENDIX V: THREAT-BASED RESOURCE MODEL

The National Guard Bureau's threat-based resource model has been used since fiscal year 2012 to help determine funding distribution percentages for the state counterdrug programs. Between fiscal years 2013 and 2015, National Guard Bureau officials stated that they determined planned funding amounts based on a combination of historical funding levels and threat-based resource model threat percentages.[56] According to officials, beginning in fiscal year 2016, funding aligned more closely with threat-based resource model threat percentages. However, National Guard Bureau officials stated that funding distribution percentages from the threat-based resource model were deemed unusable in fiscal year 2017 due to concerns they had with the amount of reporting and the quality of the data that was reported. As a result, officials stated that the fiscal year 2016 threat-based resource model funding percentages were used to distribute fiscal year 2017 funding to state programs while National Guard Bureau officials revised the model for use in fiscal year 2018. Updates to the model included expanding the number of variables to better respond to changes in drug threats, adjusting the model so that it did not treat all drug seizure incidents and amounts equally, and increasing the number of data sources. Table 10 provides threat-based resource model percentages and Table 11 funding amounts, by state, for fiscal years 2012 through 2018.

Table 10. Fiscal Years 2015 through 2018 Threat-Based Resource Model Percentages by State or Territory Program

Program	Fiscal year 2015 percentage	Fiscal year 2016 percentage	Fiscal year 2017 percentage	Fiscal year 2018 percentage
California	14.18	13.80	13.80	13.93
Texas	13.97	11.77	11.77	11.55
New York	4.66	8.11	8.11	7.88
Arizona	5.40	6.49	6.49	6.25
Florida	5.97	5.24	5.24	5.48
Puerto Rico	2.92	4.28	4.28	4.04
Illinois	3.44	3.78	3.78	3.54
Kentucky	2.23	3.59	3.59	3.32
Ohio	2.30	2.43	2.43	2.66
Tennessee	2.65	2.62	2.62	2.40
Michigan	1.96	2.14	2.14	2.38
Missouri	2.35	2.35	2.35	2.33
Pennsylvania	2.28	2.07	2.07	2.02
North Carolina	2.09	1.85	1.85	1.84

[56] According to National Guard Bureau officials, the National Guard Bureau determined planned funding amounts, in part, based on state funding requests in fiscal year 2015; states that requested an amount equal to or less than their threat-based resource model threat percentage received their full request. Where states requested less funding than requested, the National Guard Bureau redistributed leftover funds to states that had requested more than their threat-based resource model threat percentage.

Program	Fiscal year 2015 percentage	Fiscal year 2016 percentage	Fiscal year 2017 percentage	Fiscal year 2018 percentage
Georgia	2.43	1.97	1.97	1.75
Indiana	1.65	1.76	1.76	1.69
New Jersey	2.05	1.41	1.41	1.62
Virginia	1.60	1.48	1.48	1.55
New Mexico	1.04	1.24	1.24	1.43
Maryland	1.53	1.18	1.18	1.36
Louisiana	1.46	1.09	1.09	1.25
Massachusetts	1.36	1.07	1.07	1.23
Washington	1.54	0.99	0.99	1.14
Oklahoma	1.26	1.31	1.31	1.11
Arkansas	0.95	1.18	1.18	1.00
South Carolina	1.24	1.11	1.11	0.94
Alabama	1.21	1.10	1.10	0.94
Wisconsin	0.94	1.08	1.08	0.92
Oregon	1.13	0.79	0.79	0.91
Colorado	1.00	0.76	0.76	0.87
Minnesota	0.93	0.68	0.68	0.78
Kansas	1.20	0.90	0.90	0.77
Mississippi	1.01	0.66	0.66	0.76
Nevada	0.99	0.68	0.68	0.65
Utah	0.81	0.63	0.63	0.63
Connecticut	0.68	0.52	0.52	0.60
Iowa	0.98	0.67	0.67	0.57
Hawaii	0.25	0.67	0.67	0.57
Nebraska	0.79	0.55	0.55	0.47
West Virginia	0.43	0.40	0.40	0.46
Maine	0.35	0.51	0.51	0.43
Delaware	0.80	0.38	0.38	0.37
Wyoming	0.18	0.35	0.35	0.30
Washington, D.C.	0.72	0.25	0.25	0.29
North Dakota	0.12	0.32	0.32	0.27
New Hampshire	0.23	0.23	0.23	0.26
Idaho	0.35	0.29	0.29	0.25
Rhode Island	0.33	0.21	0.21	0.24
Montana	0.23	0.26	0.26	0.24
Alaska	0.27	0.24	0.24	0.20
South Dakota	0.24	0.21	0.21	0.19
Vermont	0.19	0.14	0.14	0.16
U.S. Virgin Islands	0.45	0.10	0.10	0.12
Guam	0.18	0.08	0.08	0.07

Source: GAO analysis of National Guard Bureau data. I GAO-19-27.

Note: According to National Guard Bureau officials, the threat-based resource model results were deemed unusable in fiscal year 2017 due to concerns about the amount of reporting and the quality of the data that was reported. Officials stated that fiscal year 2016 threat percentages and distribution amounts were used until changes could be made to the model to improve the reliability of the model.

Table 11. Fiscal Years 2012 through 2018 Planned Funding, by State or Territory Program (Nominal Dollars by Fiscal Year)

Program	2012 amount	2013 amount	2014 amount	2015 amount	2016 amount	2017 amount	2018 amount
California	18,357,817	24,705,866	23,308,294	22,639,065	23,073,454	20,376,127	26,286,493
Texas	15,957,648	19,244,029	18,096,454	17,478,733	19,679,316	17,378,769	21,802,655
New York	5,472,267	6,268,549	6,531,500	7,163,473	13,559,834	11,974,666	14,881,175
Arizona	8,219,187	10,200,000	14,116,892	6,643,038	10,851,211	9,582,686	11,795,194
Florida	6,886,602	11,488,199	6,320,926	6,347,694	8,761,225	7,737,022	10,347,532
Puerto Rico	4,571,199	5,501,759	3,468,617	4,563,715	7,156,115	6,319,552	7,629,059
Illinois	2,505,254	3,073,976	3,135,672	2,951,287	6,320,120	5,581,287	6,671,757
Kentucky	3,179,222	5,935,854	8,034,316	5,289,403	6,002,442	5,300,746	6,273,668
Ohio	1,887,220	3,010,295	2,443,352	2,468,261	4,062,934	3,587,970	5,010,895
Tennessee	2,448,376	3,739,148	3,595,708	3,837,808	4,380,612	3,868,511	4,532,769
Michigan	1,915,731	2,135,348	1,947,976	2,013,786	3,578,057	3,159,776	4,487,682
Missouri	2,546,394	2,516,922	2,382,271	2,992,862	3,929,175	3,469,848	4,397,509
Pennsylvania	2,634,637	2,529,808	2,914,034	2,868,961	3,461,018	3,056,419	3,812,433
North Carolina	2,566,537	1,940,725	2,064,791	1,996,380	3,093,180	2,731,582	3,472,711
Georgia	2,603,569	4,196,897	3,889,948	3,312,889	3,293,819	2,908,766	3,302,850
Indiana	1,642,761	3,317,799	3,886,980	4,207,991	2,942,701	2,598,694	3,189,610
New Jersey	2,580,733	2,799,199	2,443,663	2,123,567	2,357,505	2,081,909	3,060,327
Virginia	1,784,861	1,925,792	1,667,424	1,433,987	2,474,544	2,185,266	2,925,382
New Mexico	4,035,743	5,494,890	3,683,913	2,524,656	2,073,267	1,830,898	2,691,351
Maryland	2,142,523	2,328,565	2,763,234	2,304,829	1,972,948	1,742,306	2,561,124
Louisiana	3,938,836	2,643,873	2,396,025	1,291,725	1,822,468	1,609,419	2,365,784
Massachusetts	1,714,357	1,243,046	1,383,039	1,065,624	1,789,029	1,579,888	2,322,375
Washington	3,003,517	2,569,544	2,126,321	1,843,313	1,655,270	1,461,766	2,148,740
Oklahoma	1,504,048	1,311,812	1,497,793	1,777,016	2,190,306	1,934,256	2,101,556
Arkansas	1,591,812	2,299,258	1,786,639	1,783,881	1,972,948	1,742,306	1,893,005
South Carolina	1,819,096	1,767,728	1,819,307	1,387,388	1,855,908	1,638,949	1,780,708
Alabama	2,286,156	1,789,842	2,110,367	2,130,546	1,839,188	1,624,184	1,764,666
Wisconsin	1,584,931	1,097,283	1,367,539	1,144,083	1,805,749	1,594,653	1,732,581
Oregon	2,406,630	1,724,120	1,668,232	2,089,292	1,320,872	1,166,459	1,714,651
Colorado	1,481,252	1,117,865	1,247,416	1,403,185	1,270,712	1,122,164	1,649,538
Minnesota	1,573,084	1,357,850	1,312,450	1,387,742	1,136,953	1,004,041	1,475,902
Kansas	1,806,275	1,182,006	1,178,746	884,441	1,504,790	1,328,878	1,443,817
Mississippi	2,051,970	1,728,731	1,865,560	2,242,773	1,103,513	974,510	1,432,493
Nevada	1,474,804	1,932,798	1,478,681	1,262,081	1,136,953	1,004,041	1,226,773
Utah	1,365,684	1,735,905	1,875,157	2,104,681	1,053,353	930,214	1,189,026
U.S. Virgin Islands	1,257,392	777,544	1,256,055	841,297	750,000	750,000	1,169,731
Guam	1,233,134	647,155	563,306	632,498	750,000	750,000	1,166,431
Connecticut	1,429,129	1,198,714	1,205,451	1,311,015	869,435	767,796	1,128,631
Iowa	1,616,352	1,648,546	1,591,581	1,514,021	1,120,233	989,276	1,074,842
Hawaii	1,590,223	1,371,160	1,140,145	790,244	1,120,233	989,276	1,074,842
Alaska	1,527,606	1,589,662	0	0	750,000	750,000	1,032,337
Delaware	1,518,323	1,074,367	938,827	998,640	750,000	750,000	955,633
Washington, D.C.	1,826,712	1,034,964	1,131,791	1,166,180	750,000	750,000	925,622
Vermont	1,642,585	769,332	708,446	718,257	750,000	750,000	910,286
Maine	1,813,137	1,206,712	1,008,600	799,520	852,715	753,031	886,778

Program	2012 amount	2013 amount	2014 amount	2015 amount	2016 amount	2017 amount	2018 amount
New Hampshire	1,456,760	569,408	660,572	650,535	750,000	750,000	886,778
Nebraska	1,528,882	1,095,386	1,010,916	771,621	919,594	812,092	882,333
Rhode Island	1,415,380	945,728	750,104	944,095	750,000	750,000	875,654
Wyoming	1,259,938	732,341	577,971	596,005	750,000	750,000	869,462
West Virginia	2,129,570	1,236,452	2,998,851	2,310,368	750,000	750,000	868,178
North Dakota	1,547,566	827,367	911,218	793,178	750,000	750,000	852,578
Montana	1,509,370	925,341	936,077	754,400	750,000	750,000	808,982
Idaho	1,338,415	737,835	702,119	602,127	750,000	750,000	802,214
South Dakota	1,350,465	813,782	1,591,833	896,192	750,000	750,000	788,354

Source: GAO Analysis of National Guard Bureau data. I GAO-19-27.

Note: According to National Guard Bureau officials, final distribution amounts to state counterdrug programs may differ from planned funding amounts. Alaska did not participate in the National Guard counterdrug program in fiscal years 2014 and 2015.

APPENDIX VI: COMMENTS FROM THE DEPARTMENT OF DEFENSE

ASSISTANT SECRETARY OF DEFENSE
2500 DEFENSE PENTAGON
WASHINGTON, D.C. 20301-2500

SPECIAL OPERATIONS /
LOW INTENSITY CONFLICT

JAN 0 2 2019

Ms. Elizabeth Field
Acting Director, Defense Capabilities Management
U.S. Government Accountability Office
441 G Street, NW
Washington, DC 20548

Dear Ms. Field:

In response to the GAO Draft Report, GAO-19-27, "DRUG CONTROL: DoD Should Improve Its Oversight of the National Guard Counterdrug Program," dated October 30, 2018 (GAO Code 102249). The Department concurs with the report's recommendations and has already begun taking steps to improve the accountability of the National Guard Counterdrug Program.

Pursuant to the report's recommendations, my office will continue to work with National Guard Bureau to issue new strategic guidance, update policies and procedures, and improve staffing timelines as it relates to the management and oversight of the National Guard Counterdrug Program. The attached document outlines the steps DoD plans to take in response to the GAO's recommendations.

Thank you for the opportunity to review the draft report. My point of contact for this audit is Colonel Brent Flachsbart, 703-601-8849, brent.d.flachsbart.mil@mail.mil.

Sincerely,

Owen West

GAO DRAFT REPORT DATED OCTOBER 30, 2018
GAO-19-27 (GAO CODE 102249)

"DRUG CONTROL: DOD SHOULD IMPROVE ITS OVERSIGHT OF THE NATIONAL GUARD COUNTERDRUG PROGRAM"

DEPARTMENT OF DEFENSE RESPONSES TO THE GAO RECOMMENDATIONS

GAO RECOMMENDATION 1: The Secretary of Defense should ensure that the Deputy Assistant Secretary of Defense for Counternarcotics and Global Threats issues its counter-drug and global threats strategic framework that incorporates relevant national level strategies and reflects current drug threats and update it, as appropriate, upon issuance of the new National Drug Control Strategy.

DoD RESPONSE: CONCUR. The Deputy Assistant Secretary of Defense for Counternarcotics and Global Threats (DASD (CN&GT)) is currently staffing the draft framework with the National Guard Bureau, Combatant Commands, and other DoD components for comments and feedback. The new framework was informed by the most recently published National Security Strategy, National Defense Strategy, National Drug Control Strategy, and other relevant guidance. When published, it will provide updated foundational guidance for developing and implementing programs that support the Department's strategic goals and priorities with respect to countering illicit drug trafficking and other illicit threat networks. The goal is to publish the framework by July 1, 2019.

GAO RECOMMENDATION 2: The Secretary of Defense should ensure that the Chief of the National Guard Bureau issues interim guidance that provides detailed procedures and processes on how to operate and administer the National Guard counter-drug program.

DoD RESPONSE: CONCUR. The National Guard Bureau has begun drafting interim guidance to address detailed procedures and processes. To ensure compliance, DASD (CN&GT) has introduced a requirement for the National Guard Bureau to issue interim program guidance in the draft Fiscal Year 2020 DoD State Plans Guidance, currently in development.

GAO RECOMMENDATION 3: The Secretary of Defense should ensure that the Chief of the National Guard Bureau take steps to ensure it issues a manual to accompany Chief National Guard Bureau Instruction 3100.01A, National Guard Counterdrug Support, by June 2019.

DoD RESPONSE: CONCUR. The National Guard Bureau has begun updating Chief National Guard Bureau Instruction (CNGBI) 3100.01A to comply with the most recently published Secretary of Defense guidance and plans to expedite the issuance of the accompanying Manual. DASD (CN&GT) is working with the National Guard Bureau to ensure any updated guidance complies with changes to policy that have been included in a draft DoD Instruction (DoDI) that will govern future counter-drug program activities. When published, the new DoDI will update and consolidate published policies for DoD counter-drug and related counter-transnational organized crime support. To ensure compliance, DASD (CN&GT) has included the requirement for National Guard Bureau to update internal guidance in the draft Fiscal Year 2020 State Plans Guidance.

GAO RECOMMENDATION 4: The Secretary of Defense should ensure that the Office of the Deputy Assistant Secretary of Defense for Counternarcotics and Global Threats, in coordination with the Chief of the National Guard Bureau, assess the revised process for reviewing states' plans for their counter-drug activities and take actions based on the assessment to ensure the plans are approved by the Secretary of Defense before funding is provided to state counter-drug programs, as statutorily required.

DoD RESPONSE: CONCUR. Fiscal Year 2019 State Plans received by the DASD (CN&GT) by August 31, 2018, the published due date, were approved by October 18, 2018. As of December 3, 2018, 52 State Plans had been received. DASD (CN&GT) continues to monitor this process, with the National Guard Bureau, to ensure all 54 plans are approved accordingly. DASD (CN&GT) will continue to work with the National Guard Bureau to improve the State Plans staffing process for Fiscal Year 2020 and beyond. DASD (CN&GT) Fiscal Year 2020 State Plans Guidance will reiterate that, in accordance with statute, funding may not be provided for a State's counter-drug program until the Secretary of Defense has approved its plan.

GAO RECOMMENDATION 5: The Secretary of Defense should ensure the Chief of the National Guard Bureau incorporate the strategic counter-drug priorities, to be outlined in DOD's counter-drug and global threats strategic framework, into the threat-based resource model.

DoD RESPONSE: CONCUR. DASD (CN&GT) will work with the National Guard Bureau to support its efforts to incorporate and align DoD strategic priorities into its planning and resource allocation processes. The threats posed by drug trafficking and transnational organized crime negatively affect each state in unique ways. The Department understands the National Guard is an important asset for states' efforts to confront these threats, but that clear guidance is required to ensure planned activities align with DoD's strategic priorities with respect to readiness and threats to national security.

APPENDIX VII: STATUS OF OCTOBER 2015 RECOMMENDATIONS ON NATIONAL GUARD COUNTERDRUG PROGRAM

In October 2015, GAO issued a report on the National Guard counterdrug program titled *Drug Control: Additional Performance Information Is Needed to Oversee the National Guard's State Counterdrug Program*.[57] In that report, we made two recommendations aimed at ensuring that resources are being efficiently applied to meet the National Guard counterdrug program's objectives. Table 12 provides an update on the status of the recommendations from that report.

---

[57] GAO, *Drug Control: Additional Performance Information Is Needed to Oversee the National Guard's State Counterdrug Program*, GAO-16-133 (Washington, D.C.: Oct. 21, 2015).

Table 12. Status of Recommendations from GAO, Drug Control: Additional Performance Information Is Needed to Oversee the National Guard's State Counterdrug Program, GAO-16-133 (Washington, D.C.: October 2015)

Recommendation #1:	**Status: Implemented**
To ensure that resources are being efficiently applied to meet the National Guard counterdrug program's objectives, the Secretary of Defense should direct the National Guard Bureau in consultation with the Deputy Assistant Secretary of Defense for Counternarcotics and Global Threats to identify additional information needed to evaluate the performance of the state programs and oversee counterdrug schools' training.	Concurrence: Yes The National Guard Bureau implemented revisions to the National Guard counterdrug program to identify and collect additional information to evaluate the performance of the 54 state programs and the counterdrug schools, as GAO recommended. Specifically, in April 2016, National Guard counterdrug program officials developed a strategic framework with four goals that support counterdrug objectives of the Department of Defense, Office of the National Drug Control Policy, and Federal law enforcement. Within each of the goals, are objectives and measures to evaluate the efforts of the individual state programs and the counterdrug schools. In August 2016, each of the state programs and the counterdrug schools included the goals, objectives, and revised performance measures in their individual fiscal year 2017 plans.
Recommendation #2:	**Status: Open**
To ensure that resources are being efficiently applied to meet the National Guard counterdrug program's objectives, the Secretary of Defense should direct the National Guard Bureau in consultation with the Deputy Assistant Secretary of Defense for Counternarcotics and Global Threats to subsequently collect and use performance information to help inform funding distribution decisions to state programs and to conduct oversight of the training offered by the counterdrug schools.	Concurrence: Yes DOD's response to our report stated that it would collect and use performance information to evaluate the effectiveness of each state program to provide support and to meet its objectives. DOD also stated that it would take steps to assist states with any needed corrective-action plans. For fiscal year 2017, the National Guard counterdrug program collected performance information in its fiscal year 2017 annual assessments of state programs and counterdrug schools, but had not yet incorporated the information into funding distribution decisions. The recommendation will remain open until performance information has been included in the funding distribution process.

Source: GAO analysis. | GAO-19-27.

INDEX

A

B

C

D

E

I

J

K

L

M

U

V

W

Y